G. Penkert · H. Fansa

Peripheral Nerve Lesions

Nerve Surgery and Secondary Reconstructive Repair

Springer
Berlin
Heidelberg
New York
Hong Kong
London
Milan
Paris
Tokyo

G. Penkert · H. Fansa

Peripheral Nerve Lesions

Nerve Surgery and Secondary Reconstructive Repair

With 359 Figures

Springer

ISBN 978-3-642-07939-9
Springer-Verlag Berlin Heidelberg New York

GÖTZ PENKERT Prof. Dr. med.
Friederikenstift Hannover
Neurochirurgische Klinik
Humboldtstr. 5
30169 Hannover
Germany

HISHAM FANSA Priv.-Doz. Dr. med.
Städtische Kliniken Mitte
Klinik für Plastische, Wiederherstellungs- und Ästhetische Chirurgie
Teutoburger Str. 50
33604 Bielefeld
Germany

Library of Congress Cataloging-in-Publication Data
Penkert, G. Peripheral nerve lesions: nerve surgery and secondary reconstructive repair/G. Penkert, H. Fansa. p.; cm. Includes bibliographical references and index.
1. Nerves, Peripheral–Surgery. 2. Nerves, Peripheral–Wounds and injuries–Surgery. 3. Nerves, Peripheral–Regeneration. I. Fansa, H., 1969– II. Title. [DNLM: 1. Peripheral Nerves–surgery. 2. Peripheral Nervous System–surgery. WL 500 P41lp 2004] RD595.P466 2004 617.4'83–dc22

Springer-Verlag is a part of Springer Science+Business Media

springeronline.com

Softcover reprint of the hardcover 1st edition 2004

Illustrations: R. Henkel, Heidelberg
Cover design: F. Steinen, ᵉStudio Calamar, Spain
Product management and layout: B. Wieland, Heidelberg

24/3150 – 5 4 3 2 1 0
Printed on acid-free paper

Preface

The introduction of the microscope and microsurgery in the management of surgically treated peripheral nerve lesions revolutionized the procedure, prognosis, and results in this field. Several authors have published their vast experience, and these reports have been given preference in the present work.

The purpose of this book is not to add one more volume to the literature, but to help younger surgeons who are beginning their education to understand logically how to appraise nerve lesions and how to operate on nerves without harming them. Some experts will perhaps criticize simplifications, particularly concerning the introductory remarks or descriptions of different histological reactions to tissue trauma, but we intended to help younger physicians focus on the important theories and facts that influence preoperative decision making and the type of operative procedure to be chosen. We did not aim at total completeness but rather at clarity.

Of course, we realize that other authors have described different approaches to the various lesions, but we have tried to present our own experience over two decades with clear explanations. We may differ somewhat from other writers, which shows that different opinions are quite normal in a medical field where the surgeon sometimes has to wait more than 1 year for postoperative results. The process of learning from failures or being encouraged by good results is a long one when dealing with peripheral nerve lesions.

We probably should also acknowledge that sometimes even more detail could have been provided on certain topics, particularly on the description of the surgical approaches chosen. But it became much more difficult than initially anticipated to create a mental picture of a surgical procedure through words. Nevertheless, we hope to motivate younger surgeons to enjoy this interesting esthetic medical field, which can truly improve the quality of a patient's life. They will not only need great patience during these time-consuming operations, but also better support within their individual hospital settings and health systems.

Management of nerves requires interdisciplinary cooperation. Artificial barriers between different disciplines usually put a halt to scientific development and progress. Therefore, we intend to build a bridge between all the disciplines involved in peripheral nerve injuries and the disciplines specializing in reconstructive surgery. The possibilities offered today by microsurgery on nerves and reconstructive surgery must be part of a single worldwide concept in the future. We therefore add detailed reconstructive surgical procedures and hope that the reader comes away with a clear idea of the advice and treatment to be offered to patients. An interdisciplinary collaboration between neurologists, neurophysiologists, microneurosurgeons, and reconstructive surgeons must spread throughout the world.

Acknowledgements

My greatest gratitude and respect goes to Prof. Millesi, director of the Hand, Plastic, and Reconstructive Surgery Department of Vienna University, who became my first teacher of peripheral nerve lesions and surgery in the mid-1970s. As the pioneer of microsurgical nerve grafting, he offered me the most generous view of his remarkable experience, proved in the operating room and published in a large number of articles and books. Later, he was always available when thorny scientific questions were to be discussed and solved.

My gratitude is also extended to the foundation of Volkswagen of Hannover, Germany, which enabled me to spend 1.5 years with Millesi and his co-workers.

Once more, my greatest respect goes to Prof. Samii, director of Hannover's neurosurgical departments, who became my second teacher and, from the beginning, was very generous in allowing me to independently give advice to all patients affected by peripheral nerve lesions, to choose and provide treatment, and to document each case with top technical equipment, as well as being available on a daily basis for neurosurgical questions and problems to be solved.

Gratitude must also be extended to another member of Samii's team, Mr. S. Brinkmann, who saw to the vast number of intraoperatively acquired microphotos, only some of which were used in this book.

I must especially thank my wife, Ortrud, who spent innumerable evening hours writing and correcting this manuscript.

Great recognition goes to my colleague, Dr. Hisham Fansa, who was ready to help bridge the gap between plastic and reconstructive surgeons as well as alternative peripheral nerve surgeons such as neurosurgeons, and who thus provided a superb contribution, reflecting his capabilities as a vital complement to nerve surgery.

I also owe thanks to Springer-Verlag Heidelberg and its staff, who placed great confidence in our work. Without their cooperation and help, this book would not have reached completion.

PROF. GÖTZ PENKERT

I wish to thank Prof. Penkert for his trust and the opportunity to include a chapter on muscle and tendon transfers. Always devoted to an optimal functional outcome in his patients, Prof. Penkert never hesitated to follow the necessary interdisciplinary approach.

Great respect goes to my surgical teacher, Prof. Schneider, of the Plastic and Reconstructive Surgery Department, University of Magdeburg, Germany, who always supported me. To show my gratitude I would like to dedicate my work in this book to him.

DR. HISHAM FANSA

Contents

Part I General Considerations in Nerve Surgery

Part II Specific Types of Nerve Lesioins

Abbreviations

ADM	Abductor digiti minimi muscle
AP	Adductor pollicis muscle
APB/L	Abductor pollicis brevis or longus muscle
BR	Brachioradialis muscle
DIP	Distal interphalangeal joint
ECRB/L	Extensor carpi radialis brevis or longus muscle
ECU	Extensor carpi ulnaris muscle
ED	Extensor digitorum muscle
EDM	Extensor digiti minimi muscle
EI	Extensor indicis muscle
EPB/L	Extensor pollicis longus or brevis muscle
FCR	Flexor carpi radialis muscle
FCU	Flexor carpi ulnaris muscle
FDP	Flexor digitorum profundus muscle
FDS	Flexor digitorum superficialis muscle
FPB/L	Flexor pollicis brevis or longus muscle
IP	Interphalangeal joint
MP	Metacarpophalangeal joint
MTT	Muscle and tendon transfer
PIP	Proximal interphalangeal joint
PL	Palmaris longus muscle
PT	Pronator teres muscle
WC	Working capacity

Part I

General Considerations in Nerve Surgery

Historical Development of Peripheral Nerve Surgery

Efforts to improve peripheral nerve surgery were already under way at the end of the nineteenth century, but unfortunately did not succeed in providing sufficiently acceptable results. Only in the early 1960s was microsurgery introduced in the treatment of central nerve diseases as well as peripheral nerve lesions, although ENT surgeons were already practicing microsurgical procedures 20 years earlier. Today, the development of peripheral nerve surgery is the result of the worldwide interdisciplinary cooperation of ordinary surgeons, emergency surgeons, orthopedic surgeons, neurosurgeons, and reconstructive surgeons, in so far as microsurgical methods have been accepted and consequently applied.

The first experiment in nerve grafting was described by Phillipeaux and Vulpian in 1870, the first end-to-end suture in man by Hueter in 1873. Later, in 1885, Albert carried out the first nerve grafting in man, but he used homologous nerve grafts for bridging the defect. About 20 years later, Otfrid Foerster started to perform autologous nerve grafts, presenting his results to orthopedic surgeons in 1916. Moreover, he developed the idea of no longer sacrificing important nerve trunks to use them as grafts, but instead used small skin nerves to overcome the nerve defect. Further results on this modification were once more described by Huber in 1919. Unfortunately, for the next 40 years, the further development of reconstruction of peripheral nerve lesions completely stagnated. Only a macrosurgical view on problems of regeneration of peripheral nerves was in currency: the difference in caliber between the injured nerve trunk and the small nerve graft gained by excising small skin nerves made it possible to introduce what were called cable grafts, which were placed between the two stumps of the injured nerve trunk. In order to reach the caliber of trunks, the grafts were either glued together or wrapped in a piece of artery or vein, a method described by Brooks in 1955, Seddon in 1972, and Röttgen and Wuellenweber in 1974. However, because of the unsatisfactory results, when possible, the end-to-end suture of the two stumps of peripheral nerve trunks was preferred over cable grafts. Epineural suturing was facilitated either by mobilizing the nerve trunks over long distances or by long time-consuming flexing of the extremity joints by plastering them in certain positions. The authors believed that better results were obtained using these procedures than with cable grafts. But with these considerations in mind, the same authors should have noted the results that had already been published 15 years earlier by Nicholsen and Seddon in 1957, describing a 30% failure rate in end-to-end sutures of median nerve lesions in defects of more than 2.5 cm. Nevertheless, discussions continued on the so-called critical defect distances that should be remedied by end-to-end sutures.

Meanwhile, Jacobson introduced microsurgical techniques in peripheral nerve surgery procedures in 1963, and the more and more widespread knowledge of these microsurgical methods (Smith 1964) opened new views on the suture line: the unfortunately ongoing mechanical view of some authors advocating wrapped or glued cable grafts was consequently replaced by increasingly new biologically orientated views taking into consideration the histological aspects of nerve regeneration in grafts and at suture lines. As a result, Millesi and co-workers (1972), Samii and Wallenborn (1972), as well as Maxion and co-workers (1972) succeeded in experimentally proving that the amount of nerve regeneration after nerve suture significantly decreased with increased tension at the suture line. Their results proved a direct correlation between failures of axon sprouting and tension between sutured nerve stumps. Additionally, histological studies showed increasing scar tissue between the nerve stumps the longer the distance between the nerve ends. The above-mentioned authors thus postulated that tension at suture lines had to be avoided completely. At the same time, surgeons learned how to handle soft nerve tissue and how to succeed in microsuturing guided by the microscope. The formerly used cable grafts no longer made sense because the difference in diameter between skin nerves and main nerve trunks had lost its importance.

In the meantime, discussions started on the practicality of the different kinds of homologous nerve grafts; but rapidly autologous grafts prevailed owing to Samii's outstanding efforts during the 1970s.

Arguments for nerve tissue vascularization grew in importance: free grafted nerve tissue obviously had to be revascularized within a certain amount of time involved (Smith 1966; Penkert et al. 1988). Cable grafts of nerve trunk diameter consequently developed central necrosis because of insufficient revascularization out of their recipient bed, resulting in unsatisfactory regeneration rates, whereas small skin nerves were said to be revascularized in time, leading to the conclusion that the regenerating nerve sprouts can only be sufficiently nourished at once if they are of the diameter of skin nerves.

Considering all the above-mentioned historical facts, it is remarkable that on the one hand, excellent results achieved by new microsurgical efforts have been published (all of them described in key publications by Millesi et al. 1975, 1976, 1977), while on the other hand, discussions on critical defect distances of nerve gaps continued in Europe for some time.

Today, however, the microsurgical handling of nerves and the repair of nerve defects with autologous grafts with no tension has been accepted as the treatment of choice. Nevertheless, this kind of time-consuming surgery did not find appropriate recognition in our health system, hospital departments, and in the general public.

Anatomy and Histological Reaction of Traumatized Nerves

2.1 Macroscopic Anatomy of the Peripheral Nerve System

A special comparable system of nerve trunks passes through the upper and lower limbs, which must be thoroughly understood by every physician treating peripheral nerve lesions. It is astonishing that the ramifications of nerves and the special muscles innervated by these nerves are totally comparable between the upper and lower limbs (▶ Fig. 2.1). Imagining this comparability facilitates the clinical investigation of patients suffering from incomplete or complete nerve lesions. Anatomically and functionally comparable are the axillary (circumflex) nerve and obturator nerve, the musculocutaneous nerve and femoral nerve, the median nerve and medial plantar nerve, the ulnar nerve and lateral plantar nerve, the radial nerve and common peroneal nerve, as are the individual ramifications of the radial and common peroneal nerves, that is, their superficial branch as well as their deep branch (posterior interosseous nerve in the lower arm). Important ramifications may vary depending on their possible levels; these variations must be taken into account in nerve surgery, but most of them are not of great importance, for example, the ramification of the sciatic nerve into the tibial and peroneal nerves as well as the ramification of the tibial nerve into the medial and lateral plantar nerves. However, there are three ramifications of the upper limb nerves that cannot be mentioned often enough, which will raise serious problems in the assessment of certain lesions during surgery. For example, motor fibers innervating the thenar muscles, which are normally found within the median nerve, may remain located within the ulnar nerve (Riche-Cannieu anastomosis), a fairly frequent situation in humans. These motor fibers leading to the thenar muscles may arise from the ulnar nerve fibers at different unknown levels and then join the median nerve fibers. In some cases, the motor branch of the thenar muscles even leaves the ulnar nerve at the palm level. In such cases, actually not all that rare, a complete loss of continuity of the median nerve trunk would not result in thenar muscle paresis, and a surgically reconstructed median nerve could not restore any real thenar function.

On the other hand, fibers supplying the hand's intrinsic muscles, normally expected to run with the ulnar nerve, may also vary in so far as they run with the

Figure 2.1

Scheme comparing nerve ramifications of upper and lower extremities

▼

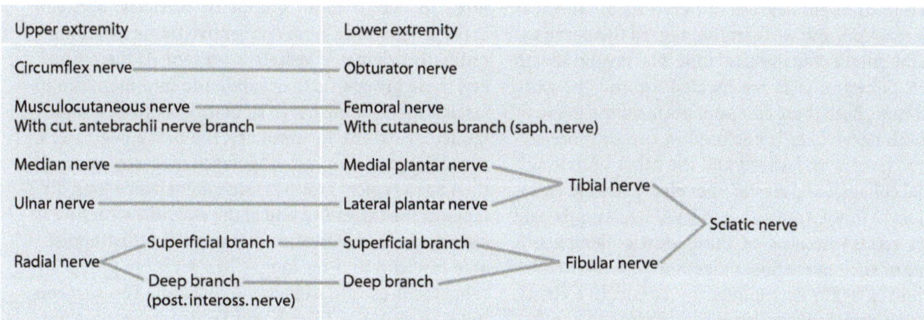

median nerve first, then change at different forearm levels to the ulnar nerve (Martin-Gruber anastomosis; see also Chaps. 5, 6). Sometimes they even use the anterior interosseous nerve for interchange (see Chap. 5).

The ramification of the lateral cord into the median nerve trunk and the musculocutaneous nerve may be situated much more distally at the level of the middle third of the upper arm, i.e., all fibers of the musculocutaneous nerve arise from the median nerve only at this level and its ramification into motor branches already starts after a short musculocutaneous segment. Special reconstructions dealing with the musculocutaneous nerve, particularly reconstructions of brachial plexus lesions, might lead to certain difficulties resulting from such low-situated ramifications, because in all cases of brachial plexus lesions, the main target structure remains the biceps muscle and its musculocutaneous nerve. Thus, the surgeon is suddenly confronted with a situation requiring nerve grafts much longer than expected, resulting in a shortage of grafts for the necessary additional reconstruction.

In conclusion, the above-mentioned variations may produce severe confusion, and one should be aware of their possible existence and resulting clinical consequences. For instance, a median nerve transsection that was believed to be complete may surprisingly be associated with preserved thenar muscle function, but nevertheless need nerve repair. On the other hand, a median nerve transsection may be associated with an additional loss of intrinsic hand muscle function, almost simulating an ulnar nerve lesion.

2.2 Microscopic Anatomy of the Peripheral Nerve System

A certain simplification is necessary in a first approach to different degrees of nerve lesion and scar tissue reaction, and we therefore regard the nerve axon as the smallest anatomical unit. The myelin sheath and its Schwann cells are located around the axon membrane. Both these components form the nerve fiber. Each nerve fiber is enclosed in two or more layers: one layer with latticed and the other with longitudinal collagen and elastic fiber elements (the endoneurium). If we transect a nerve, its stumps will always retract because of these elastic elements. A bundle of such nerve fibers together with their endoneurium is again surrounded by connective tissue, and these grouped structures are referred to as a fascicle. This is a true surgical unit that can be easily visualized under the microscope.

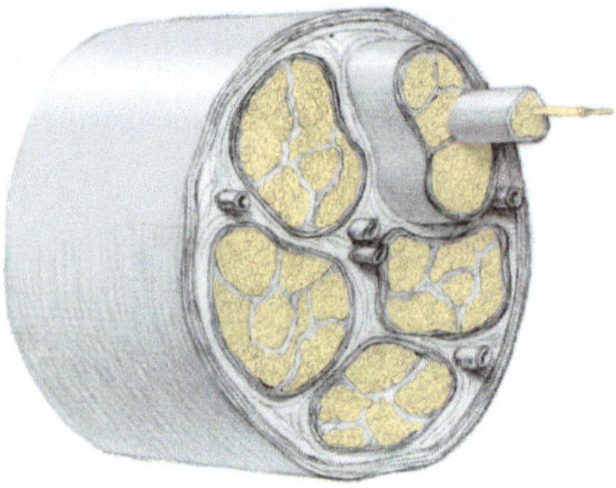

Figure 2.2

Group arrangement of a peripheral nerve: bundles of fascicles in close proximity, forming a fascicle group separated from other groups by a slightly wider interfascicular space of vessels and connective tissue. Epineurium surrounds the trunk, perineurium the fascicle groups and fascicles

Numerous fascicles of each nerve are arranged into groups of fascicles (▶ Fig. 2.2), again surrounded by a few layers of connective tissue (the epifascicular perineurium). According to Sunderland's studies, this group arrangement changes its distribution from central levels to the periphery (▶ Fig. 2.3). Additionally, individual cross-connections between these fascicles and groups of fascicles exist (the plexiform structure, according to Sunderland), which are endangered during microsurgical dissection (Sunderland 1991).

Nerve roots, at their central level, consist of fewer but thicker fascicles divided into sectors by small membranes, whereas more toward the periphery, the nerve takes on its typical group arrangement with three to five or more groups of fascicles. Between these groups, only loose connective tissue with longitudinally orientated vessels is present. At the periphery, these groups further subdivide into many small fascicles so that the nerve structure acquires a multifascicular nature. In summary, the nerve begins as a monofascicular or an oligofascicular structure, it then has a typical group arrangement over a long distance of the extremity, and at the end, this structure is abandoned in favor of multiple small indistinguishable fascicles and no longer has a visible group arrangement (multifascicular structure). The surgeon must be aware of this changing arrangement. A mi-

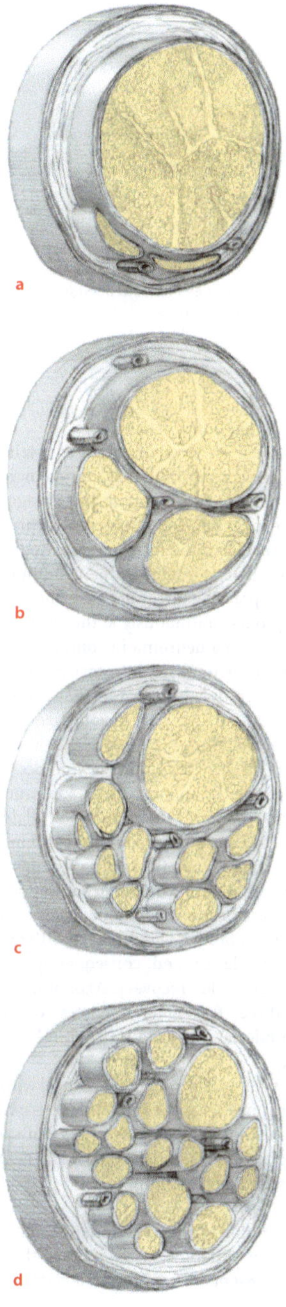

◀ Figure 2.3a–d

Changing of the interfascicular nerve pattern from proximal to distal levels (according to Sunderland's studies). a At beginning levels, monofascicular pattern; b oligofascicular pattern; c group arrangement, typical of main nerve trunks, here there are three fascicle groups; d polyfascicular pattern at the peripheral end

crosurgical separating dissection (microneurolysis) is only possible and allowed in the segments with a group arrangement, while at the root level, dissection between fascicles would damage their integrity.

Following nerve damage or even transsection, all the elements constituting the nerve fiber degenerate from the level of the lesion to the periphery. Only the Schwann cells remain viable and able to reconstruct a new myelin sheath when new axons find a pathway to outward growth. All surgical efforts currently aim at establishing the best conditions possible so that the axon's sprouting process achieves its former target.

2.3 Types and Degrees of Nerve Lesion

Two different principal mechanisms usually lead to nerve trauma: blunt or transecting injuries to the limbs. The former may be affected by crushing or traction or indirectly by radiation or heat, the latter by bone fractures of the limbs or by open penetrating injuries.

As a result of these destroying effects on nerve tissue, we distinguish between lesions with and without loss of continuity. In almost all cases, the question of continuity of the injured nerve at first remains unanswered. In order to identify what kind of lesion is present, two systems describing the degrees of lesion have been developed.

In 1943, Seddon established the well-known concept of neurapraxia, axonotmesis, and neurotmesis, according to the degree of compressing and injuring forces. In neurapraxia, the lesion leads to a partial or total functional block of electrical conductivity due to myelin sheath degeneration within the affected nerve segment, clinically meaning a 3- to 4-week temporary stage of functional deficit, the amount of time needed to restore the myelin sheath after removing the causal factors. Cases of axonotmesis are defined as a complete interruption of axon continuity associated with Wallerian degeneration in the distal part of the nerve. The regenerating process starts early in the proximal part of the injured nerve if the microanatomical situation allows it: potentially, its fibers are

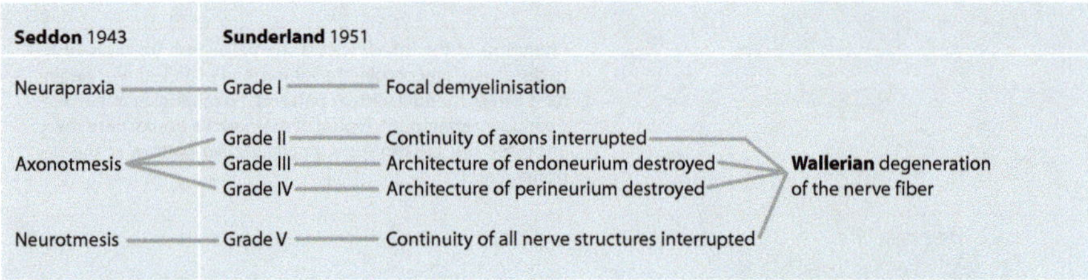

Figure 2.4

Scheme to distinguish classifications of nerve lesions according to Seddon (1943) and Sunderland (1951). Seddon's axonotmesis consists of three additional types of connective tissue damage that influence recovery chances

able to resprout into the periphery, but depending on the distance to their former target, they need a few months to develop new contacts. Additionally, around these fiber sprouts, individual myelin sheaths are reformed by Schwann cells alive during the regenerating process. Neurotmesis, contrary to the two former types of lesion, means a complete interruption of the nerve trunk resulting in a total lack of spontaneous recovery.

First published in 1951, Sunderland distinguished five degrees of lesion (▶ Fig. 2.4). We consider this latter classification to be much more detailed and more suitable than Seddon's categories for visualizing and understanding the different types of disturbing events and the consequences that may occur within the nerves. We believe that it should still be considered valid:

Grade I: Sunderland's grade I lesion is nearly identical to Seddon's neurapraxia. The myelin sheath is the most sensitive part of the nerve fiber; thus, focal demyelination occurs first. The rearrangement of the myelin sheath takes 3–4 weeks. After this short period, the nerve can almost regain its normal function.

Grade II: As a result of higher compressing forces, the axons undergo Wallerian degeneration. Nevertheless, each axon remains enclosed by its basal membrane and endoneurium so that, during axon sprouting, each fiber succeeds in regaining its former muscle end-plate. Although this process lasts for some months because of the distance, the end result may come close to a restitution ad integrum.

Grade III: In this degree of lesion, the endoneural structures of the nerve fibers are progressively destroyed so that motor axons can sprout into a sensory pathway or vice versa. This situation leads to a certain amount of mis-sprouting later followed by extensive functional deficits.

Grade IV: Because of now disarranged perineural structures, the amount of mis-sprouting increases, effectively ensuring, for example, that antagonistic muscles are innervated simultaneously. This situation again increases the resulting functional deficit in comparison to grade III lesion. Additionally, ongoing compressing forces are even able to block the axon sprouts continuously at the lesion, a situation resulting in a neuroma in continuity. This is comparable to a total nerve interruption. Thus, grade IV and grade V lesions, together, present the same poor prognosis as far as spontaneous recovery is concerned.
The quality of regeneration, the number of resprouting axons, the amount of mis-sprouting, and the quality of the final functional result all depend on the potential disintegration of the original fascicle group arrangement because of damage and eventual incomplete recovery. According to Sunderland's classification, Seddon's idea of axonotmesis now contains a wide field of different degrees of nerve lesion and, consequently, of quite different chances for recovery. Axonotmesis thus contains three further subdegrees of lesion, namely, Sunderland's grade II, III, and IV lesions (▶ Fig. 2.4).

Grade V: A grade V lesion is again identical with Seddon's neurotmesis, i.e., a complete interruption of the entire nerve trunk, with no chance of spontaneous recovery and leading to a terminal neuroma at the proximal nerve stump.

Comparing Seddon's and Sunderland's historical classifications of different nerve lesions, the latter classification presents a few simple advantages. On the one hand, the notion of different types of risks and chances for recovery resulting from traumatic forces on nerve tissue goes into much more detail. On the other hand, Sunderland's efforts have led to a more reasonable explanation as to why spontaneous recovery and functional recurrence cannot be expected as a rule, nor why operative treatment does not always improve nerve function, but may even lead to unexpectedly poor results despite time-consuming microsurgical neurolysis procedures. The surgeon might also underestimate the degree of lesion and not operate appropriately.

However, additional factors influencing the regeneration process, often negatively, still exist: first, the ongoing process of muscle atrophy can become more and more irreversible roughly 6 months after the lesion, and second, secondary reactions of the connective tissue following nerve damage (see Sect. 2.4).

2.4 Scar Tissue Reactions Following Nerve Lesion

Regarding Seddon's and Sunderland's classifications of peripheral nerve injury, we should regularly expect more or less nerve regeneration within a period of either a few weeks or a few months. Unfortunately, however, each trauma causes connective tissue reactions, histologically well-known processes starting after the trauma, such as the necessary waiting period of a few weeks before the complete picture can be histologically assessed. This process is referred to as fibrosis and produces compressing forces on the axon sprouts. In case of a grade I lesion, the temporary stage of functional deficit would turn into a steady stage if an ongoing compression remains. The same holds true for axonotmesis (Sutherland's grades II–IV), which is associated with Wallerian degeneration in the distal part and regeneration from the proximal part of the nerve. Despite a primary optimal regenerating process, scar strangulation can secondarily decrease or prevent electrical conductivity by disturbing the rather sensitive myelin. If the amount of scar strangulation further increases, the outgrowing process of axon sprouts itself can remain primary or become secondarily blocked.

Considering all these secondary effects, Millesi (1992) established a classification of fibrosis types resulting from nerve injury. It was taken from a surgical point of view, as he microscopically noted that the fibrosis could originate from quite different parts of the connective nerve tissue:

Type A: Fibrosis of the epineurium
In this case, the surrounding layer of the epineurium is involved to the point that scar strangulation compresses the entire nerve trunk. Theoretically, this type of fibrosis can occur in all cases of grade I, II, or III lesions, according to Sunderland's classification. It is important to note that, independent of these types of lesion, chances of spontaneous recovery remain significantly decreased as long as axon compression is present. Therapy should therefore aim at opening the epineurium.

Type B: Interfascicular fibrosis
The connective tissue between the fascicle groups is involved. Each fascicle group is individually affected by compressing forces. This type of fibrosis should decisively influence the following surgical treatment if compared with type A fibrosis. A simple opening of the fibrotic epineurial sheath would be insufficient because compressing forces on fascicles would continue.

Type C: Intrafascicular fibrosis
According to Sunderland's classification, this type of fibrosis can take place only in grade III or IV lesions. The fibrosis involves the connective tissue of the endoneurium of each fascicle, with the nerve in great danger of developing a neuroma in continuity. Chances of spontaneous recovery disappear completely and surgical options must be even more radical.

Clinical Presentation of Nerve Lesions

3.1 Management of Diagnosis

In peripheral nerve surgery, treatment planning must begin with an accurate anatomical and neurological assessment in order to judge which nerve or combinations of nerves have been injured. We have found it helpful to bear in mind the comparability of the nerve ramifications of the upper and lower limbs (see Chap. 2). Each nerve of the arm corresponds to a special nerve of the leg and significant distinctions do not exist, with the exception of levels of ramification. Thus, clinical investigation will clearly assess which nerve is actually involved. Unfortunately, however, this examination will reveal nothing about the chances of spontaneous recovery: the time span between nerve lesion and potential and expected regeneration often lasts several months. During this period, we can test the behavior of the axon sprouts only by eliciting the Tinel sign. Palpation and percussion of the affected nerve trunk at different points will trigger an electric-current-like pain that is individually experienced in the sensitive area previously belonging to the injured nerve. The maximum point where the physician can effect such a triggered pain derives from the location of the maximum number of outgrowing axon sprout ends. If the trigger point moves downward during a period of some months, axon outgrowth is occurring, a positive prognostic factor. If the trigger point stops at the same level over several investigations, the outgrowth of axon sprouts is completely blocked, indicating surgical intervention. Under special circumstances, the trigger point of the Tinel sign may even return to the lesion during a short follow-up period, thus indicating increasing compressing forces by scar tissue strangulation mentioned in Chap. 2. According to Seddon's classification, in all cases of axonotmesis, the Tinel sign is the only real aid in decision making.

Electrophysiological testing, with measurements of electrical conductivity of motor and sensitive pathways as well as electromyography, will also make it easier to determine the extent of nerve lesion. However, it should be kept in mind that all types of electrical conductivity are already destroyed in cases worse than grade I in Sunderland's classification (with the exception of nerve root avulsion including the spinal ganglion). Electromyography reveals signs of complete denervation (pathological spontaneous activity, recruited by muscle fiber activity only) starting after a period of 4 weeks; it is then helpful when making the decision to know which nerve or combination of nerves is disconnected from nerve supply. An undetermined period of time follows, during which electromyography does not help answer the most important question about eventual spontaneous recovery and potential out-growth of axon sprouts into the periphery. Only if reinnervation potentials occur within the muscles do we obtain information that axons have regained contact to the muscle end-plates and that nerve continuity has been preserved. Considering the above-mentioned process of muscle atrophy, we often have to make our decision about nerve repair earlier than reinnervation eventually occurs.

3.2 Surgical Types of Nerve Lesion and Treatment Modalities

3.2.1 Entrapment Syndromes

Entrapment syndromes are lesions in anatomically narrowed regions, i.e., the carpal tunnel, the supinator channel, the thoracic outlet or the tarsal tunnel. In typical situations, they do not present sudden onset of symptoms, but nerve function decreases very slowly, and electrophysiologically, nerve conductivity remains preserved even in the most severe cases, but of course, with reduced velocity. They initially belong to Sutherland's grade I lesions. Compressing forces of scarred epineurium, interfascicular or even intrafascicular scarring occur only in a few cases, which are then associated with Wallerian degeneration and sometimes with increased blocked regenerating forces.

The surgical treatment of entrapment syndromes predominantly consists of a simple decompression of the narrowed region. However, if the patient presents a preoperative severe loss of function or an unexpected loss of electrical conductivity and intraoperatively, an unusual thickening and hardening of the nerve tissue, the surgeon must immediately decide whether to start a stepwise microsurgical dissection. As a first step, the hardened epineurium must be incised and opened in a longitudinal direction. The second step involves removing the epineurium from the entire circumference. Lastly, under higher magnification, clearly visible fascicle groups are gently separated from each other. After that, the perineural sheath of some fascicle groups can be incised again in a longitudinal direction. These microsurgical steps are referred to as epineurotomy, epineurectomy, and interfascicular neurolysis.

Scientific discussion is still ongoing on stepwise neurolysis with entrapment syndromes. We must take into account the plexiform structure of nerves that Sunderland's studies have shown. During separation of fascicle groups, cross connections between them are automatically destroyed, followed by small neuromas after a period of 8 weeks. This procedure may result in an extremely painful nerve lesion for the rest of the patient's life. The surgeon must decide during the operation what should be done with such chronically entrapped nerves showing advanced functional deficits and possibly presenting with severe pain; however, the operation must be the last one if at all possible. Reoperations carry a high risk of worsening the situation significantly because new scar tissue may form around the nerve. Thus, the first surgeon bears the entire responsibility. Of course, microsurgery should only be undertaken in advanced cases. The stepwise procedure is the best, and it should be stopped immediately as soon as the microscope shows that fascicles are expanding similarly. The different steps of neurolysis must not be engaged at any price so as to prevent painful intraneural neuromas.

3.2.2 Traumatic Nerve Lesions in Continuity

The traumatic nerve lesions in continuity originate for the most part in a crush injury or a nerve traction. Theoretically, the first four grades of lesion according to Sunderland's classification and all three types of scarring according to Millesi's classification can be present and even mixed within one affected nerve trunk. It is often difficult to determine with the naked eye whether or not the nerve fascicles and nerve fibers are in continuity within such a nerve trunk. A thickening and hardening of the nerve trunk itself is still not sufficient proof of a neuroma. Fibrotically altered connective tissue can imitate such a neuroma, and it can cause a pseudoneuroma. It is impossible to distinguish between these two types of neuroma macrosurgically. However, with magnification, the epineurium in the intact part of the nerve proximal and distal to the injured area can be incised longitudinally. After that, the external sheath of the epineurium must be removed again at the proximal and distal area. Individual groups of fascicles are also exposed and slightly separated from each other (▶ Fig. 3.1). As one approaches the injured segment, one should be able to continue the above-mentioned steps of neurolysis in Millesi's type A or B lesions, eventually revealing a pseudoneuroma. If the scar-

Figure 3.1

Principle of interfascicular neurolysis. The epineurium is incised and removed, the fascicle groups are gently separated. The perineurium can be incised in the longitudinal direction only if really necessary

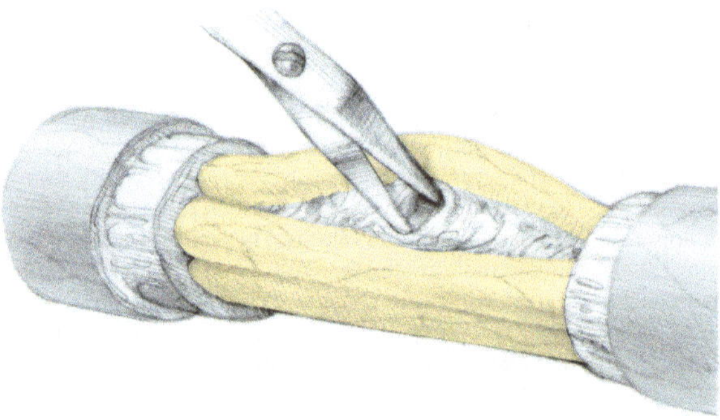

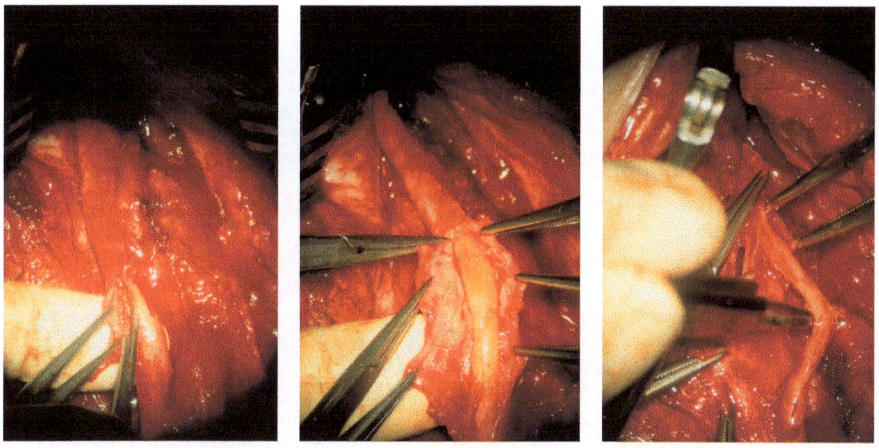

a–c

Figure 3.2 a–c

Example of epineural neurolysis, here of the radial nerve after distally located humerus fracture. a, b Epineurotomy; c epineurectomy

ring also involves the endoneurium (type C), neurolysis aiming to preserve the visible microstructures becomes increasingly difficult as the attempt to dissect within the fibrotic center progresses; this situation leads to a neuroma in continuity. This special and very delicate situation of scar tissue reaction, mainly a fibrosis of the endoneurium only (Millesi's type C), may indeed lead to dissectible fascicle groups if severe epi- and interfascicular fibrosis is missing; however, when trying to palpate them between two finger tips, they feel completely hardened and fibrotic at the end of the neurolysis, revealing several small neuromas in continuity at the same nerve segment running side by side.

Our goal is always to achieve sufficient decompression in order to enable the axon sprouts to overcome the lesion and reach their target. Depending on the amount of damage, an epineurotomy and epineurectomy may be sufficient (▶ Fig. 3.2). In the case of a pseudoneuroma, stepwise microsurgical neurolysis is the treatment of choice (▶ Fig. 3.3), but in the case of a true neuroma or even several neuromas in one segment, resection and restoring of nerve continuity must be carried out (▶ Fig. 3.4); consequently, grade III or IV lesions with type C fibrosis need repair despite preserved nerve trunk continuity.

If there is doubt, intraoperative nerve stimulation is fundamental to confirm fascicles and fascicle groups that are still anatomically and even functionally intact. This method requires that the anesthesiologists raise the patient's level of muscle relaxation for a short time, and requires preserved axonal continuity to the muscle target to derive directly the potentials from muscles. Independent of peripheral muscle reactions is the use of intraoperative nerve action potentials (NAP), in other words, nerve stimulation proximal and deduction of potentials distal to the questionable nerve segment, a method that is entirely credited to Kline and Hudson and co-workers (1995). Special equipment and experience in evaluating the resulting potential quality are of course necessary.

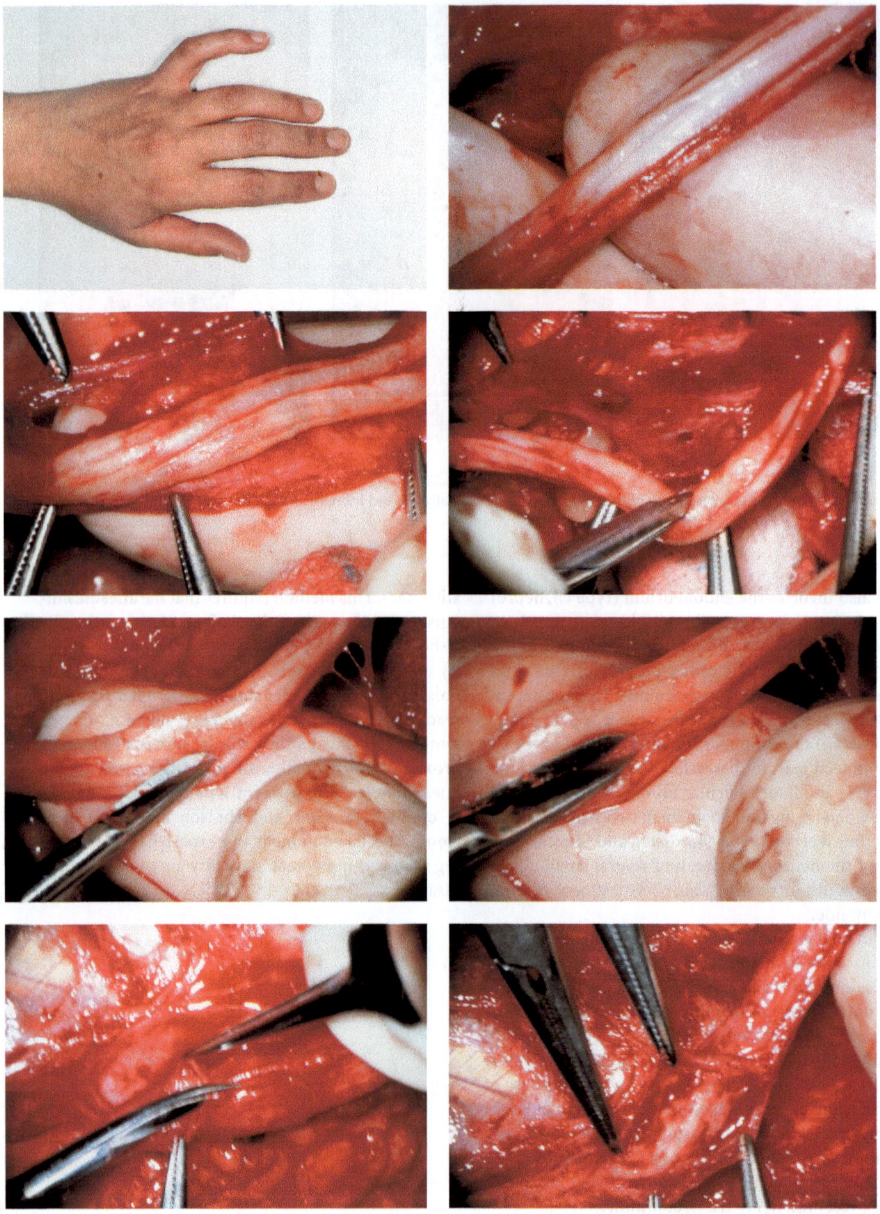

a b
c d
e f
g h

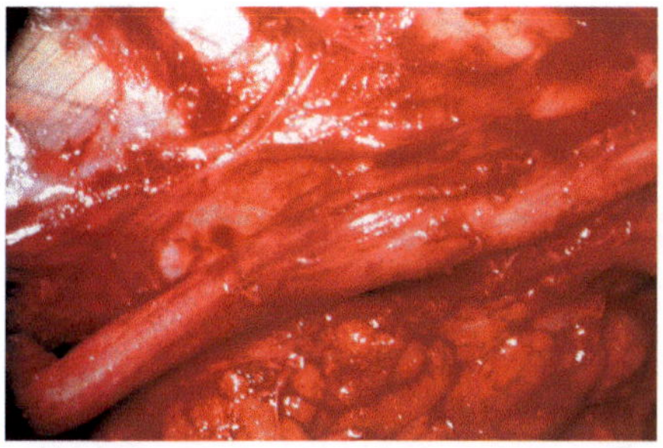

i

◀ **Figure 3.3 a–i**

Example of interfascicular neurolysis, here of the ulnar nerve after elbow fracture. a Severe signs of the nerve lesion; b epineurotomy; c, d epineurectomy; e–h interfascicular neurolysis; i end result

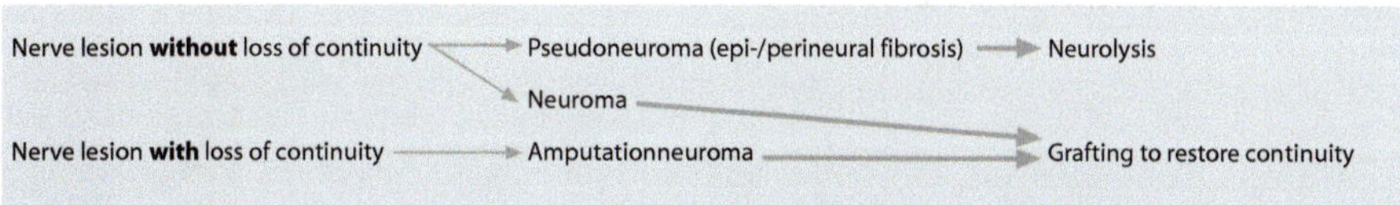

Figure 3.4

Scheme to distinguish different types of therapy, depending not on nerve continuity but rather on different soft tissue reactions weeks after the injury

3.2.3 Traumatic Nerve Lesions Without Continuity

Traumatic nerve lesions without continuity include all cases of neurotmesis in Seddon's classification and grade V lesions according to Sunderland. But as mentioned in the preceding section, severe cases of grades III and IV lesions with Mellesi's type C fibrosis must also be included.

The different kinds of nerve repair that have to be implemented on these lesions have recently changed, as described in Chap. 1. Nowadays, three important factors must be kept in mind if nerve repair is sought:

1. The quality of nerve fiber growth depends on an accurate approximation of the nerve stumps. The former technique for nerve repair was the epineural end-to-end suture. Histological studies have shown that, despite an exact epineural suture, accurate approximation of corresponding fascicles could not be achieved in each individual case (Edshage 1964). Although the nerve ends seemed to be accurately connected from an external point of view, histological studies proved the existence of unsatisfactory fascicular alignment at the suture line. Today, and because of tension at the nerve stumps, grafts are used to restore nerve continuity. For nerve grafting, size and distribution of the fascicular structures of the nerve stumps can be taken into consideration. If a fascicle is of the same diameter as the nerve graft, it can be dissected, isolated, and anastomosed with one nerve graft. A fascicle group of about double the caliber of the graft, resisting division, should be connected to the distal fascicle groups using two grafts (▶ Fig. 3.5). In the case of a polyfascicular nerve with only little interfascicular tissue, the nerve stumps may not be divided into different fascicles or fascicle groups. Several grafts may be sutured side by side with the nerve end so that the whole surface of the nerve stump is covered. The same technique is used if the nerve stump consists of only one large fascicle, such as at the root level of the brachial plexus or sometimes in higher radial nerve levels. As already mentioned, there is also a change in size

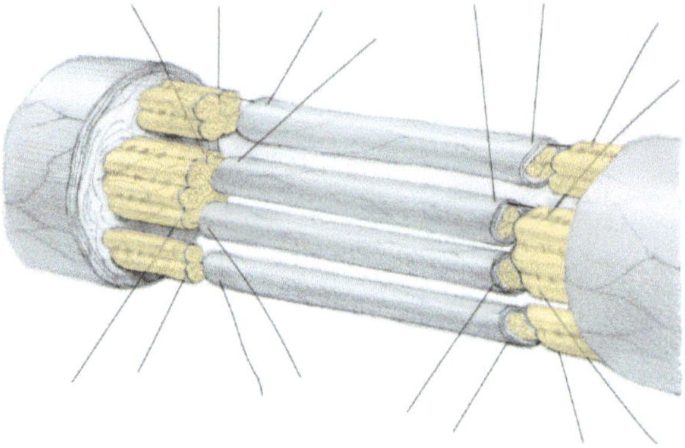

Figure 3.5

Principle of the interfascicular grafting technique (according to Millesi's technique). Sural nerve segments are adapted to corresponding fascicles or fascicle groups. Suture material: 10–0 nylon. Stitches through epineurium of the graft and epineurium or perineurium of the fascicles or fascicle groups

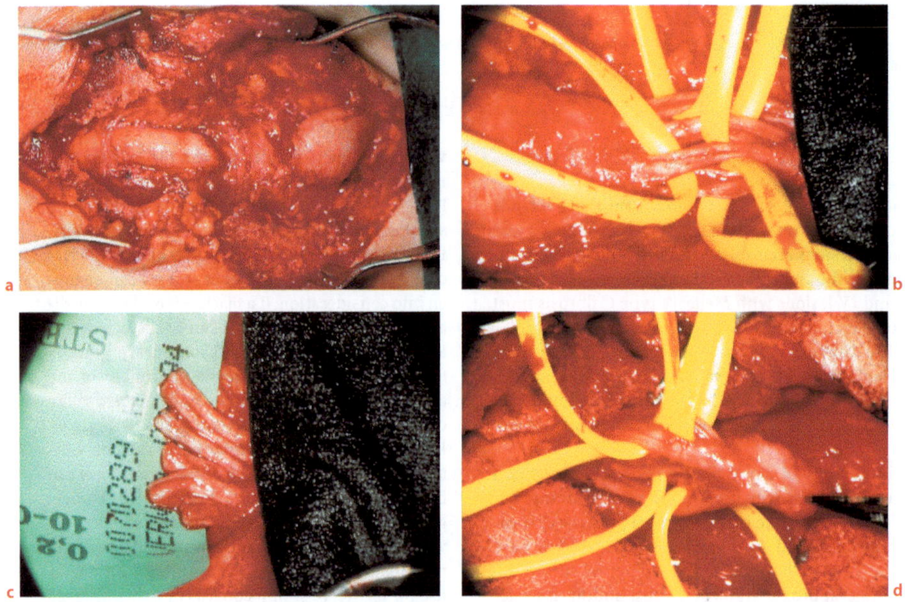

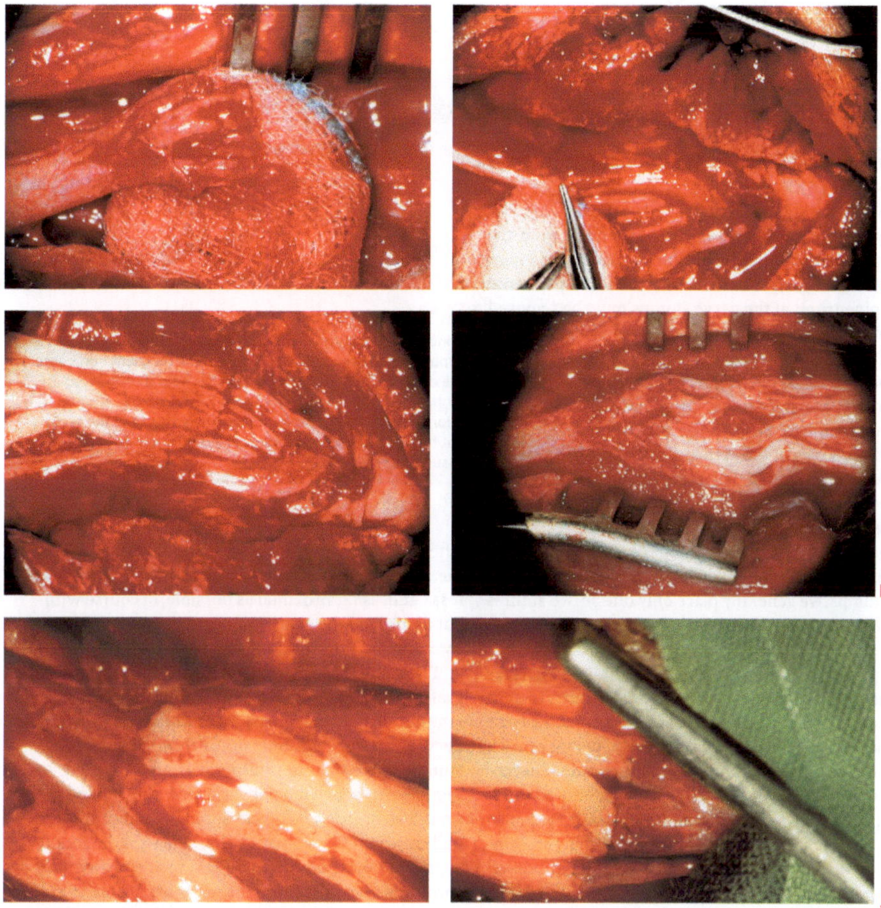

Figure 3.6 a–j

Example of interfascicular nerve grafting, here caused by a median nerve lesion at wrist level. a Both nerve stumps, neuroma on the right (proximal); b interfascicular separation proximally; c individual transsection of separated fascicles; d interfascicular separation distally; e transsection of fascicles distally; f first stitch between graft and fascicle proximally; g end result of the proximal coaptation; h the same situation distally; i, j interfascicular anastomoses with high magnification and distribution of the fascicles within a certain distance of a nerve trunk, resulting in differences in the particular pattern of the proximal and distal nerve stumps. The surgeon's task is to establish an accurate approximation of the nerve grafts with special components of the distal and proximal nerve stump regarding these differences (▶ Fig. 3.6).

2. A second important factor is that the histologically defined process of fibrosis originates from the epineurium of the nerve stumps (Sunderland 1991, Millesi 1992). The already fibrotically altered epineurium at the nerve stumps must be removed over a short distance for two reasons: first, it produces compressing forces and therefore blocks the outgrowth of the axon sprouts and their ingrowth into the distal stump; second, different cells involved in the fibrosis process originate from the outer layers of the epineurium.
3. Attention should be paid to the graft's length, which should be a little longer than the nerve defect, in order to avoid tension at the suture line and guarantee optimal adaption. For the adaption and fixation of the individual graft ends at the nerve stumps, we generally place only one or two sutures with 10-0 suture material. Depending on the circumstances, in a single case epineural, perineural, epiperineurial, or interfascicular tissue structures are individually used to secure the suture. In general, one suture through the epineurium of the nerve graft and through the perineurium of each fascicle group is sufficient to ensure individual coaptation, to avoid harmful tension, and to minimize resulting foreign body granulomas. Fibrin glue induces a local inflammation and in time hinders the ingrowth of vascular sprouts at the sutured segments (Penkert et al. 1988).

The sural nerve should be the first choice of a nerve graft because of its approximately 40-cm length in adults. Both sural nerves may be removed without any significant harm to the patient. Long nerve defects and defects of very thick nerve trunks may be an exception. For bridging such defects, we need not only both sural nerves, but also the cutaneous brachii and antebrachii medialis nerves. Very rarely, the lateral femoral cutaneous nerve or the superficial branch of the radial nerve can be used as a graft. For removal of the sural nerve, the first skin incision is done behind the lateral malleolus; the nerve is then exposed somewhat behind or beside the saphena parva vein. Thus, the nerve can be looped, and by slide pulling, it can be palpated in the proximal direction.

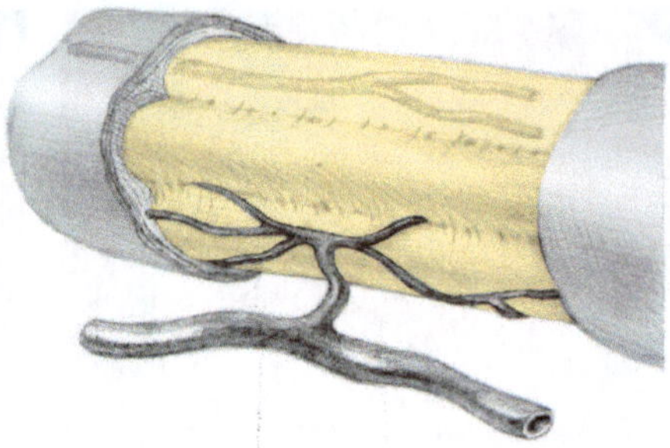

Figure 3.7

Principle of the revascularization of a free nerve graft (author's experiments). Sprouting vessels from the recipient bed enter the epineurium from the third day after operation onward (regional) and from the nerve stumps the fourth day after operation (longitudinal). There must be no ischemia of the recipient tissue, and contact to bones or ischemically damaged soft tissue must be avoided

After one or two more short transverse skin incisions, the sural nerve can be prepared up to the popliteal fossa and, as far proximal as possible, of course without damage to the nearby tibial nerve trunk, it is gently extracted through the skin incisions.

The success of this type of free autologous nerve grafting depends on prompt nutrition and revascularization of the transplants. Revascularization of the nerve graft does not only occur through both nerve stumps to which the transplant is anastomosed. In 1951, Hiller experimentally showed that the nerve graft also receives its blood supply mainly from the bed in which the transplant lies. We experimentally supported these findings (▶ Fig. 3.7) and proved that sprouting vessels occur in the nerve graft after 3 days, independent of the graft's length (Penkert et al. 1988). It can be emphasized that the sciatic nerve of the rabbit used in these experiments was of approximately the same diameter as the human sural nerve that we usually use for nerve grafting, so that the experimental preconditions for revascularization were the same as in humans.

In conclusion, the majority of nerve lesions without continuity must be repaired by nerve grafting so as to guarantee:

- The most accurate alignment of individual structures with comparable diameters (▶ Fig. 3.6 a–j)
- The possibility of completely preventing tension at the suture line (▶ Fig. 3.8) so that the patient's own fibrin glue can eventually prove to be sufficient to

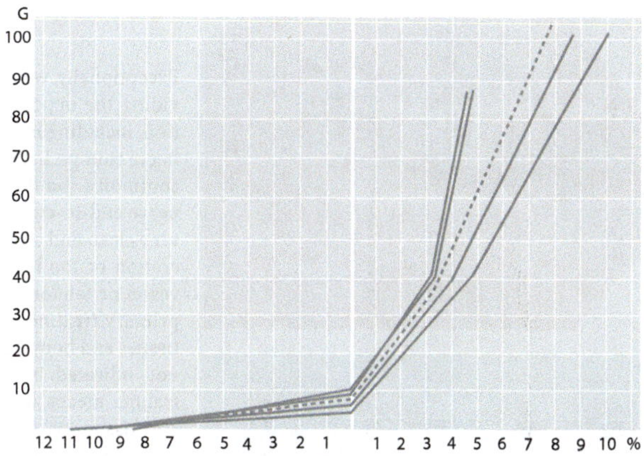

Figure 3.8

Relationship between nerve defect and tension (according to Millesi's experiments on rabbits). *Vertical axis,* force in grams needed for the adaptation of the nerve stumps. *Horizontal axis,* gap in percentage of the whole nerve trunk length. *Left side,* defect after retraction of stumps due to elasticity; *right side,* situation with increasing defects after nerve stump resection

maintain coaptation, a procedure with good outcomes according to our experience

- The possibility of regeneration even if rather long nerve defects have been repaired, a situation frequently encountered following extensive damaging traction forces
- The ability to resect secondary fibrotic nerve stumps without causing harm until soft tissue is observed under the microscope (▶ Fig. 3.6), allowing optimized sprouting after restoration of continuity
- The sufficient and quick renourishment and revascularization of grafts (▶ Fig. 3.7) independent of their length (former arguments against the use of long free nerve grafts are no longer valid)

In a very few selected cases, nerve stumps can still be sutured end to end, placing the stitches through their epineurium. Nevertheless, retracting forces at the nerve ends may hinder tension-free adaptation, particularly if lacerated sectors of the nerve were previously removed. Therefore, only fresh clear-cut injuries, with no contamination and laceration of the surroundings, come into consideration to spare grafting.

3.2.4 Nerve Rotation

Single observations of exceptional cases with rotated nerve segments (rotational distortion) have to be mentioned (Portilla Molinar et al. 1998). Small nerves such as the anterior and posterior interosseous, suprascapular, and axillary (circumflex) nerves, but also the radial nerve trunk at the level where it pierces the lateral intermuscular septum distal of the spiral groove are affected. Repeated lateral and rotatory displacements, for instance, caused by pro- and supination movements, together with cyclical compression caused by sharp structures, can be the origin of such lesions. In small nerves, an inspection guided by magnification is advisable so as not to overlook these rare lesions, particularly as diagnosed anterior and posterior interosseous nerve entrapment disturbances with sudden onset should be assumed to belong to this exceptional group of lesions needing microscopic control.

What kind of microsurgical treatment should be provided? First, the fascicles have to be made visible by means of an epineurotomy and inspection under high magnification. A careful derotation should be the next step. The single case of radial trunk rotation that we have seen needed resection of the affected segment and repair by grafting (▶ Fig. 3.9); recovery was unsatisfactory because it was carried out too late after the lesion's onset. In 1994, Vispo Seara and Lanz reported recovery following simple derotation, but in small nerves. In general, neurolysis and derotation after epineurotomy or, alternatively, resection and repair, are the treatment modalities advised. Reliable advice on the etiology and type of surgery is still needed.

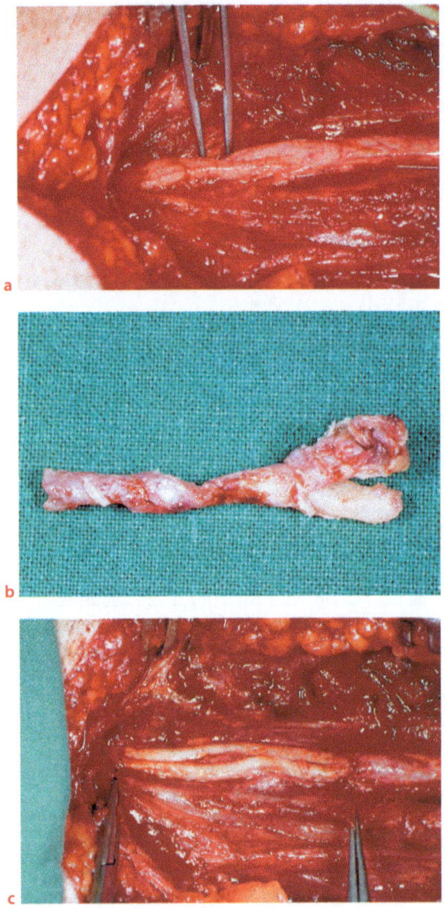

Figure 3.9a–c

A case of nerve rotation. a Radial nerve of the upper arm; b resected nerve segment; c nerve repair by grafts

3.3 Timing of Operation

Exceptionally, we may encounter open wounds, providing the opportunity for primary wound inspection, including immediate identification of nerves or nerve stumps. In our opinion, primary repair of nerve continuity should be considered at this time; then nerve end-to-end suture is allowed only in cases of a very clean and sharp nerve transsection without laceration of the involved nerve stumps. A coexistent vessel or tendon injury is not a contraindication to primary treatment, but in cases of contusion of soft tissues and bony damage, primary nerve treatment is not indicated, because the extension of such nerve trauma means we must expect the development of scar tissue , particularly involving the nerve stumps. According to Millesi's considerations, they cannot be estimated during primary nerve repair. It has also been argued that secondary treatments on bones or tendons, and the risk of insufficient wound healing or even of inflammation depending on the origin of damage, would endanger nerve sutures or grafts from primary interventions.

The advantage of early secondary treatment, about 4–6 weeks subsequent to the injury, now almost always requiring grafting, is the terminated scar reaction that the surgeon can still estimate. Thus, it is now possible to act on the nerve fibrosis appropriately. All the nerve grafts can be placed in and between healthy tissue without risking further surgery.

In conclusion, we believe that most theoretical considerations and practical experience favor early secondary nerve reconstruction when compared with primary repair.

If the patient has sustained a closed lesion, there is no available information on the continuity of the theoretically involved nerves, the degree of the lesion, and the tendency for secondary fibrotic reactions within the nerve. Nerve conductibility may be blocked because of segmental demyelination or Wallerian degeneration. Recovery, if it does start, may take a few weeks or several months, depending on the extent of the lesion and the distance to be overcome from the lesion to the target. Circular compressing forces around or within the nerve may hinder nerve regeneration (Sunderland 1991; Millesi 1992). Unfortunately, most cases present with a primarily unclear nerve lesion. To date, we could only advise repeated clinical, neurographic, and electromyographic examinations. However, time should not be neglected considering the irreversible process of muscle atrophy after several months.

If the evaluations fail to reveal any sign of nerve recovery, only the downward migration and the main trigger point of the Tinel sign could help in decision making. If migration has stopped or never occurred, a late secondary operation is indicated not later than 6 months after the injury, if possible, but a few months earlier is preferred: approximately 6 months after the injury, there is a significant drop in the extent of regenerative forces because of degenerative processes within the muscles. In patients who were operated on later, the axon sprouts reached targets that had sustained excessive irreversible atrophy. After long intervals between trauma and the decision to operate, chances of recovery are considerably reduced. It must also be remembered that the process of outgrowing axon sprouts takes several months, a time span to be added to the preoperative waiting time. Patients who were operated on late increasingly needed simultaneous or secondary reconstructive surgery for satisfying functional results to be achieved. Some nerve lesions affecting nerves with rather poor regeneration prognosis such as lesions of the common peroneal nerve should never be repaired later than 6 months after the injury for the patient to have motor recovery. If the intention is to restore sensitivity, surgery can be planned at any time.

Several new reports on ultrasound investigations have shown surprising possibilities to overcome the time factor in the diagnostic dilemma of cases requiring a decision on early or late secondary exploration: in 2001 Peer and co-workers, and more recently in 2003 Kele and co-workers, found that nerve neuromas and nerve discontinuity were easily detected with ultrasound in relatively superficially located nerves. Further experiments will determine how reliably this method can work on deeply situated nerves such as the axillary (circumflex) nerve. If this turns out to be reliable, it will revolutionize the decision for and timing of operations.

3.4 Operation in a Bloodless Field

The use of an occluding cuff to produce a bloodless operating field is very common and repeatedly advised in plastic and reconstructive surgery. In 1992, Millesi advised using a cuff during the dissection of all structures of the lower arm and lower limb. Without doubt, this facilitates the exploration of nerves, tendons, and vessels, especially in an area where former lacerations and scar tissue adhesions have changed the anatomical situation. In his opinion and experience, a close cuff should even be allowed over a period of 2 h with no harm to postoperative nerve function. According to Birch and co-workers in 1998, paralysis was always produced after occluding a cuff more than 30 min. In their opinion, paralysis always spontaneously recovers within a few minutes after the release of pressure. But the same authors sometimes noted a much longer-lasting paralysis, and they also described rare occurrences of permanent paralysis. A reversible paralysis is said to be due to transient ischemia. The longer-lasting paralysis seems to result from damage to the myelin sheath and requires roughly 4 weeks to recover. However, permanent paralysis is necessarily caused by complete damage to all elements of the nerve and results in a severe postoperative deficit. Additionally, reflex sympathetic dystrophies were described by Birch (1998). In 1995, Kline and Hudson observed a tourniquet-related conduction block over a period of 20 min or more by intraoperative recordings of nerve action potentials.

Do we really need a bloodless operating field? The following reasons could be used to argue against the use of occluding cuffs:

- The truly difficult explorations, dissections of the brachial plexus, thoracic outlet, facial and spinal accessory nerves, circumflex (axillary) nerve, radial nerve after humerus fractures, and nerves within the buttocks cannot be managed with aid of a tourniquet. If the surgeon has experience on these nerves, a tourniquet is no longer helpful, with the exception of special indications on hand surgery such as during the exploration of the deep branch of the ulnar nerve in the palm (see Chap. 5).
- Tourniquet-related nerve conduction blocks are of no great importance as long as they remain reversible, as is usual. However, both irreversible damage and reflex dystrophy are dreadful complications that would not be a desirable surgical outcome.
- If the nerve exploration revealed a situation needing nerve repair or even nerve grafting, diffuse bleeding following release of cuff pressure can make it difficult to regain control for a short period. After microsutures, wound compression would completely displace all microsurgical adaptations. Thus, great patience is needed to individually coagulate the great number of small vessels.

It must be realized, however, that arguments in favor of operating in a bloodless environment are overridden by esthetic considerations on the one hand, but particularly by a facilitated and safer soft tissue separation and a safer dissection under microscope on the other hand, all important arguments for use of a preliminary tourniquet in cases of lesions located distal to its placement. Nevertheless, one must remain aware of the above-mentioned risks. There is no doubt that a tourniquet is mandatory in surgical procedures within the palm. In cases of carpal tunnel or distal ulnar nerve release, opinions may differ. At the moment, harm to digital nerves when entrapments in the hand were operated on without a bloodlessness environment might produce litigation more easily than tourniquet-related nerve damage.

3.5 Postoperative Treatment

First of all, wound closure is a procedure potentially displacing grafts and coaptation lines and causing redevelopment of a neuroma at the suture line. Therefore, the surgeon must ensure gentle and adequate wound closure. Postoperatively, it should be routine to immobilize the affected extremity for 8–10 days with a plaster bandage after nerve suture or nerve grafting. The bandage must be placed in exactly the same position that the limb had during the operation, and applied as gently as the wound closure had been done. Experimental studies have demonstrated that the stability of nerve suturing or grafting without tension achieved the tensile strength of a healthy nerve within 7 days after the operation (Samii and Penkert 1998). Therefore, there should be no need for immobilization of the limbs for longer periods than this. Two weeks after surgery, we start with physiotherapy in order to avoid inactivity of the neighboring joints.

Following either neurolysis or nerve repair, we are again confronted with a long period of time without knowing whether regeneration is really taking place. During this time, the downward migration of the Tinel sign is once again the only indication of sprouting axons. Clinical and electromyographic studies every 3 months are also important. Often seen earlier in electromyography than clinically, signs that reinnervation is beginning appear, but depending on the distance, most still appear after several months.

The value of the postoperative electric stimulation of the paralyzed muscles has remained unclear until today. There have been reports that this kind of therapy provides better results than without electrical stimulation, but scientific proof is lacking. It is very important to stop the stimulation therapy when signs of reinnervation occur and then immediately to start active training of the reinnervated muscle groups. Without question, this training should be undertaken as often as possible.

Ongoing clinical evaluations and electromyographic studies may reveal a simultaneous innervation of antagonistic muscles. Mis-routing after nerve damage or repair is the origin of this phenomenon. Muscle or tendon transfers should be tried as a solution to improve functional results. Reconstructive surgery procedures provide additional help to patients (see Chap. 10), particularly in cases of complete lack of recovery, when this type of surgery should be advised.

Scientific Outlook

The evidence that the sprouting process of axons after nerve damage and nerve repair complies with a natural law still raises a great number of questions: the individual amount of mis-routing and how to optimize this situation, how to support the growing forces of the sprouts pharmacologically, and how to minimize muscle fiber atrophy. Unfortunately, solutions that enable us to manage these questions remain elusive. Clinical and experimental research to date has only contributed a few small hints.

New methods of diagnosis and follow-up examination are evolving. Besides the valuable clinical examination and the common neurophysiological techniques, these include motor-unit estimation and twitch force superposition, making it possible to quantify degeneration and regeneration objectively (Fansa et al. 1997; Lenz et al. 2001).

Stimulating degeneration to allow faster axonal ingrowth and stimulating regeneration are other avenues of exploration. Growth factors are widely administered (mostly locally) to achieve this type of stimulation (Fansa et al. 2002). However, systemic pharmacological treatment that would have no side effects in humans would facilitate matters considerably. Several drugs such as nonimmunosuppressive compounds derived from FK 506 (Tacrolimus) are in still the experimental stage. In hand transplants, FK 506 was shown to accelerate nerve regeneration rapidly (Fansa et al. 2000). Additionally, there are drugs available that keep the deinnervated muscle intact and then allow a faster regeneration (Frerichs et al. 2001).

Third, the neuromuscular junction zones should be more closely studied in the future. By means of immunofluorescence, these areas can be made experimentally visible since they consist of special recipient structures at the muscle fiber surface. These structures have to be reoccupied by axon sprouts after neurolysis or nerve repair. In experiments, we found a considerable disparity between the pre-existing and the amount of finally reconnected neuromuscular junctions. This finding might lead to an important source of functional deficits, again in addition to factors such as mis-sprouting, different kinds of scar tissue reactions, and the progressive muscle atrophy mentioned in earlier chapters. Furthermore, neuromuscular junctions in these experiments are not reestablished in the presence of the approaching axon sprouts, but pre-existing recipient structures are always reoccupied by the axons (indirect neurotization, Becker and Penkert 2000). Further experiments, which unfortunately have not yet been published, revealed that the axon sprouts are even able to find these junctions with no connection to a distal nerve stump (direct neurotization). Thus, they are able to find their path between muscle fibers simply led by neurotropic factors, which was empirically proven two decades ago (Millesi and Walzer 1981) and should therefore be advised in special injury situations (see Chaps. 6 and 13). In our opinion, the region of the neuromuscular junctions and the process of their reoccupation by axon sprouts need more attention to influence and improve the regenerating process.

A different topic is the engineering of peripheral nerves to overcome eventual problems of autografting. The autologous nerve graft is still the gold standard; however, limited availability and quality of donor nerves necessitate the search for alternative grafts. Nerve allografting is currently limited to special cases due to the necessity of immunosuppressive drugs. A possible alternative could be the tissue-engineered nerve, made from the patient's own viable Schwann cells that support regeneration and a biocompatible matrix that serves as a scaffold. In a series of experiments, we were able to show good regeneration through grafts made from cultured Schwann cells and scaffolding basal lamina (Fansa et al. 2001). But we must not forget that nerve defects and regeneration distances in animal experiments are essentially shorter, respectively, than the nerve defects to be overcome by axon sprouts in humans.

Part II

Specific Types of Nerve Lesions

mediately. There are two exceptional cases where restriction is needed but no real immobilization: cases with meralgia paresthetica and tarsal tunnel syndromes (see Sects. 5.12 and 5.18). Electroneurographic postoperative studies may serve as proof of successful decompression, and electromyography may reveal improvement indicated by increasing reinnervation potentials or normalization of the potential configuration.

Sometimes, contrary to normally expected improvements, ongoing denervation potentials after surgery can suggest insufficient decompression. Even further deterioration, probably due to proceeding intraneural compressing scars, is also possible. If reoperation on such cases is then considered, the surgeon runs a high risk of inducing additional scar tissue around the nerve trunk; a particular risk arises on the nerve fascicle if an interfascicular separation was done before or is intended at this time. Therefore, it must be repeated again and again that each operation should be the first and last one.

5.1 Thoracic Outlet Syndrome

The group of thoracic outlet syndromes remains controversial worldwide. Etiology, difficulties in diagnosis, and two different approaches to surgical treatment are still in discussion.

First, this syndrome has to be defined as an irritation syndrome caused by structures in place since birth. Neither a narrow tunnel nor an unfavorable location of the affected nerves can be the origin of the irritation. The onset itself may be spontaneous and unrelated to any trauma but associated with for the most part slight chronic deterioration. Very rarely, the patient is able to remember a sudden onset related to a particular incident. The patient's history may disclose, for example, a participation in a move, playing cards without interruption over a period of several hours, carrying heavy shopping bags, but also car accidents, particularly without any severe trauma. At the beginning, the patient sustains symptoms comparable to the electric-current-like sensations of the Tinel sign. On the other hand, this is the only real aid in reaching the diagnosis because it indicates not only degenerating and regenerating processes, but much more importantly, the involved nerve segment. The patient is able to localize the Tinel-like pain to a particular area of the upper extremity or to one or two neighboring dermatomes, allowing the clinician to refer back to the affected nerve trunk. These are nearly always the medial and the lower trunks of the supraclavicular part of the brachial plexus.

We have never operated on patients in whom the typical Tinel sign in the supraclavicular groove could not be elicited: its existence is a prerequisite to surgery. Neither electrophysiological tests nor imaging investigations such as three-dimensional CT or magnetic resonance imaging, even when a cervical rib was revealed, proved really helpful to establish a firm diagnosis. Of course, by means of imaging studies, cervical disc ruptures, and electrophysiological studies, more peripherally located entrapment syndromes producing comparable symptoms must be excluded before operation. Thus, the diagnosis of thoracic outlet syndrome is finally made after excluding all other remaining options. Women with a thin and high neck are predominantly affected.

The often associated functional stenosis of the subclavian artery can be revealed by digital subclavian arteriography, but even this does not lead to a firm diagnosis because such a stenosis is not regularly combined with nerve irritation and vice versa. The same holds true for the Adson maneuver. In terms of diagnosing thoracic outlet syndromes, we believe that a stenosis of the artery, if revealed either clinically or with ultrasound or X-ray, cannot be taken as proof of automatically associated neuroirritation.

Structures causing nerve irritations include fibrous edges within the scalene muscles, additional scalene muscles, fibrous bands between an elongated lower cervical transverse process, the first or an additional cervical rib, or a bony structure alone. Unfortunately, all the fibrous soft tissue structures cannot be revealed by imaging investigations, the main reason why the assessment of the final diagnosis remains so difficult. The surgeon must be aware that these structures underlie not only the primary trunks of the brachial plexus but also the subclavian artery with its branches: the transverse colli artery. In addition to these fibrous or bony structures, a hypertrophic suprapleural membrane is able to trap the inferior trunk. If the surgeon opens this membrane, the intrapleural space is penetrated, which may cause pneumothorax, secondary hematothorax, or chylothorax. The supraclavicular groove contains a plexus of small venous and chylous vessels associated with the often enlarged lymph nodes. These small vessel systems can be injured during exploratory surgery and postoperative complications may occur such as occult late venous bleedings or fistulas of chylous liquid into the supraclavicular groove or even into the pleural space. Therefore, an effective postoperative suction drainage for a few days is advisable, but

Figure 5.1a–c

Thoracic outlet syndrome on the right side. a Skin incision; b exploration of the lateral neck triangle, external jugular vein ligated; c inferior trunk in view after moving aside phrenic nerve, scalene muscles, and subclavian artery – a situation revealing inferior trunk irritation between artery and first rib

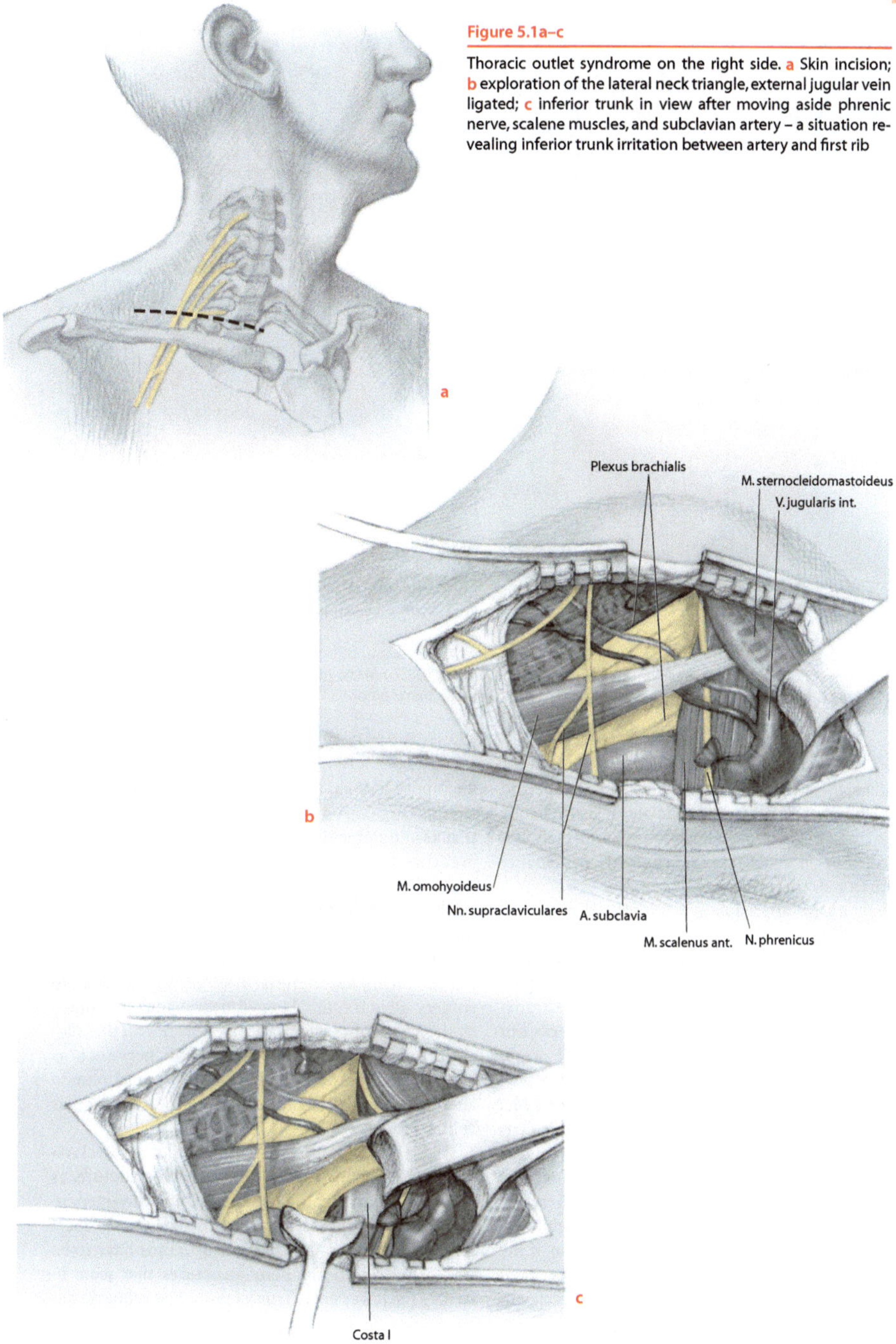

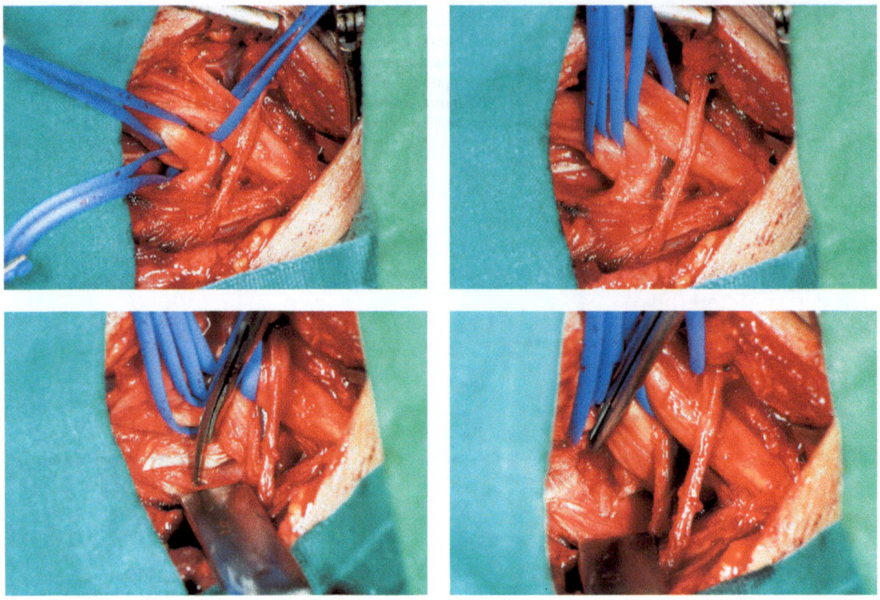

Figure 5.2a–d.

Thoracic outlet syndrome on the left side. a Identification of roots and trunks; b fibrotic structure under the inferior trunk; c transsection of the fibrotic medial scalene muscle; d released situation after transsection

it is nevertheless not a guarantee against unexpected complications. We prefer thoracic outlet surgery only on patients who have been hospitalized for a few days, with the option to observe them 24 h after removing the suction drainage.

The surgical approach is still debated and even leads to litigation. Two different surgical approaches are debated: the supraclavicular and the transaxillary approaches. Both of them are characterized by particular complications. A precondition of the transaxillary procedure is the removal of the first rib, but this endangers the C8 or T1 root just at their origin within the sulcus of the associated transverse process. These iatrogenic lesions are mostly irreversible. On the other hand, the supraclavicular approach endangers the small phrenic nerve. It has such a small caliber that it can easily be harmed or even kinked by the surgeon or by the instruments, and therefore must be kept away from the scalene muscles while exploring the roots. Nevertheless, in our opinion, if the patient sustains the typical electric-current-like pain indicating nerve irritation, we prefer the supraclavicular approach, which provides a better view on the irritating structure (▶ Fig. 5.1). First, however, nerve trunks and nerve roots, the subclavian artery with its branches, the scalene muscles, and particularly in the beginning the phrenic nerve must be dissected and even isolated over a long distance, and the surgeon must gently set aside each individual structure; in summary, a very delicate approach. We avoid looping nerves during decompressive surgery, in contrast to surgery after trauma. Looped nerves may be kinked by the assistant surgeon, as can be seen with the inferior trunk in ▶ Fig. 5.2a, b. The phrenic nerve acts as an important borderline: all dissections must remain lateral to it so as not to injure the internal jugular vein.

A small skin incision 5–6 cm parallel to the clavicle gives enough space to explore each structure, as well as to set aside individual nerves and the artery to find the traumatized structure, situated at the deepest level of the exploration. Soft tissue bands have to be transected, additional bony structures that seem to irritate the lower nerve trunks should be subperiosteally skeletonized and removed bit by bit with a punch. It is especially important in this step to observe all nerves and vessels in the vicinity. Bleeding has to be stopped immediately by bipolar coagulation, but if trying to do so, the origin of the bleeding has to be made visible and the bipolar forceps have to be placed on the individual vessel stump, again observing the surroundings. The surgeon should have experience in this supraclavicular area. The patient will surely note damage to the phrenic nerve when starting sports activities. The restrictions caused by hemiparalysis of the diaphragm are irreversible.

The possible risk of a phrenic nerve transsection makes many thoracic surgeons prefer the transaxillary approach with first rib resection. When clinical symptoms of repeated functional stenosis of the subclavian artery arise, in other words, when the patient's radial pulse disappears when working with the arm elevated, when the hand and fingers get cold in this position, and when the typical signs of nerve irritation are more or less absent, the transaxillary approach might be more effective because, with functional stenosis, one could expect compression between two bony structures, one of them the first rib.

On the other hand, during exploration, especially in women with a high and thin neck, we have frequently found an anomalous cranial convex curved segment of the subclavian artery. In these cases, preoperatively diagnosed functional stenosis was associated with predominant neurogenic symptoms. The affected nerve trunks were always slightly compressed between the artery and the underlying disturbing fibrous structure. We think that this anatomical combination can be highly dangerous when managed by the transaxillary route because the irritation is located far from the first rib. We must keep in mind that, in all cases of thoracic outlet irritation, but especially in the latter one, a complete disappearance of neurogenic symptoms depends mainly on removal of disturbing fibrous structures (▶ Fig. 5.2), not on removal of bony structures.

A postoperative suction drainage is mandatory, independent of the approach, as it works against the development of pneumothorax, chylothorax, or hematothorax, risks that require hospitalization for 3–4 days.

Nevertheless, when there are neurogenic symptoms, we believe that the supraclavicular approach is superior to the transaxillary route.

5.2 Costoclavicular Syndrome

The most important question is whether costoclavicular syndrome is ever able to cause neurological symptoms or even casualties. The narrowed space between the clavicle and the first rib usually causes vascular symptoms as first described by Falconer and Weddell in 1943. In their description, soldiers complained of symptoms in their arms when standing at attention and carrying heavy loads on their shoulders. Interestingly, these costoclavicular compression syndromes were not associated with a positive Adson maneuver, meaning a disappearance of the radial pulse by passive elevating of the arm and turning the head to the opposite side.

We have never had a case of a real nerve irritation syndrome located at the costoclavicular space, with the exception of one case that developed callus after a fracture of the clavicle. The treatment consisted of reduction of the callus only.

5.3 Hyperabduction Syndrome

The question must be raised of whether hyperabduction syndrome really does exist or whether it is able to cause a neurogenic irritation. The first observations were described by Wright in 1945. The symptoms were reported to occur in patients who had to keep their arms hyperabducted during their work.

We have only seen one such case, a young man who presented the typical neuroirritation downward into the sensitive area of the radial nerve as an indication that the posterior cord was involved. The location of the irritation was the attachment of the pectoral minor muscle tendon at the coracoid process of the scapula. In an attempt to determine the location, the characteristic Tinel sign could be elicited in the infraclavicular area.

The treatment consists of infraclavicular exploration with a 90° incision angled to the clavicle and downward toward the axilla, dissection of the pectoral major and the deltoid muscles, as well as the cephalic vein between both muscles. Then the fed tissue and the overlying fascia must be opened to reveal the transverse fibers of the pectoral minor muscle. This muscle should first be dissected in its entire circumference and then transected (▶ Fig. 5.3). Wound closure requires a suction drain.

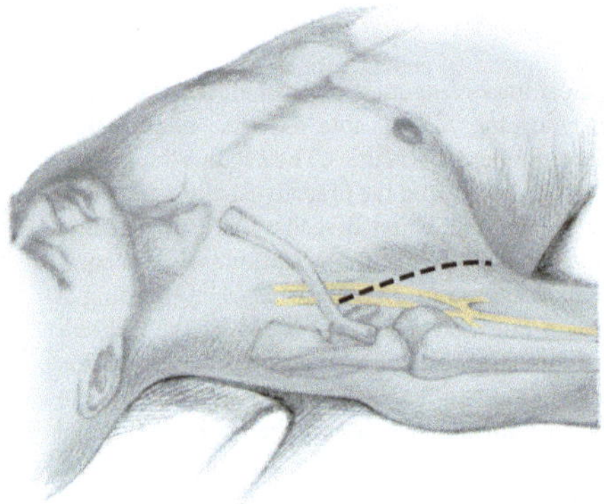

a

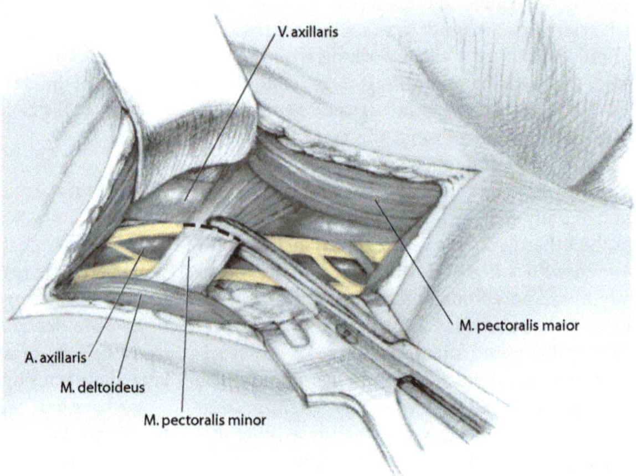

b

Figure 5.3 a, b

Hyperabduction syndrome. a Skin incision; b transsection of the pectoral minor muscle tendon

5.4 Suprascapular Nerve Entrapment

The suprascapular nerve contains motor fibers supplying the supraspinatus and infraspinatus muscles as well as sensitive fibers leading to a skin area behind the scapula. Therefore, its entrapment causes pain in this area, numbness, and in advanced cases, weakness and atrophy of the supra- and infraspinatus muscles. Clinically, the supraspinatus muscle is responsible for the first 15° of abduction of the shoulder and the infraspinatus muscle is responsible for the external rotation of the upper arm, both functions easily tested by asking the patient to perform one of these functions against resistance.

Reliable electroneurographic measurements do not exist but electromyography may reveal denervation potentials in the muscles. Testing the infraspinatus muscle is reliable, whereas results from the supraspinatus muscle may be deceptive because of the overlying trapezoid muscle fibers which, of course, in case of a denervation of the supraspinatus, remain intact. The Tinel sign is provocative at the suprascapular notch where the entrapment is located.

The Tinel sign and pathological electromyographical findings are mandatory to exclude an injury to the rotator cuff of the shoulder, which can closely mimic a suprascapular entrapment, especially when the patient presents with sudden onset. The tendons

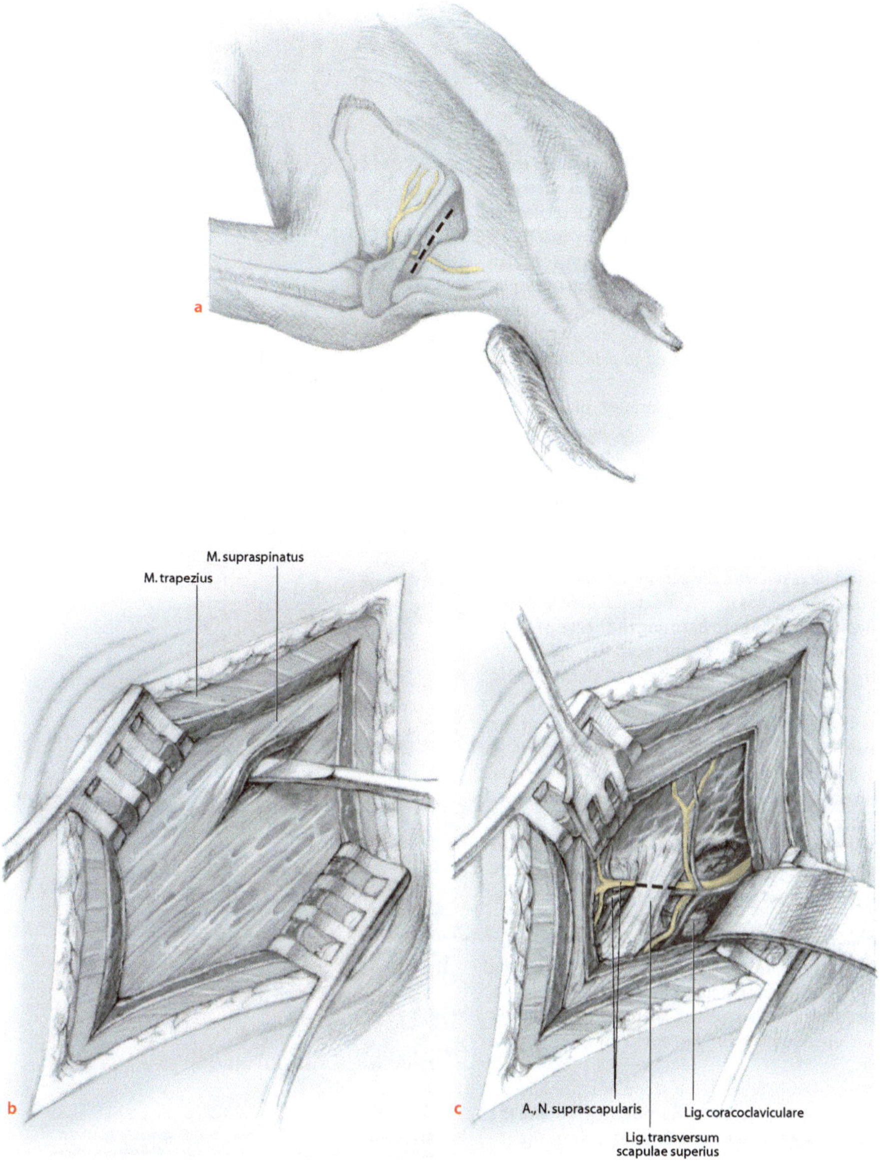

Figure 5.4 a–c

Suprascapular nerve entrapment on the right side (patient in prone position). a Skin incision; b transmuscular approach into the fossa supraspinata; c exploration and transsection of the transverse superior scapular ligament of the supraspinatus and infraspinatus, along with the subscapular and teres minor muscles, blend into the fibrous capsule of the shoulder joint, thus forming the rotator cuff. When, in the case of a cuff lesion, these muscles contract, they appear to be weak because parts of their insertion are unstable and cause severe pain. Nevertheless, their potentials in electromyography remain normal, and typical denervation potentials never occur in these muscles. However, after a certain time, atrophy caused by inactivity does appear, yet again mimicking the suprascapular nerve involvement. To add to the confusion, some patients, after a shoulder injury, may have both a rotator cuff tear and a suprascapular nerve lesion. An MRI study of the shoulder is required to establish or exclude an injury to the cuff.

The treatment of nerve entrapment must aim at transecting the transverse scapular ligament and, rather rarely, the more proximally situated coraco-clavicular ligament. A sometimes existing proximal branch to the supraspinatus muscle as well as a small artery running alongside may arise from their main trunk proximal to the transverse scapular ligament. Care must be taken with the suprascapular artery because injuring it leads to severe arterial bleeding that is difficult to stop without harming the nerve. We prefer an incision parallel to the scapular spine and slightly above it (► Fig. 5.4). Fibers of the trapezoid muscle and fibers of the supra-spinatus muscle are split without transecting them. At the bottom of the suprascapular groove, the suprascapular nerve and artery must be dissected gently. This procedure may present many more problems than expected because, firstly, nerve and artery are both located more laterally than often expected, and secondly, the crucial part of the operation takes place at a considerable depth, making magnification or even a microscope necessary (► Fig. 5.5).

After an earlier trauma affecting the scapular bone, a few patients have presented with a narrowing of the suprascapular notch itself, requiring not only a transsection of the transverse scapular ligament but also an enlargement of the notch by means of a punch.

The incision parallel to the scapular spine also allows an approach into the infraspinatus groove in the very rare cases presenting with weakness of the infraspinatus muscle, as well as with a normally functioning supraspinatus muscle.

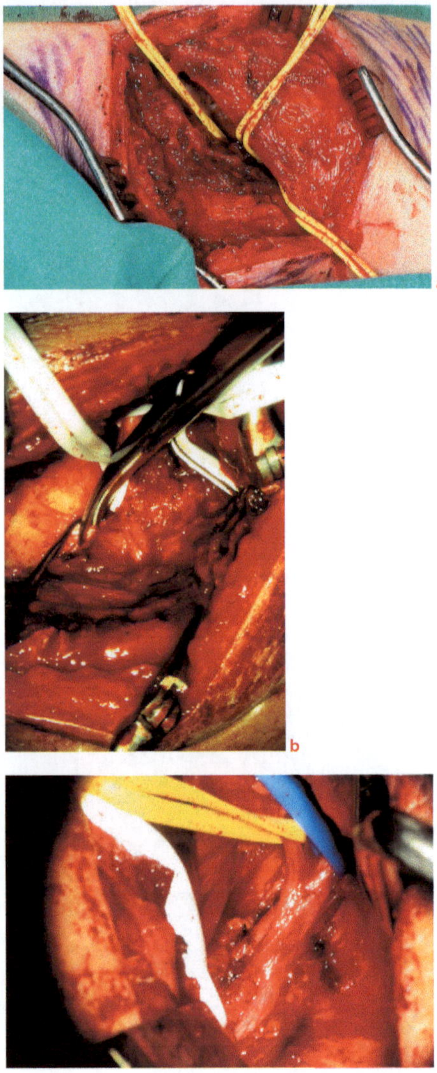
a
b
c

Figure 5.5 a–c

Suprascapular nerve entrapment on the left side (patient in prone position, view from patient's head). a Exploration of the fossa supraspinata; b transsection of the transverse superior scapular ligament under magnification; c ramification of the suprascapular nerve in view after ligament transsection

5.5 Ulnar Nerve Entrapment at Elbow Level

At elbow level, the ulnar nerve is unfavorably located within a small groove between the olecranon and the medial epicondyle. The aponeurotic roof of that groove more or less compresses the nerve depending on the position of the elbow joint. At the entrance into the groove, the aponeurosis forms a U-shaped arch that sometimes sharply compresses the nerve. The 1.5-cm nerve segment above this compressing level is often edematously swollen. On the other hand, in more advanced cases, the nerve segment located under the aponeurotic roof develops a slightly increasing scar tissue reaction, more frequently involving the interfascicular tissue than the epineurium. This situation leads to a classic pseudoneuroma if it has not been released early enough.

A different point of nerve compression is located at a more distal nerve segment within the original cubital tunnel: between the origins of the two heads of the flexor carpi ulnar muscle. Between these small muscle bellies, the surgeon must open a thin fascia, situated under the muscle fibers, again forming a sharp edge at the entrance point of the nerve.

An extremely rare level of nerve compression, affecting not only the ulnar nerve but also the median nerve in some cases, is Struther's arcade, normally tendon-like fibers of the triceps muscle crossing the ulnar nerve, but occasionally a fibrotic ligament originating from a bony outcropping of the humerus and distally running toward the medial epicondyle, first described by Struthers in 1854.

The symptoms depend on the degree of nerve lesion; they mostly start with irritation and numbness over the hypothenar muscle and over the flexion side of the one and a half ulnar fingers. The area of numbness includes a small region at the dorsoulnar aspect of the wrist and hand, representing the small dorsal skin branch supply leaving the ulnar nerve 3–4 cm proximal to the wrist. This area will help clinically distinguish between ulnar nerve entrapments at elbow and wrist levels.

The pathognomic Tinel sign can be elicited at the individual maximum point of compression so as to distinguish between the few possible etiologies of entrapment at the elbow level. Some patients complain of decreasing myokinetics of the small hand muscles. Very characteristic is the inability to adduct the thumb without flexing the tip of the thumb (sign according to Froment). In very advanced cases, patients sustain atrophies of the thumb adductor and the hypothenar muscles, the latter associated with inability to abduct and adduct the fifth finger. All these symptoms most often start spontaneously without any special incident or even accident in the patients' history, but nevertheless, very rarely, a sudden onset of all these symptoms has been noted. These patients' histories showed extended computer work with the angled elbow on a desk or a sudden onset after sleeping one night lying on one side with the angled elbow under the body.

Ulnar nerve entrapments with sudden onset and without severe trauma in the patient's history may rapidly disappear spontaneously if the patient is able to avoid specific movements or positions that compress the ulnar nerve, in other words, long periods flexing the elbow. If the symptoms do not improve but remain unchanged or even deteriorate, as in all widespread slowly progressing cases, surgery is mandatory.

In Europe, the appropriate surgery is being debated. Several surgeons now prefer a small longitudinal incision over the distal segment of the bony ulnar nerve groove leading between the two heads of the flexor carpi ulnar muscle, for the most part used to treat classic cubital tunnel syndrome. If this incision is extended in a proximal direction, the entire aponeurotic roof of the bony groove is transected. In this situation, the nerve is free of compression but the elongating forces during flexion of the elbow joint continue. This would also occur with the scar tissue reaction of the interfascicular tissue if it had already started before surgery. In this case, the result would be unsatisfactory and the patient would require reoperation. Other patients may complain of exaggerated electric-current-like pains when the operated area is resting on top of a desk, indicating a loss of the sheltering roof over the nerve. These patients may request additional surgery. For this reason we prefer to transpose the nerve above the medial epicondyle into a position ventral to the elbow joint. However, we have seen the results of operations where the nerve was not transposed far enough so that it remained situated near the medial epicondyle and a bit ventral to it. The continued oversensitivity of this region following insufficient transposition has led some surgeons to transpose the nerve back into the bony groove where the elongating forces restart and the nutrition of the nerve surrounded by bony structures remains questionable, as are situations where the gliding surface of the nerve has been completely lost due to external scar tissue reaction. Summarizing all these experiences, it is our opinion that a sufficient transposition of the ulnar nerve over a distance of 12 cm or more seems to be the most sufficient and satisfying procedure if the intention is that the patient not complains of residual symptoms. Nevertheless, as recently reported by Spinner in 2000, in very rare cases, the medial portion of the triceps may offend the sufficiently transposed nerve when its fibers also insert at the medial epicondyle. This must be noted as a rare cause of failed transposition when reviewing the literature; we have had no experience of this sort, and therefore continue to argue for transposing the ulnar nerve as described below.

We start the incision medial to the epicondyle in an inverse U-shaped manner and extend the incision about 3 cm over the upper arm and 4 cm over the lower arm so that the incision finally is shaped like three counter-rotating curves (▶ Fig. 5.6). After the operation, no scar tissue contraction can hinder the elbow flexion and extension. A flap of skin and subcutaneous tissue is then prepared, revealing the fascia of the muscles and the epicondyle. The muscle fascia is at first incised parallel to the expected nerve, proximal to the elbow; the nerve should be identified by palpation with a fingertip within the muscles, the gliding tissue surrounding the nerve is then incised longitudinally over a few centimeters so that the nerve is identified with certainty. The further dissection starts in a distal direction, opening the roof of the bony groove between the olecranon and the medial epicondyle. When following the nerve between the two heads of the flexor carpi ulnar muscle, first the external fascia of the muscles has to be opened, then both heads of the muscle must gently be split, and finally the incision of the deep fascia overlying the ulnar nerve must be long enough. After this surgical step, the nerve can be raised out of the bony groove; all the adhesions up to the entrance into the forearm muscles must be transected, but at this level, the surgeon must be careful not to damage the several small branches leaving the nerve at different levels and entering the muscles. These small branches may be mobilized by longitudinally opening the outer layers of the ulnar nerve epineurium. This procedure can sometimes gain 4 cm or more in length in these branches, and the branches can be separated from the residual main nerve so that it can be transposed far enough, first to prevent later kinking during elbow movements, and second, to preserve all muscle branches. Only the one sensory branch to the joint should be transected. Proximal to the elbow joint, the medial intermuscular septum between the triceps and the brachial and biceps muscles has to be isolated, incised, or even partially excised to prevent later nerve kinking over its sharp edge. We then transpose the nerve as far as possible and at the distal part, we incise the fascia over the forearm muscle bellies that

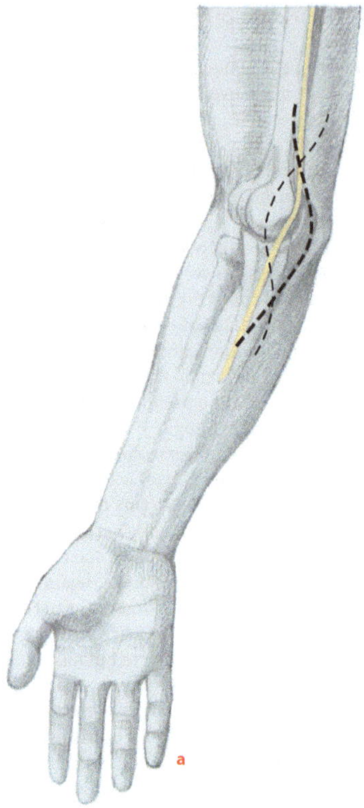

Figure 5.6 a–d

Ulnar nerve transposition (right arm). a Skin incisions used; b skin flap; c nerve release; d nerve transposition with preservation of all proximal motor branches

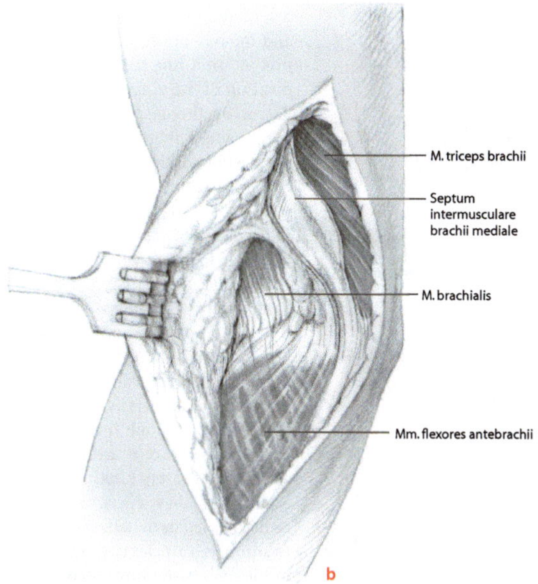
M. triceps brachii
Septum intermusculare brachii mediale
M. brachialis
Mm. flexores antebrachii

b

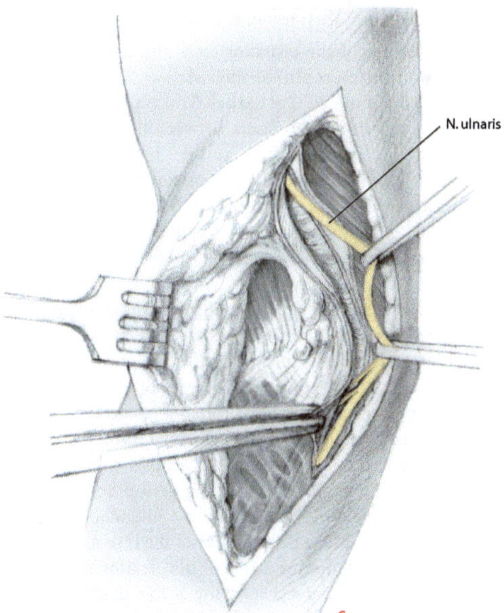
N. ulnaris

c

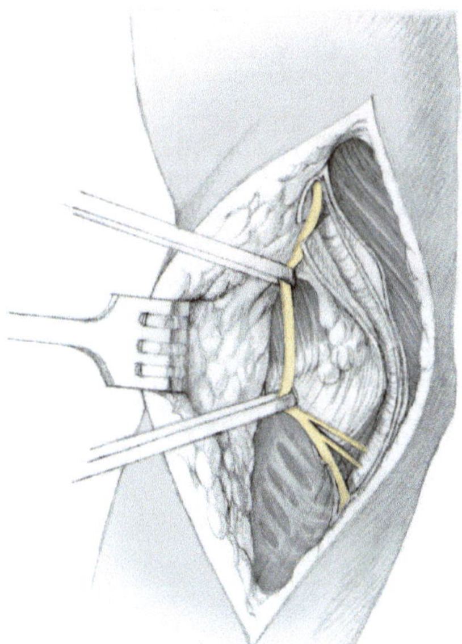

d

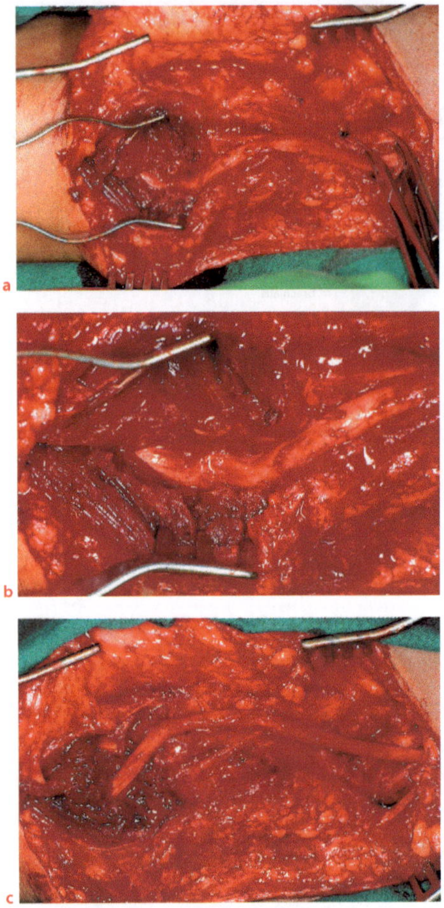
a b c

Figure 5.7 a–c

Insufficient ulnar nerve transposition (right arm, elbow level). a Intermuscular septum preserved; b kinking of the nerve because too closely situated beside the elbow joint; c corrected situation

originate from the medial epicondyle (pronator teres and the two heads of the flexor carpi ulnar muscle); this incision line runs parallel to the expected new position of the ulnar nerve. Between the muscle bellies, separating fascias are again identified by feeling them using a fingertip. These fascias are incised between the muscle fibers so that the transposed ulnar nerve will not be irritated by these sharp-edged structures. All the soft-structured muscle fibers themselves are preserved because they do not irritate the transposed nerve.

Submuscular transposition of the ulnar nerve has been described to be associated with a partial resection and repositioning of the medial epicondyle (e.g., King and Morgan 1959). In 1995, Kline and Hudson found that nerve transposition is associated with a partial proximal transsection of the pronator teres muscle and the one head of the flexor carpi ulnar muscle, which are resutured. This method seems to completely prevent kinking by later joint movements, as illustrated in ▶ Fig. 5.7 a, b. Nevertheless, our experience has led us to believe that a subcutaneous transposition is sufficient when three preconditions are fulfilled: first, the transposition has to lead into a recipient bed a few centimeters away from the medial epicondyle (▶ Fig. 5.7 c); second, the proximal intermuscular septum has to be incised or even partially excised (▶ Fig. 5.6 d); and third, the separating fascias between the bellies of the pronator teres and flexor carpi ulnar muscles must also be incised.

Exclusively, the pure cubital tunnel syndrome, the compression under the deep fascia between the two heads of the flexor carpi ulnar muscle, naturally makes it possible to avoid the transposition procedure. Quite a few surgeons prefer this method, particularly when working in private practice. But how can we distinguish preoperatively or perhaps intraoperatively that we are exclusively dealing with this special entrapment localization? Further discussions are needed to answer this question. We are still influenced by severely painful postoperative situations following procedures in which nerves were not transposed but simply decompressed, probably resulting from disregarded irritations above the cubital tunnel.

If a stepwise microneurolysis on nerves that have been chronically entrapped over a long period and that have developed a pseudoneuroma is intended, and the patient presents with atrophies of the intrinsic hand muscles, one must be aware of the plexiform structure of the ulnar nerve, especially at the elbow level. If the patient does not suffer from pain but mainly from severe paresis, more aggressive action may be appropriate than if the patient's complaint consists only of the usually local irritation and radiating pain. In the latter case, a separating dissection between fascicle groups or fascicles is of no use because this procedure regularly produces small individually painful neuromas originating from all previously transected cross-connections. However, in each case of advanced symptoms, we would advise surgeons at least to open the epineurium in a longitudinal direction and to remove parts of the epineurium, thus finishing with an external microdecompression. As already mentioned in Chap. 1, the decisions involved during the different operating steps in neurolysis depend on the experience of the surgeon, and the predominance of specific symptoms.

Several resolvable stitches can be used to fix the nerve within the recipient bed between the muscle fascia and subcutaneous tissue; the nerve must remain unstrangulated and longitudinally movable behind these stitches. A suction drainage is placed in the area where the ulnar nerve was formally located. Immobilization of the elbow joint is not needed, and movement exercises done by the patient are started at least 1 week later. Most patients already try to move their joint the second day after operation. We manage the ulnar nerve surgery as out-patient treatment.

5.6 Median Nerve Entrapment at Elbow Level

If we compare our own experience with reports recently published in the United States and Great Britain, compression neuropathies of the median nerve at elbow level seem to occur very rarely (see Stern and Fassler 1991; Kline and Hudson 1995; Birch et al. 1998). Etiological factors can be a Struthers ligament, the biceps tendon, the lacertus fibrosus, the two heads of the pronator teres muscle, especially if an aponeurotic arch between the two heads is present (pronator teres syndrome), and finally a fibrous band within the pronator teres itself.

During clinical investigation, paresthesias and numbness in the distribution of the entire median nerve are found, which help clinically to distinguish between lesions at elbow and wrist. The usually slight weakness involves all the median innervated forearm muscles and the radial lumbrical and thenar muscles of the hand, so that flexion of the three radial fingers, the opposition of the thumb, and the flexion of the wrist are involved together. The Tinel sign is positive at the individual level of compression, but unfortunately, after giving some branches to the pronator teres muscle, the nerve goes very deep into this muscle and the Tinel sign may remain hidden, and surgical exploration is difficult. When the compression is caused by the tendon or aponeurosis of the biceps, the pronator teres muscle also shows denervation potentials in the electromyography. Electroneurographic and electromyographic tests are reliable in establishing the diagnosis.

As the median nerve runs parallel to the brachial artery, the course of the nerve between the biceps muscle and the brachial muscle is well known. The nerve passes under the biceps tendon and aponeurosis, then the pronator teres muscle. The main belly of this muscle has to be lifted up, branches leaving the main nerve trunk to the pronator teres have to be preserved, the pathway between the two heads of the pronator teres has to be explored, and if necessary, the ulnar head of the muscle should be transected (▶ Fig. 5.8), particularly if a fibrous band or an aponeurotic arch crosses the nerve fibers. The surgery has to be completed by a suction drain and there is no need for immobilization.

We have had only one case in which paresthesias and weakness developed overnight in a cachectic patient. During exploration, the median nerve was fibrotic over a distance of 3–4 cm before entering deep under the forearm muscles, making it clear that a chronic compression under the biceps aponeurosis had preceded.

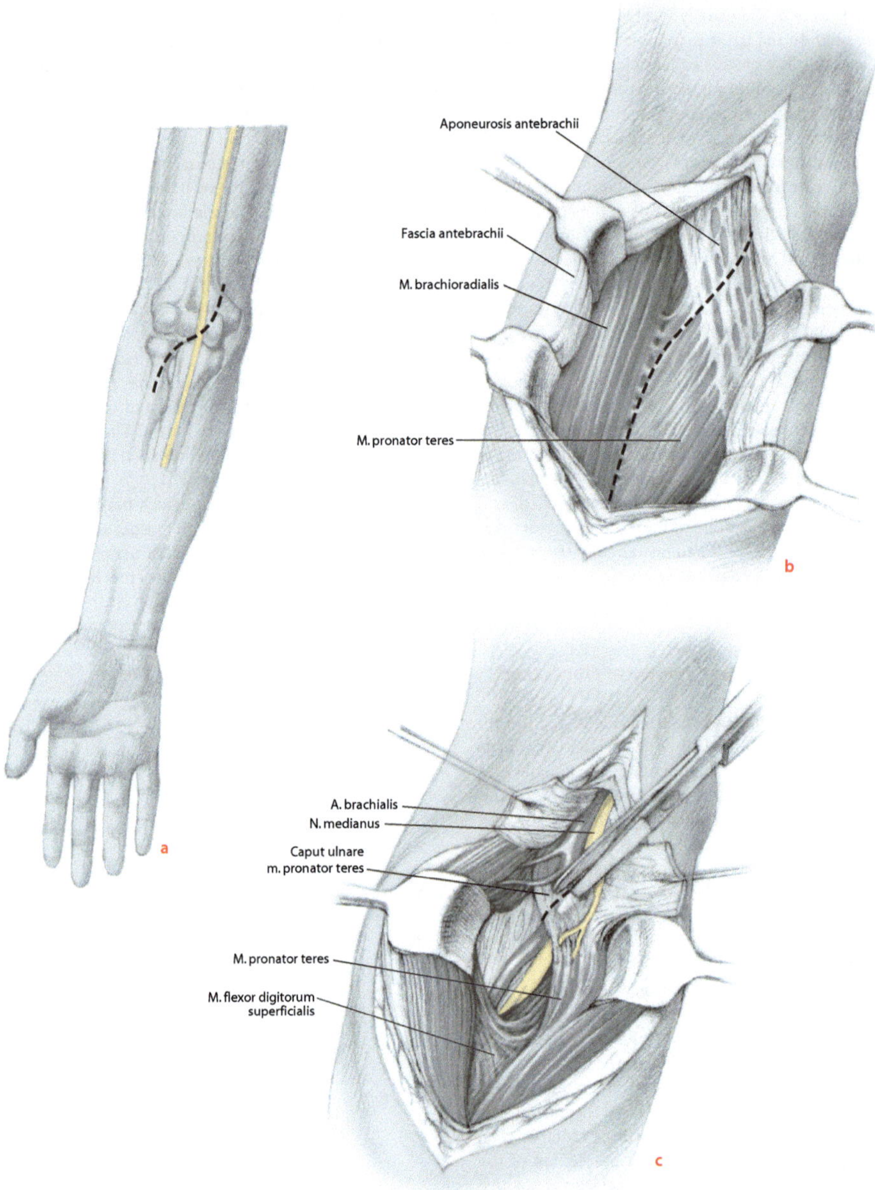

Figure 5.8a–c

Median nerve entrapment at elbow level (right arm). a Skin incision; b superficial situation; c nerve exploration between pronator teres and brachioradial muscles first, then superficial and deep flexor digitorum muscles split, ulnar head of the pronator is to be divided

5.7 Anterior Interosseous Nerve Entrapment

The entrapment of the anterior interosseous does not occur more often than the entrapment discussed in the preceding section, but reliable experiments with intraoperative findings have not been published. The syndrome was described by Kiloh and Nevin in 1952. The nerve supplies the long flexor of the thumb and the radial part of the deep flexor of the index. It also supplies the pronator quadratus muscle, and it has no cutaneous sensory distribution. The latter explains why a Tinel sign is completely absent in these cases. Rarely, the anterior interosseous contains the Martin-Gruber anastomosis fibers as well (see Chaps. 2 and 6). The etiology of a compression of the small nerve under the radial head of the superficial flexor muscle or a sudden arterial thrombosis is currently being discussed. New single observations described three cases of a monofascicular and oligofascicular rotation of the small nerve (Vispo Seara et al. 1994).

With sudden onset and pain completely absent at night, the anterior interosseous palsy presents with functional loss of the flexor pollicis longus and flexor indicis muscle and an inability to flex the end phalanges of the first and second finger (▶ Fig 5.9 a, b). Patients only note palsy when trying to hold a cup of coffee between these two fingertips or when using a pocket lighter. Thus, the idea of a real entrapment seems rather questionable, because the symptoms, which are similar to paralysis, start at night. If the nerve contains Martin-Gruber fibers, the intrinsic muscle weakness of the hand causes more severe troubles. Characteristic is the absence of any sensory deficit. In the six cases we have observed, no initial or additional pain appeared. However, in 1986, Gaitzsch and Chamay described three cases of special presentations of paralytic brachial neuritis, or Parsonage-Turner syndrome, mimicking anterior interosseous nerve compression. But it must be pointed out that their cases started with an acute episode with severe pain in the arm and forearm followed by the typical palsy.

Although the sudden palsy means a dramatic functional loss for the entire hand, surgical exploration again is questionable in our opinion. Nobody is able to explain reliably why there is frequently a sudden onset, which structure seems to act as a causing factor, and why spontaneous recovery with and without surgery and complete failures despite surgery occur.

The operation starts with a skin incision over the mid forearm and slightly proximal, the bellies of the flexor carpi radial and pronator teres muscles are

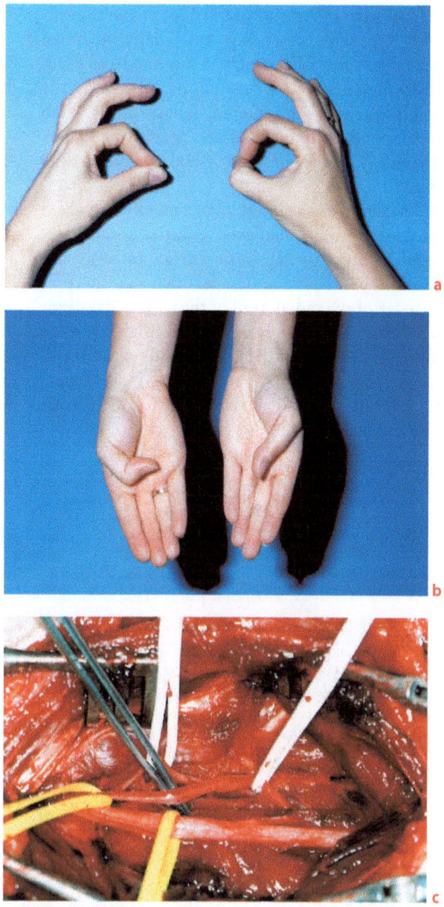

a

b

c

Figure 5.9 a–c

Anterior interosseous nerve entrapment (left arm). **a, b** Paralysis of the flexor pollicis longus and flexor indicis muscles on the left hand; **c** exploration of the nerve (anterior interosseous nerve at forceps, median and interosseous nerves at the *yellow loops*, interosseous anterior artery at the *white loops*) split from each other, and the surface of the superficial flexor muscles is then exposed. Finally, the radial origin of the superficial flexors is retracted and separated from the flexor pollicis longus belly. Thus, the deep compartment is entered, where the median nerve is found, with the ulnar artery crossing underneath and the anterior interosseous nerve arising from the median nerve at its radial aspect and running downward on the interosseous membrane, again crossed under by a smaller artery, the anterior interosseous artery (▶ Fig. 5.9c). Particular care must be taken to predispose anomalies such as a sharp fibrous edge of the radial head of the superficial flexor or a slippage of a muscle fascia that might trap the small nerve. Because of the unexpected possibility of the above-mentioned nerve rotation cases, an inspection of the very small nerve with the microscope should not be forgotten.

5.8 Posterior Interosseous Nerve Entrapment

Comparable to the anterior interosseous nerve, the posterior one mainly contains motor fibers. It has a very small sensory skin distribution on the dorsal aspect of the hand between the first and second fingers. As with the anterior interosseous lesion, an entrapment syndrome of the posterior interosseous nerve may present severe weakness, but no numbness, with the exception of the small area mentioned, and usually no pain. A Tinel sign is absent. Still proximal to the elbow level, the division of the radial nerve starts in the superficial and deep branches. The latter goes deep into the supinator muscle. At the entrance point of the supinator tunnel, a fibrotic arch belonging to the aponeurosis of the supinator muscle crosses the deep branch (arcade, according to Frohse). This is the

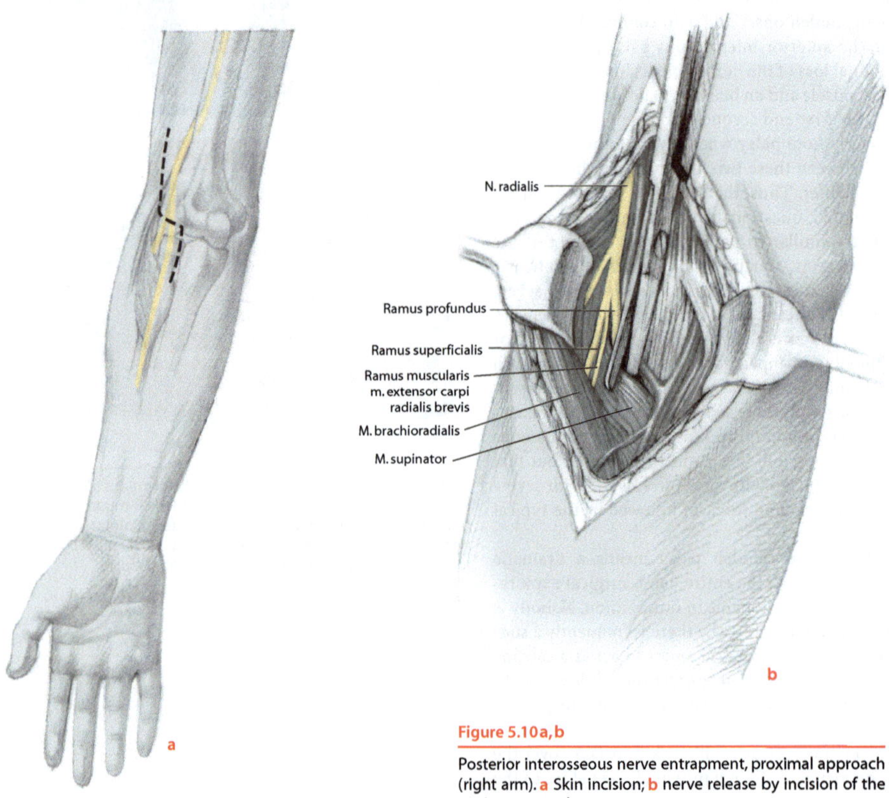

Figure 5.10a, b

Posterior interosseous nerve entrapment, proximal approach (right arm). a Skin incision; b nerve release by incision of the supinator muscle point from which, in our opinion, all chronically proceeding entrapments and the occasionally sudden ongoing compressions (sometimes associated with injections against a radial epicondylitis) originate; consequently, there is no doubt that this syndrome requires an approach from a proximal direction (▶ Fig 5.10).

One very important small motor branch leaves the superficial radial nerve approximately 3–4 cm before the supinator channel supplying the short extensor carpi radial muscle (▶ Fig. 5.11a). Characteristic of the posterior interosseous entrapment presentation is the preservation of this muscle function so that the patient can extend the wrist but then keep it in radial abduction. In contrast, the ulnar wrist extensor and the remaining extensors develop a weakness.

The clinical diagnosis consists of the observation of the above-mentioned pareses in combination with a preserved wrist extension, but only in radial abduction. Distal motor latency testing and electromyography complete the examination.

Operation seems to be rather simple if compared to surgery on the anterior interosseous nerve (▶ Fig. 5.10). The skin incision is best S-shaped using the elbow crease, starting at the distal lateral upper arm area. Great care has to be taken with the very small branch to the extensor carpi radial muscle from the beginning, because the patient may subsequently sustain additional severe deficit. Therefore, intraoperative electric stimulation equipment is mandatory to identify the nerve as early as possible. The arcade of Frohse must be incised (▶ Fig. 5.11b), some fibers of the supinator muscle can be transected, but of greater importance is incising the aponeurotic surface of the supinator muscle so that muscle fibers and the posterior interosseous nerve together gain space. There is no need to transect the supinator muscle itself completely. Just in front of the entrance point into the supinator channel, small arteries and veins cross the deep radial nerve branch. They have individually to be tied by bipolar forceps and transected. Nevertheless, if bleeding suddenly occurs, one should not coagulate without the individual origin of the bleeding in view because of the above-mentioned small motor branch and the risk of late rebleedings. Single observations of rotatory displacements or rotational distortions of the small nerve at the entrance level into the supinator channel were first described by Wilhelm in 1976 and later by Poritlla Molinar in 1998, and a microscopic inspection to exclude these rare findings is advised (see also Chap. 3). A suction drainage for 24 h is mandatory. There is no need for postoperative immobilization.

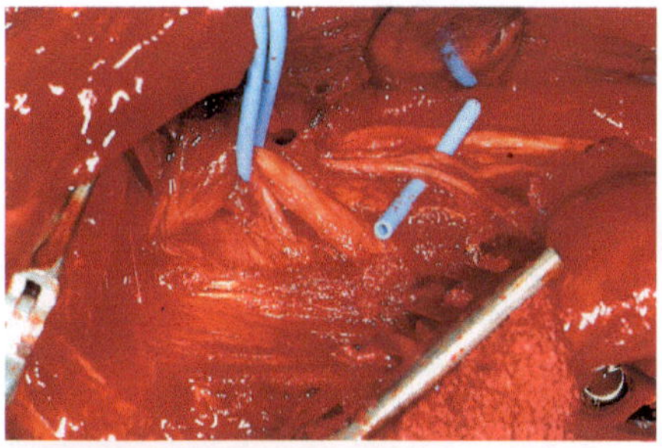

a

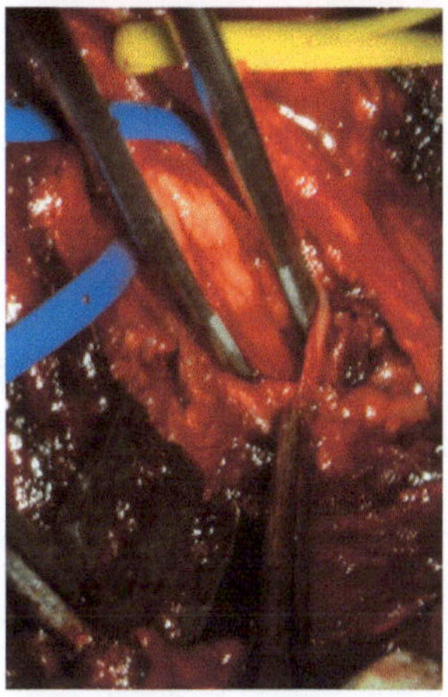

b

Figure 5.11 a,b

Posterior interosseous nerve entrapment, proximal approach (left arm, view from the medial side). a Exploration of the deep (*blue loop*) and superficial radial nerve branches, small motor branch to the short radial wrist extensor in between (piece of loop underneath); b arcade of Frohse

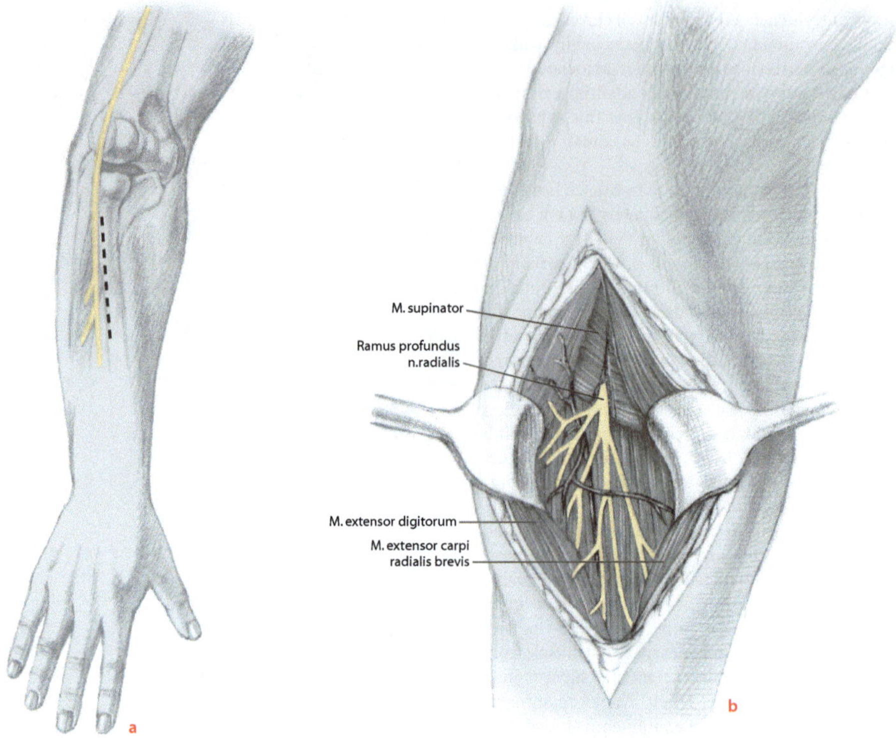

Figure 5.12 a, b

Posterior interosseous nerve entrapment, distal approach (right arm). a skin incision; b exploration of the deep branch and its numerous motor branches after splitting the extensor muscles. (Note that differences of figures result from the fact that patients lie supine with their hand in pronation, whereas in an anatomical atlas, bodies lie prone with hand in supination)

In the literature and from our experience, another approach to the posterior interosseous nerve passes through the extensor muscles toward the interosseous membrane (▶ Fig. 5.12). After forearm trauma, a combination of this approach with the initially mentioned proximal approach is indispensable. However, in the case of entrapments, two disadvantages of the distal approach must be considered: (a) the origin of the entrapment, the arcade of Frohse, will come into view just at the end of the dissection after a complete transsection of the supinator; (b) this approach endangers several branches to all the forearm extensors (▶ Fig. 5.13). The only exception would be cases of posterior interosseous entrapment associated with lipomas under the supinator muscle. If a resistance can be palpated within the extensors, MRI is necessary. We have observed four such cases and succeeded in removing these tumors using the dorsal approach.

The dorsal approach starts with a longitudinal skin incision of approximately 5 cm just over the dorsal extensors; the bellies of the common finger extensor and the ulnar wrist extensor are separated, thus opening a deeper compartment, where fibers of the deep flexors should be split until the posterior interosseous nerve, located on the interosseous membrane, and its motor branches, which have to be dissected and preserved, come into view. The nerve has to be followed proximally by incising the aponeurosis of the supinator and splitting its muscle fibers. The overlying flexors are simply retracted and, of course, completely preserved. Wound closure requires suction drainage and no postoperative immobilization.

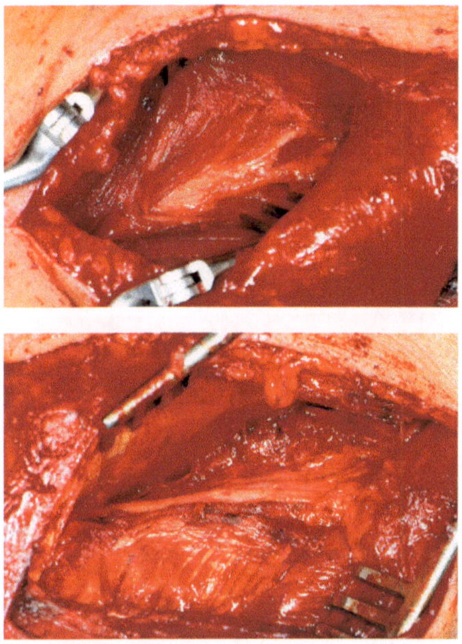

Figure 5.13 a, b

Posterior interosseous nerve entrapment, distal approach (left arm). a Exploration distal to the supinator muscle; b transsection of the supinator muscle

5.9 Superficial Radial Nerve Entrapment

Rare cases of painful compression of the small superficial branch of the radial nerve are noted in addition to entrapment of the deep branch, which is not usually painful. On the one hand, an irritation syndrome caused by the brachioradial muscle tendon may occur, as described by Millesi in 1992; on the other hand, nerve branch irritation may result from habitually wearing overly tight watch bands or bracelets. Only the truly spontaneous entrapment can be solved by a small exploration where the Tinel sign can be evoked, whereas the cuff-like compression only requires a change in the patient's behavior.

These purely superficial radial branch lesions are rather rare, and the symptoms may be misleading and misdiagnosed as De Quervain's tenosynovitis. However, the nerve lesion can be revealed by showing an abnormality of the superficial radial sensory potential, especially if compared with the results of the contralateral nerve.

5.10 Median Nerve Entrapment at Wrist Level

The entrapment of the median nerve at wrist level is known as carpal tunnel syndrome (CTS), the most widespread spontaneous nerve compression syndrome that exists in humans. Contrary to all of the irritation or compression locations discussed thus far, the carpal tunnel is a narrow channel existing since birth. Additional anomalies aiding diagnosis are absent here, with some rare exceptions. Therefore, a reliable etiology remains unknown in the majority of cases. Amyloid sedimentations, gravidity, fractures of the distal head of the radial bone, or perilunate luxation are known to induce a situation that additionally confines the carpal tunnel. Quite rarely, additional muscles or a persisting median artery play an etiological role. On the other hand, in normal cases with usually spontaneous onset, the real individual causative factors can be considered, for instance, chronic inflammatory or rheumatoid tendovaginitis.

The clinical differential diagnosis between lesions at elbow level and wrist level depends on the involvement of the median innervated forearm muscles, particularly the superficial and deep long flexors, which continue working in CTS cases.

We believe that a preoperative electroneurographic verification is mandatory. Besides a disk rupture at the C6/7 level, thoracic outlet irritation and even subacromial impingement belong to alternative syndromes that may cause similar symptoms and, particularly, similar pain. It is not rare that we receive patients who have had surgery for CTS but nevertheless suffer from ongoing pain within their arm involving a few fingers, especially during the night. Palpating the supraspinatus tendon or the long biceps tendon provokes a severe lancing pain radiating into several fingers. These patients sometimes also sustain paresthesias such as fingers becoming numb, although nerve involvement is absent. The same holds true with symptoms of the radial or medial epicondylitis.

As the patient cannot enlarge the space within the carpal tunnel by his or her own behavior, sometimes possible in ulnar nerve compression cases at elbow level, surgery is mandatory with the few exceptions of CTS associated with gravidity. Trauma and especially fracture-related CTS cases are emergency situations. Transecting the transverse carpal ligament is the major goal.

This may sound very simple but is the source of debate on small or large skin incisions as well as open versus endoscopic surgery. The one critical point is the motor thenar branch and its anomalies, as well as the sometimes disturbing scar between thenar and

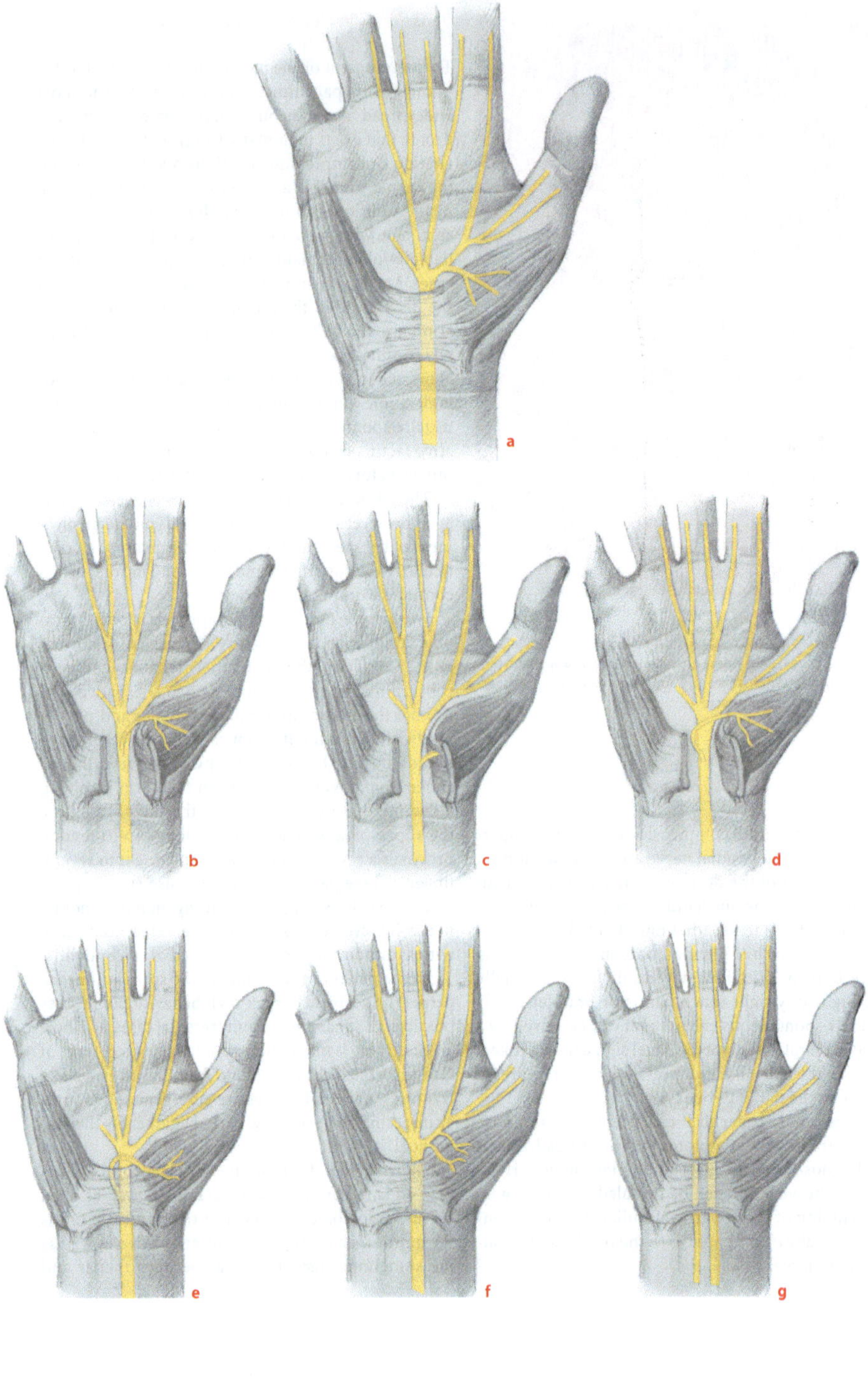
a
b
c
d
e
f
g

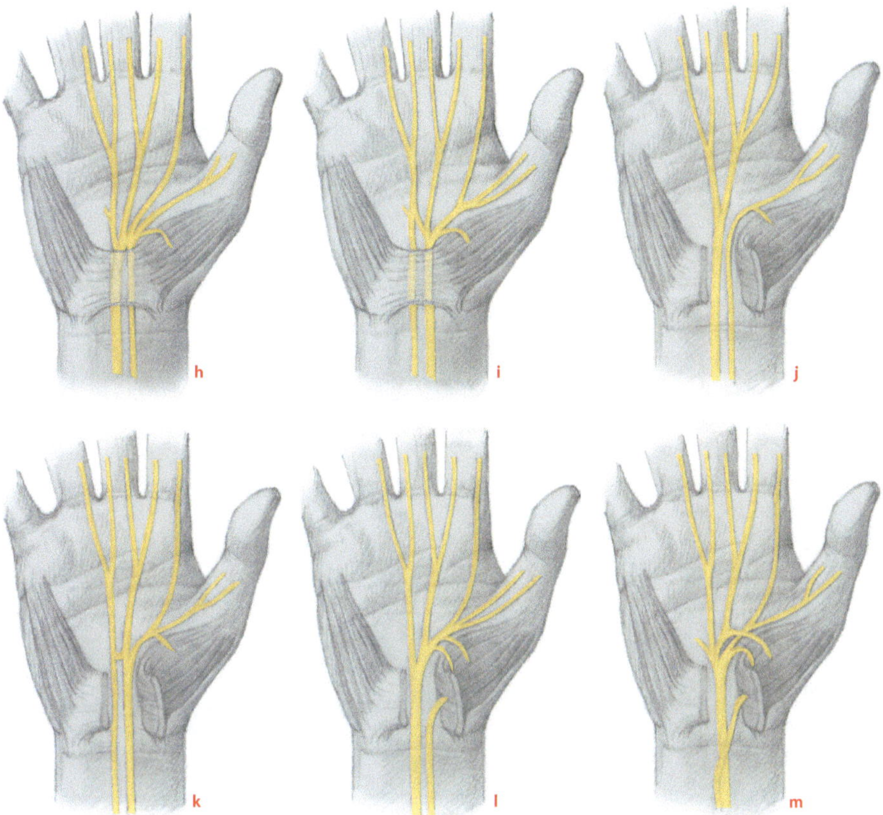

Figure 5.14 a–m

Thenar branch variations. a Normal situation; b–m different variations according to Lanz

hypothenar muscles, possibly prolonging the disability, and lastly the reliable radicality of the ligament transsection. Details on one-portal and two-portal techniques of endoscopic surgery, their advantages and disadvantages, their risks and data on their recurrence rate, their indications and contraindications have recently been described in detail and shall therefore not be repeated here, except for the final statement. "Two-portal endoscopic carpal tunnel release offered neither advantages nor disadvantages compared with the open two-incision technique," a surgical technique developed by Millesi using two open incisions preserving the skin between thenar and hypothenar structures (Girsch et al. 2001).

It is extremely important to be aware of the variations in the thenar branch, which were described in 1977 by Lanz (▶ Fig. 5.14), such as a transligamentous course, an extraligamentous recurrent course, a branch leaving the median nerve trunk at its ulnar aspect and then crossing over the median nerve, or the coexistence of accessory branches. We have seen a branch that left the ulnar nerve at the metacarpal level and crossed through the palm into the thenar space as part of a Riche-Cannieu anastomosis (see Chaps. 2 and 6). Historically, open surgery started with small transverse incisions using a wrist crease, resulting in an intolerable morbidity concerning the thenar branch. Hand surgeons reacted with large incisions of

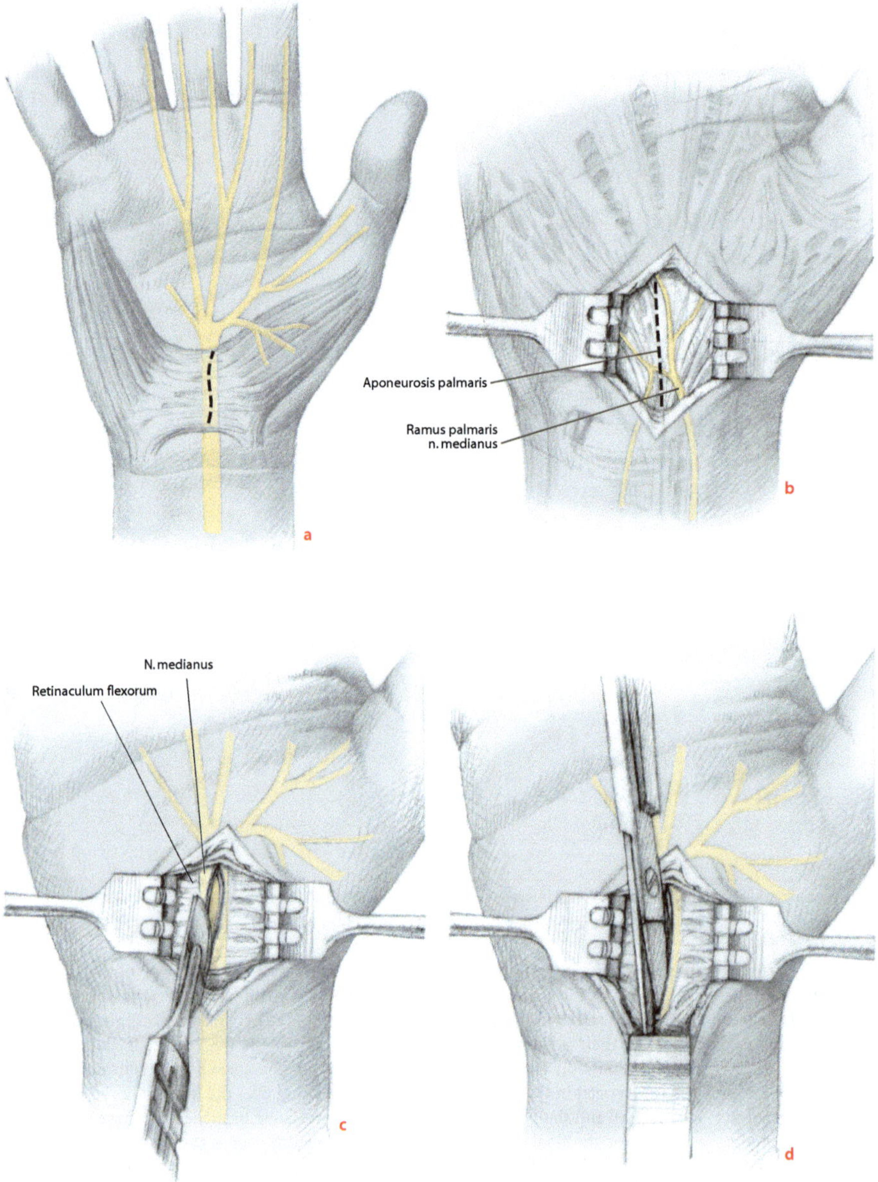

Figure 5.15 a–d

Carpal tunnel syndrome. a Skin incision; b palmar aponeurosis to be incised; c transverse ligament to be incised; d additional incisions to the proximal part including parts of the lower arm fascia, and to the distal part

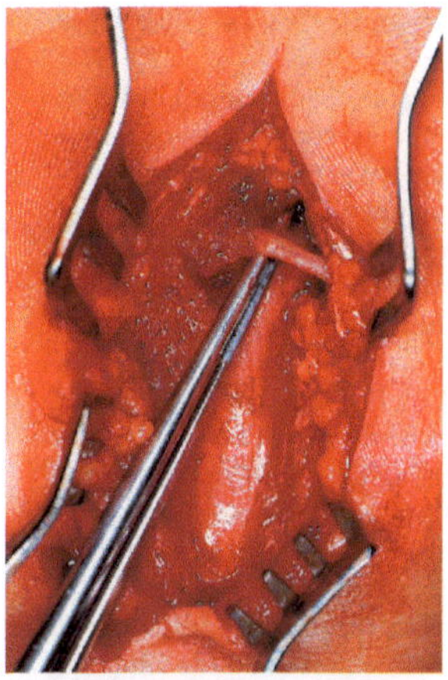

a

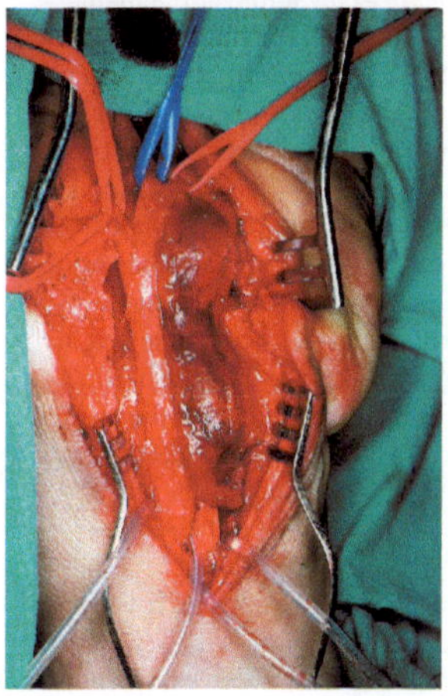

b

Figure 5.16 a, b

Anomalous cases of carpal tunnel syndrome. a Thenar branch crossing over the median nerve, originating from the ulnar nerve (right hand); b hematoma within the carpal tunnel

about 5 cm, working in a bloodless field, firstly dissecting the sensory branches to all three and a half radial fingers, then identifying the thenar branch, and only then releasing the tunnel by transecting the ligament. Discussion on the value of microsurgery after the release began with Curtis and Eversmann's report in 1973, but did not continue.

Because we are more certain to detect and preserve anomalies, we prefer open surgery rather than endoscopic approaches. We use a 1.5-cm incision between the thenar and hypothenar spaces (▶ Fig. 5.15). We believe that this involves less risk, especially for younger surgeons, than an endoscopic surgical attempt: thenar branch anomalies are better viewed with open surgery (▶ Fig. 5.16). On the other hand, new reports on ultrasonic investigations of carpal tunnels seem to make it easier to detect nerve anomalies preoperatively. This might facilitate future decisions on whether difficulties are to be expected with endoscopy.

After the skin incision, a self retractor is placed; the bulging fat tissue should be completely retracted on both sides, the aponeurosis of the palmaris longus muscle is split, the underlying palmaris brevis muscle fibers are transected, leading to the deep compartment, covered by the carpal ligament, which is gently incised transverse to its fibers and parallel to the expected content of the carpal tunnel using a small knife, until the longitudinal running structures below it become visible. This procedure is the most difficult part of the operation. Nevertheless, finishing the operation at this stage would be insufficient and cause a recurrence. Nerve decompression has to be extended far enough into the palm and has to include a short distance of the ventral surface of the forearm (▶ Fig. 5.15d). By means of a manual retractor, the skin under the incision edges is lifted up so that the thenar branch and the vessel arch are safely preserved during extension of the decompression.

Microsurgical stepwise neurolysis may be exclusively indicated in CTS cases related to substantial trauma, particularly if severe paresis or atrophy of the thenar muscle occurred early. This atrophy indicates intraneural compressing scar tissue, which would remain in place after a simple external release. Microsurgery is the only procedure allowed and indicated when motor deficits provide the strongest indication to surgery. Occasionally an isolated entrapment of the motor thenar branch can occur, but only at its entrance into the thenar muscle. Sensory deficits may be missing, which should raise suspicion of this isolated lesion. In this case, the procedure should review the thenar branch course.

CTS is frequently accompanied by a tendovaginitis stenosans of flexor tendons of the affected hand. No difficulty is involved in simultaneously releasing the carpal tunnel and opening the proximal circular band of the affected tendon via a small additional transverse incision at level of the MP joints. Special care must be taken with the sensitive digital nerves on each side of the tendon, especially on the radially located nerve of the thumb, which may be situated more or less on the tendon. Of course, the distal circular band of the involved tendon must remain intact in order to preserve it as hypomochleon.

Wound closure includes a drain without suction for 24 h. It should run out of the wound proximal to the most proximal skin stitch. We completely avoid subcutaneous stitches so that no strangulation is caused within the wound. There is no need for immobilization. The skin stitches remain at least for 12 days.

5.11 Ulnar Nerve Entrapment at Wrist Level

Comparable to the median nerve within the carpal tunnel, the ulnar nerve together with the ulnar artery passes through a rather narrow fibrous channel called Guyon's canal. With the cross-section of this channel in view, the border surfaces are shaped by fibers of the ulnar ligament as a roof, and at the lateral side by the pisiform bone. About 1 cm distal to it, a small but the most important branch leaves the ulnar nerve at its lateral aspect, turns lateral or ulnar first, then medial, where it curves around the hamate bone and passes transverse above the heads of the metacarpal bones, there supplying the intrinsic muscles and finally the adductor pollicis, first described by Hunt in 1908.

First, the differential diagnosis between entrapments at elbow level and wrist level is of great importance. The dorsal cutaneous nerve arises from the ulnar nerve about 5 cm proximal to the wrist crease. The distribution area of this cutaneous nerve may not be involved in distal nerve compression. The patient complains of numbness only over the flexion side of the one and a half ulnar fingers and the hypothenar branches, and of myokinetic disturbances of the small hand muscles. The syndrome occurs rarely, but must be kept in mind, especially after a patient's report of a long bicycle ride or leaning on the extended wrist during several recreational activities. The Tinel sign is positive at wrist level because of the sensory fibers within the nerve. The diagnosis can easily be completed by electroneurography and electromyography. The latter study must reveal normal function of the forearm flexors because they are ulnar nerve innervated.

With the exception of cases with sudden onset, in other words, cases with a recognizable causative event, surgery is mandatory and comparable to carpal tunnel surgery. Compression syndromes related to one of the above-mentioned traumas may recover spontaneously and should be observed for a short period of time whether or not they improve spontaneously. If surgery is decided, however, exploration is more difficult than in CTS. Because skin incisions that simply cross over skin creases must be avoided, we prefer an incision starting between the hypothenar and thenar eminences, and after that using one of the wrist creases to lead the incision to the head of the ulnar bone. Lastly, we extend the incision 1.5 cm proximal and slightly lateral to the expected ulnar nerve and artery (▶ Fig. 5.17). The nerve and the ulnar artery running alongside are easily found at the medial aspect of the ulnar flexor carpi tendon and the head of the ulnar bone (▶ Fig. 5.18 a), and beginning from that point, both structures are dissected to the palm by retracting the triangled skin flap over the hypothenar eminence. The ligamentous roof of the channel is completely incised longitudinally; the nerve must be explored until the deep motor branch comes into view. This branch is again in danger of being compressed by a small fibrotic arch that acts as the origin of the flexor digiti minimi muscle (▶ Fig. 5.18 b–d). In this context, it must be remembered that the deep branch at first arises in the ulnar direction, then turns radial and crosses under the remaining nerve. The above-mentioned fibrotic arch must be incised to ensure motor recovery.

In 1992, Millesi advised a lateral approach with a far lateral skin incision. Skin incisions which lead into the hypothenar skin should be avoided completely.

Rarely, exclusive involvement of the associated deep motor branch with no sensory loss as well as intact hypothenar muscles may be encountered. In these cases, the patient usually presents with a history of a crush trauma. These cases only require special exploration of the point where the deep motor branch arises. This branch turns slightly lateral at first, then medial, where it crosses under the skin branches. A skin incision can be chosen within a crease over the medial aspect of the hypothenar muscle. In this situation, a bloodless field during the operation is advisable. Exploration of the entire wrist nerve segment to the motor branch provides greater safety, especially for surgeons with less experience.

In wound closure, we avoid subcutaneous stitches because they may develop new transverse strangula-

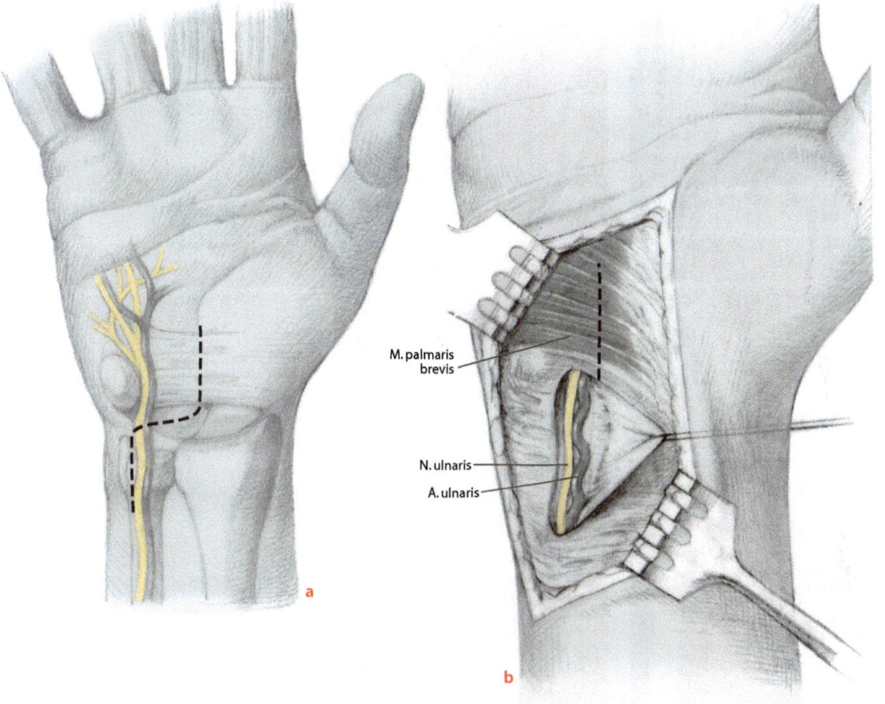

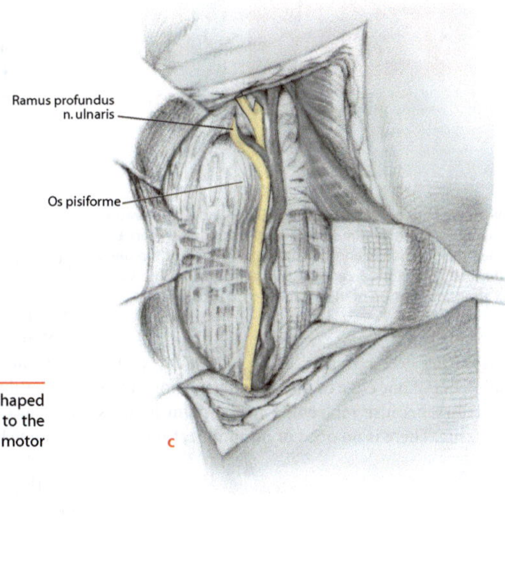

Figure 5.17 a–c

Ulnar nerve entrapment at wrist level (right hand). a S-shaped skin incision; b exploration of nerve and artery medial to the pisiform bone; c additional exploration of the deep motor branch

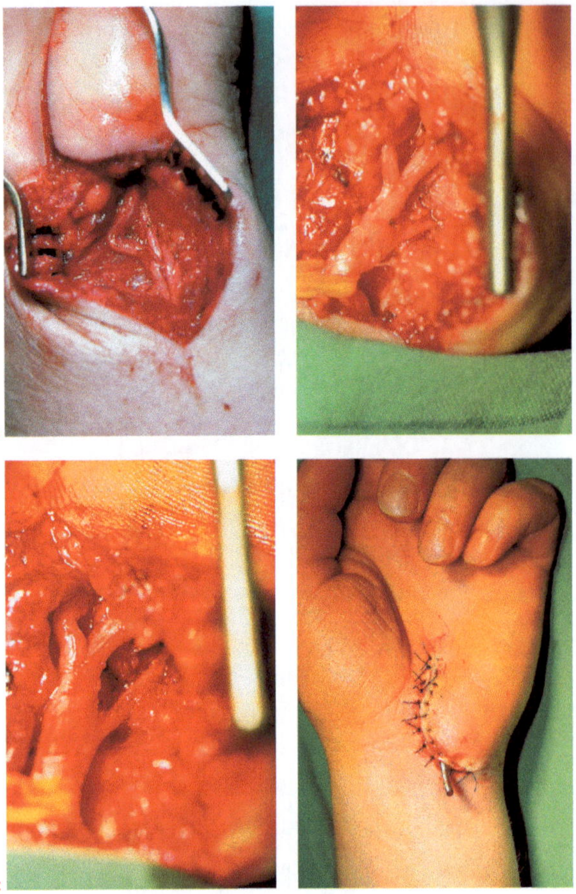

Figure 5.18 a–d

Ulnar nerve entrapment at wrist level (left hand). a Exploration of Guyon's channel, wound ulnar artery beside the nerve, S-shaped skin incision; b another case: exploration of the deep motor branch, fibrotic arcade transverse to its course; c situation after transsection of the arcade; d skin incision used

tions on the decompressed nerve. A small drainage leading out of one edge of the skin incision for 24 h is mandatory because rebleeding in the palm induces scar tissue. There is no need of immobilization.

5.12 Lateral Cutaneous Nerve Entrapment of the Thigh

The entrapment of the lateral cutaneous nerve of the thigh is located at the level of the inguinal ligament (meralgia paresthetica). The nerve arises from the L2 root and remains within the retroperitoneal space. It exits the pelvis just beside the anterior superior spine of the iliac bone. At this point, it angulates sharply downward and passes medial to the anterior superior spine between several portions of the inguinal ligament. At first, the nerve remains below the fascia of the thigh and runs medial to the sartorius muscle deep to the iliacus fascia, then it pierces the fascia a

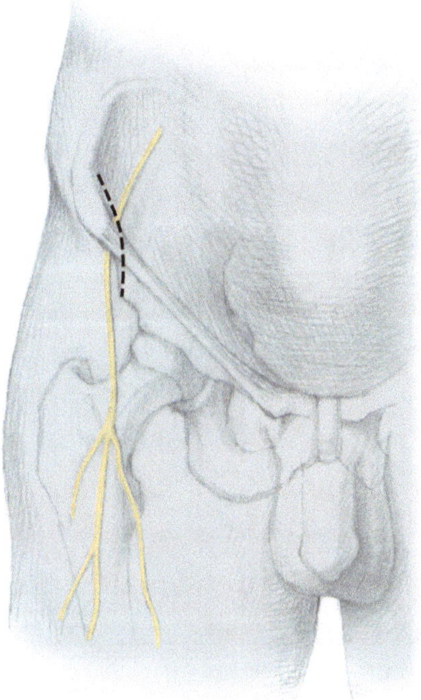

a

Figure 5.19a–c

Lateral cutaneous nerve entrapment (right side). a Skin incision; b identification of the iliac spine; c exploration of the nerve after fascial splitting, just beside the spine, and underneath the inguinal ligament. Parts of the ligament are to be incised

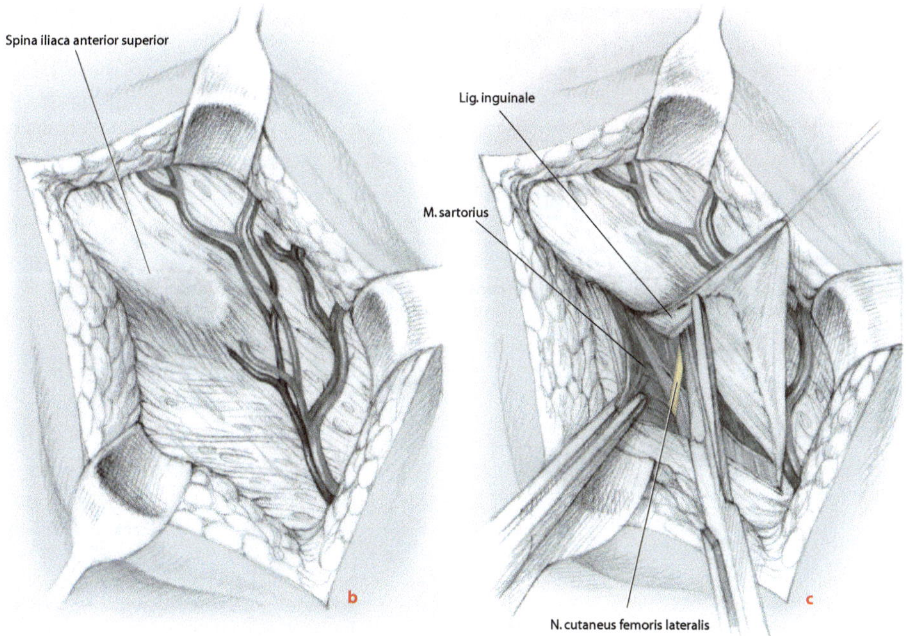

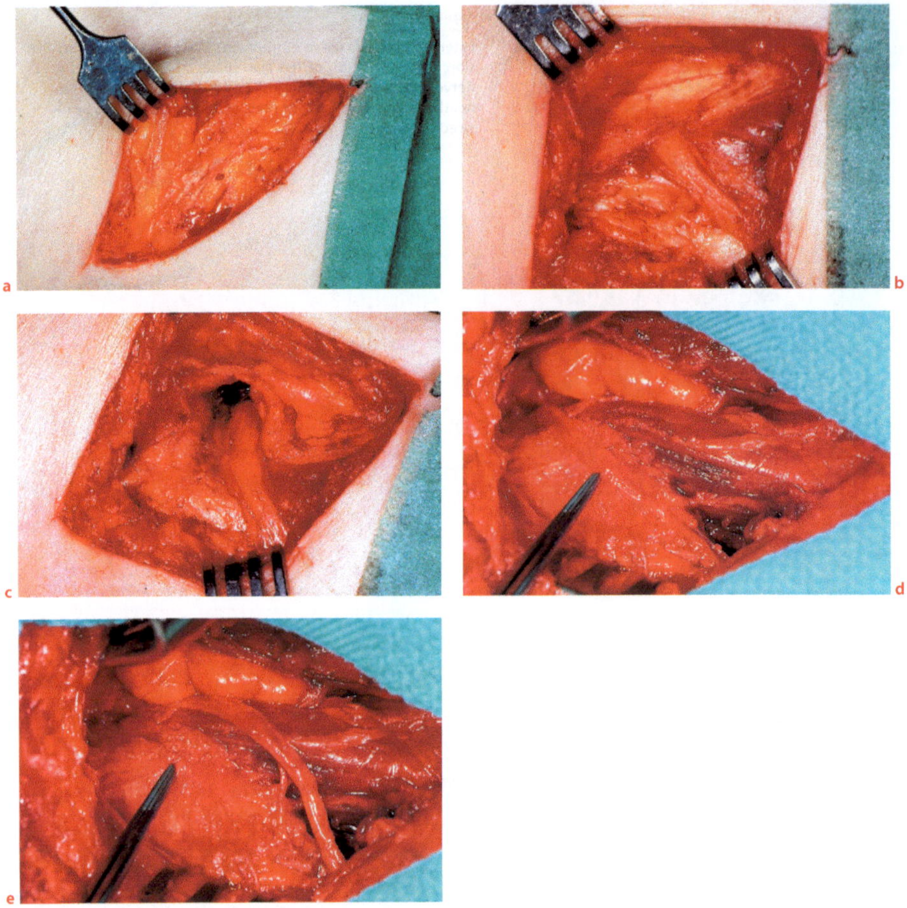

Figure 5.20 a–e

Lateral cutaneous nerve entrapment (left side). a Incision; b nerve between inguinal ligament fibers; c situation after external neurolysis; d another case (right side), anomalous nerve course, crossing over the spina; e situation after nerve transposition few centimeters below the spine to supply the lateral thigh skin via several small branches.

The symptoms are often electric-current-like pain, suddenly radiating into the distribution area of the entire nerve worsened by standing and walking, and relieved by rest with a flexed hip joint. If the symptoms persist long enough paresthesias and alterations of the sensation affecting the lateral side of the thigh are also part of the patient's history. These alterations unfortunately indicate advanced intraneural scar tissue and decisively worsen the prognosis if operated on, according to our experience. It is useful to explain this thoroughly to the patient before operation.

The electric-current-like pain radiation can be provoked by deep palpation immediately medial to the anterior superior spine. The pain completely disappears if local anesthesia is injected at the same point. Both of these tests are pathognomic and serve as proof of the meralgia paresthetica.

Surgery consists of neurolysis with transsection of some portions of the inguinal ligament, so that the small nerve is completely released at its turning point (▶ Fig. 5.19 c). We avoid neurotomy so as not to induce the development of a painful neuroma that could be more troublesome than the meralgia. This may sound simple, but the dissection of the nerve under the fascia may be difficult: on the one hand, the nerve is rather thin, making it difficult to identify and preserve it (▶ Fig. 5.20 a–c), and on the other hand, we may find anomalies in its course such as associated small nerves that pass between other portions of the inguinal ligament or an anomalous nerve course (▶ Fig. 5.20 d–e). For this reason, we prefer the approach starting below the inguinal ligament in order to identify the small nerve far from possible anomalies. Therefore, the skin incision runs from the anterior superior spine, or slightly medial to it, straight downward over a distance of about 5 cm. As a next step, the fascia of the thigh is longitudinally incised downward, and beside the medial border of the sartorius muscle, the affected nerve, of a caliber no larger than the sural nerve, must be identified. Nevertheless, irreversible damage to the nerve does not seem to be completely avoidable, and a numbness of the former painful skin area may result. We would advocate trying neurolysis first, with nerve preservation in any case, as recently described by Mirzai et al. in 1993.

In case of recurrence, to be expected in at least 20% of cases, reneurolysis is often unsatisfactory. In such situations, a neurotomy proximal to the inguinal ligament, resulting in a loss of sensitivity in the nerve's distribution, may be preferable. However, painful terminal neuroma remains possible.

Because of bad experiences after managing this surgery as outpatient treatment, we now prefer hospitalization for a few days. The surgical area becomes rather heavily loaded by the abdominal content, particularly if portions of the inguinal ligament have been transected. The area may even develop a femoral hernia, an argument to preserve at least parts of the ligament. Also important is to remain reserved during the patient's mobilization to avoid new strangulations of the nerve within the freshly operated region. A suction drainage is mandatory because of the risk of rebleeding. A compression bandage is impossible.

5.13 Pudendal Nerve Entrapment

We have seen three instances of entrapment of the pudendal nerve, two in women and one in a man. The nerve arises from the 2nd to the 4th sacral roots. It soon leaves the pelvis through the great sciatic foramen but re-enters it below the sacrospinal ligament. Between this ligament and the sacrotuberous ligament, it enters the perineal region, supplying the perineal skin by small sensory branches leaving to the midline, whereas the main branch supplies the genital region.

The entrapment is located at the sharp edge of the transverse running sacrotuberous ligament.

Test infiltrations provide the diagnosis, and the typical Tinel sign is found at the special entrapment level, roughly 2–3 cm behind the anus.

The surgery is very simple through an incision approximately 3 cm beside the anus and a little bit dorsal to it (▶ Fig. 5.21). The trapping ligament should rapidly be palpated with a fingertip. In the case of the man, we succeeded in releasing the nerve by surgery with partial transsection of the sacrotuberous ligament; in the two women, only transvaginal steroid infiltrations were used.

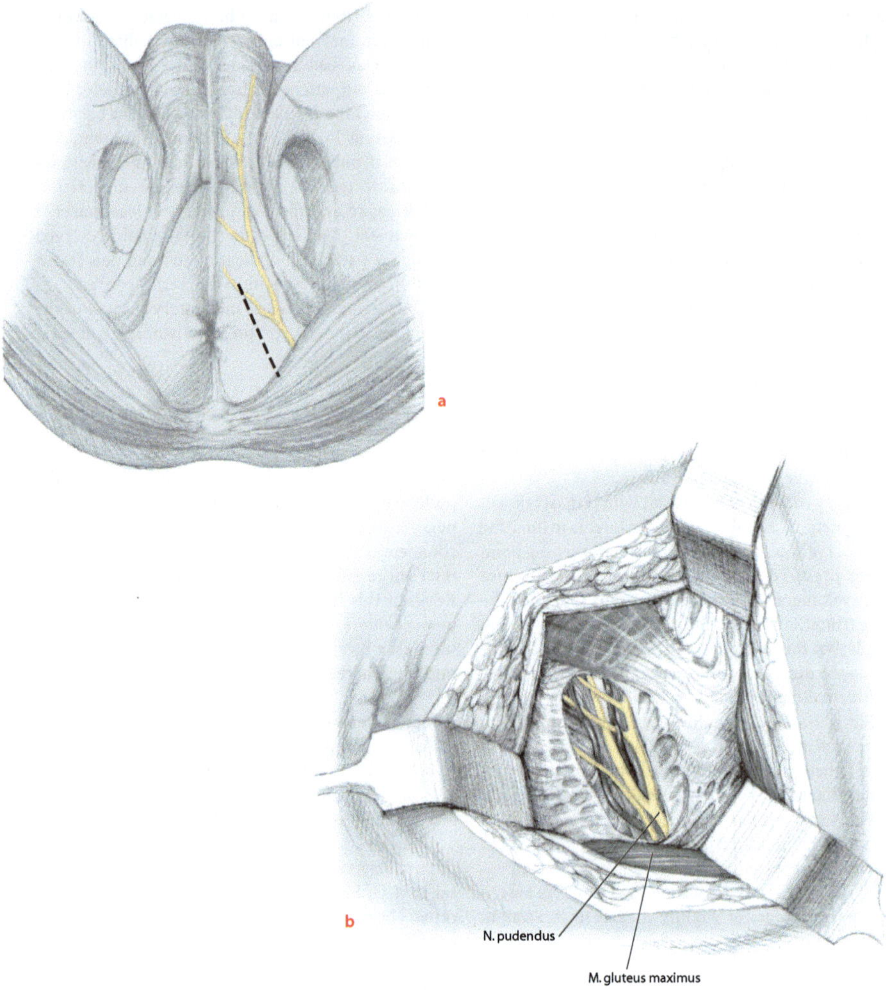

Figure 5.21 a, b

Pudendal nerve entrapment. **a** Skin incision; **b** nerve exploration, the sacrotuberal and sacrospinal ligaments under the gluteus muscle fibers are to be incised for nerve release

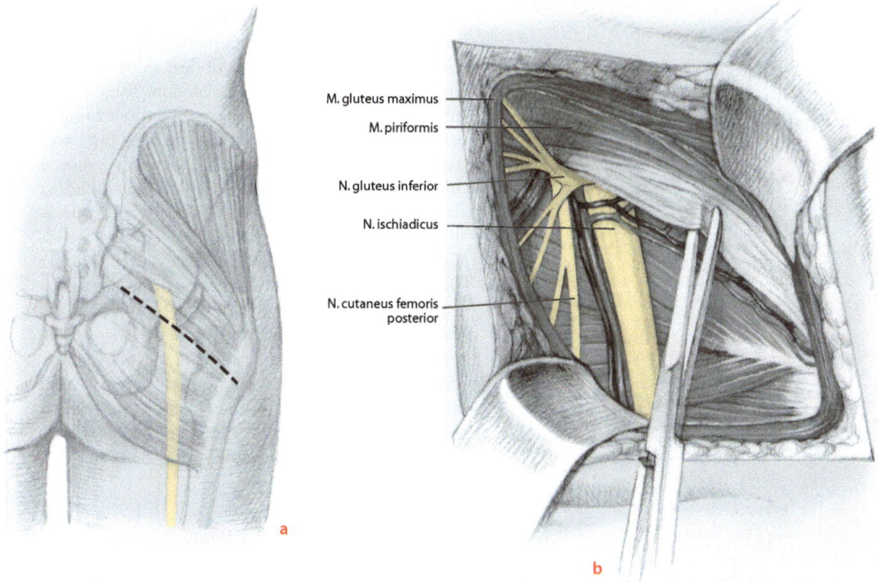

Figure 5.22 a, b

Sciatic nerve entrapment at the pelvic outlet, patient in prone position (right side). a Skin incision; b piriform muscle tendon to be divided

5.14 Sciatic Nerve Entrapment at the Pelvic Outlet

The sciatic nerve leaves the pelvis through the lower part of the great sciatic foramen, which is divided into a higher and lower opening by the transverse running piriformis muscle. Comparable to the thoracic outlet, at the level of the pelvic outlet, similar irritation syndromes rarely occur but if they do so, they cause an extensive electric-current-like pain radiating into the entire distribution area of the sciatic nerve. MRI or CT scans should exclude lumbar disk herniations at the L4/5 and L5/S1 levels, as well as tumors such as neurinomas within the pelvis. Sometimes additional CT scan-guided periradicular injections with steroids are necessary to exclude symptoms arising from a narrowed root recess. If a Tinel sign or an electric-current-like radiating pain beside the tuber ischiadicum can be elicited by forced and deep palpation a sciatic irritation at that point is fairly certain. Test infiltrations could be used, but because of the side-by-side running inferior gluteal artery, these punctures are not without risk, so we would advise not using these infiltrations. The decision for surgical exploration needs time and several detailed explanations. The patient should decide without being influenced by the surgeon.

We have had five cases leading to surgery and each time chose an incision line parallel to the expected fibers of the gluteus maximus muscle, then the muscle fibers were split, separated to both sides, and manually retracted (▶ Fig. 5.22). The fibers of the gluteus medius muscle can be lifted up slightly; then the sciatic nerve can be felt within, far medial to the great trochanter. At the exit point, the nerve is covered and sometimes even divided by a sharply edged tendon of the piriformis muscle (therefore referred to as piriformis syndrome). If a nerve division exists, the higher portion consists of peroneal fibers, whereas the lower portion contains the tibial nerve fibers (▶ Fig. 5.23 a). Because the piriformis tendon is to be expected the origin of all the irritation, as Yoemans described in 1928, it should be completely transected transverse to its fiber course (▶ Fig. 5.23 b). It is important not only to preserve the inferior gluteal artery, but also the inferior gluteal nerve, which turns

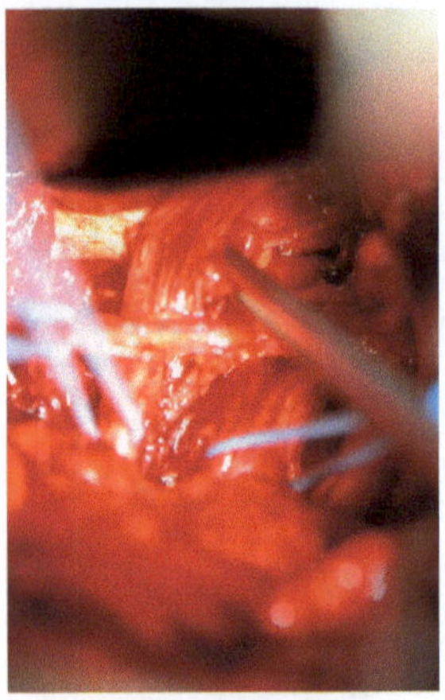

a

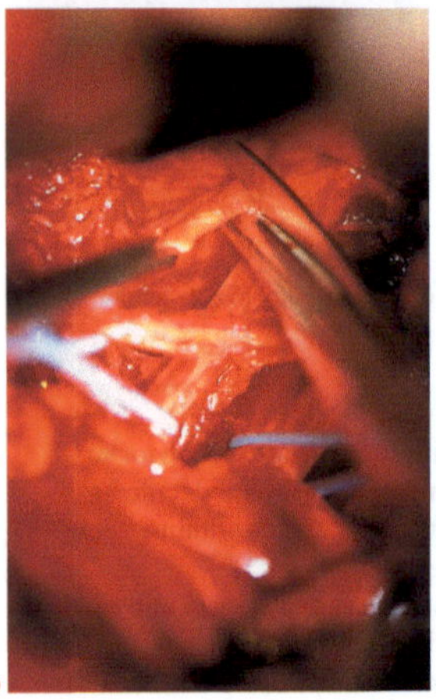

b

Figure 5.23 a, b

Sciatic nerve entrapment at the pelvic outlet, patient in prone position (right side). a Peroneal and tibial parts of the sciatic nerve separated by the piriform muscle and its tendon; b released situation after transsection of the muscle

around the low edge of the piriformis muscle and runs upward. Parallel to the inferior gluteal artery, there is an additional nerve, the posterior cutaneous femoral nerve. Occasionally, large veins cross over the sciatic nerve. They have to be individually tied and transected so that disturbing intraoperative bleeding or postoperative rebleeding is avoided as far as possible. Exploration requires suction drainage but no postoperative immobilization.

The four cases we have operated on completely improved by exclusively transecting the piriformis muscle, but in one case, there was no clear evidence of entrapment by this muscle or its tendon. Thus, we extended our surgery in a manner comparable to cases of thoracic outlet syndrome by enlarging the lower edge of the sciatic foramen. The bone was removed bit by bit by several punches, with all surrounding structures in view at all times. This patient preoperatively presented with a subtotal foot drop at the affected side and an additional weakness of the plantar flexion. His pain rapidly disappeared and he experienced lasting recovery of his muscle function. Because of the encouraging results, we enthusiastically advise this kind of exploration if the above-mentioned more proximal located diseases are excluded and if a positive Tinel sign can reliably be derived. Of special importance is that the typical electric-current-like pain is truly evocable.

5.15 Obturator Nerve Entrapment

The obturator nerve originates from the anterior divisions of the L2, L3, and L4 roots. It runs to the medial border of the psoas muscle and takes a vertical course toward the obturator foramen. Still proximal to the entrance, the nerve divides into two branches, a superficial one, which supplies the adductor longus and gracilis muscles, and a deep branch, which supplies the adductor magnus and obturator externus muscles. A skin branch distributes a small area at the proximal medial aspect of the thigh where the pain is located in case of entrapment.

The diagnosis mainly consists of test infiltrations with local anesthesia just at the point where the pain can be elicited by deep palpation. The nerve is covered by the long adductor and pectineal muscles and consequently a Tinel sign may remain hidden.

Surgical exploration is done via a longitudinal skin incision from the medial aspect of the inguinal ligament and downward, running about 5 cm (▶ Fig. 5.24). It allows an approach between the long adductor muscle and the pectineal muscle. The nerve is accompanied by two branches of the obturator artery, which also pass through the obturator channel.

Figure 5.24 a–d ▶

Obturator nerve entrapment (right side). a Skin incision; b approach between pectineal and long adductor muscles; c exploration of the nerve and its branches; d enlargement of the bony nerve exit

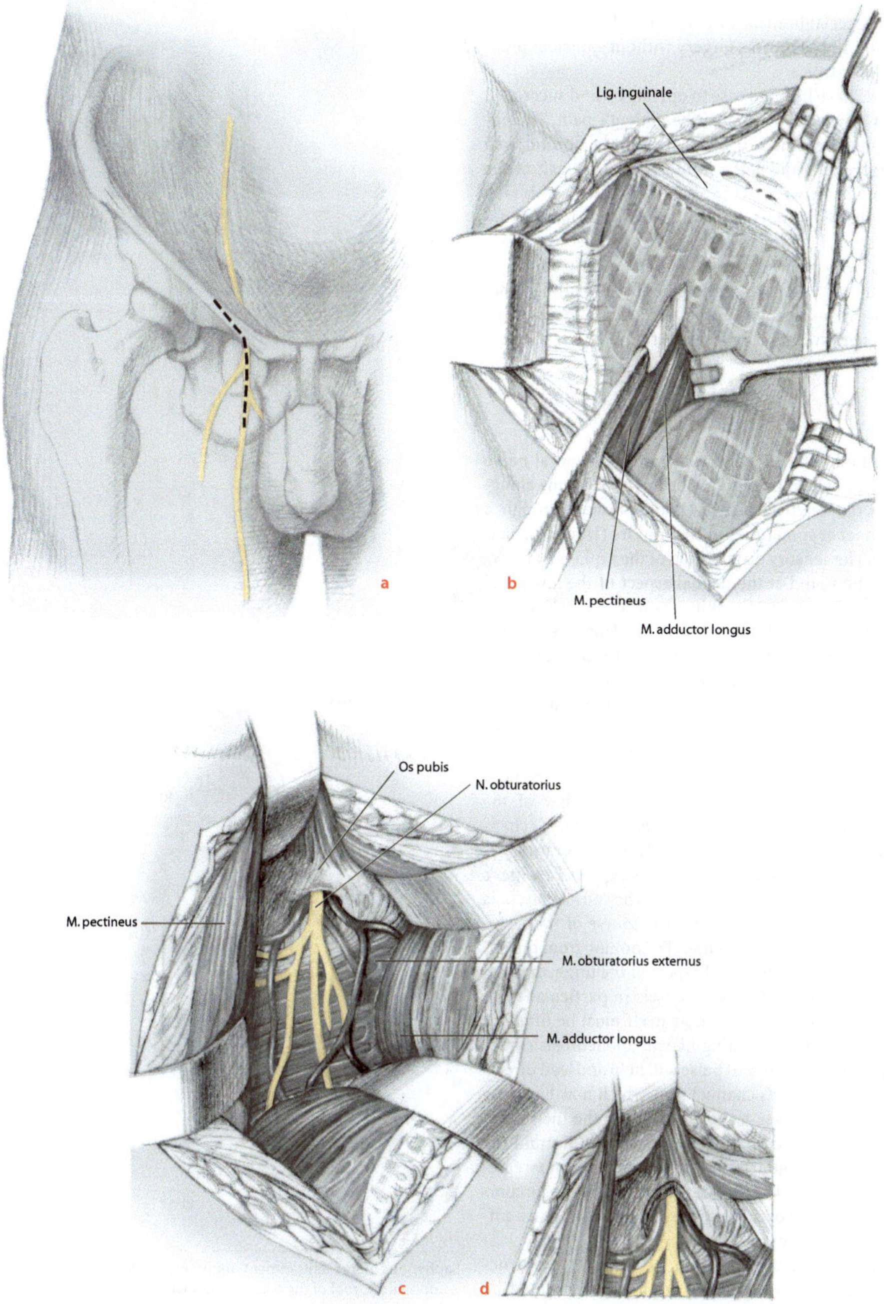
Lig. inguinale
M. pectineus
M. adductor longus
Os pubis
N. obturatorius
M. pectineus
M. obturatorius externus
M. adductor longus
a
b
c
d

The arterial branches would cause disturbing bleeding if injured during surgery without sufficient proximal control.

We have had one case to operate on and succeeded in a satisfactory relief of the patient's pain. The entrapment seemed to originate from a fibrotic arch compressing the nerve from above at the exit of the foramen. As with all the other entrapments, this arch was incised. Unfortunately, the literature does not detail typical etiologies of the rare spontaneous obturator nerve entrapment. "Spontaneous" obviously means that alternative etiologies by special space-occupying lesions within the pelvis were excluded by preoperative imaging investigations.

5.16 Saphenous Nerve Entrapment

The saphenous nerve arises from the femoral nerve 2–3 cm below the inguinal ligament and runs alongside the relatively large femoral artery through a channel of sometimes 10 cm or more (Hunter's channel). The sensory distribution of the saphenous nerve is to be found at the medial aspect of the lower leg. This region covers the skin area where pain has to radiate, especially if the region of the Hunter's channel is palpated. On the contrary, pain at the medial aspect of the thigh is not pathognomic and does not ensure diagnosis. Test infiltrations to confirm the diagnosis involve a high risk of inducing bleeding from the usually large-caliber accompanying artery.

Surgery on saphenous entrapment is slightly more difficult than expected because the caliber of the nerve is comparable to the sural nerve, Hunter's channel is far away and relatively deep. Exploration requires an incision as long as the expected Hunter's channel, 10–12 cm (▶ Fig. 5.25). The muscle fascia is incised parallel to the expected course of the nerve parallel to the sartorius muscle. Looking from the opposite side on the medial aspect of the thigh, the lower border of the sartorius muscle in particular must be dissected, and the muscle itself must be lifted up until a structure looking like an aponeurosis comes into view. The femoral pulse will help and lead directly to this Hunter's channel roof, which now has to be incised transverse to its fibers, as for the incision of the transverse carpal ligament, keeping in mind the underlying large artery and the comparably extremely small nerve. The roof of the channel has to be completely incised over the entire distance to obtain a sufficient release of the nerve.

Usually during operation, no pathological structures such as an anomaly are found that could be

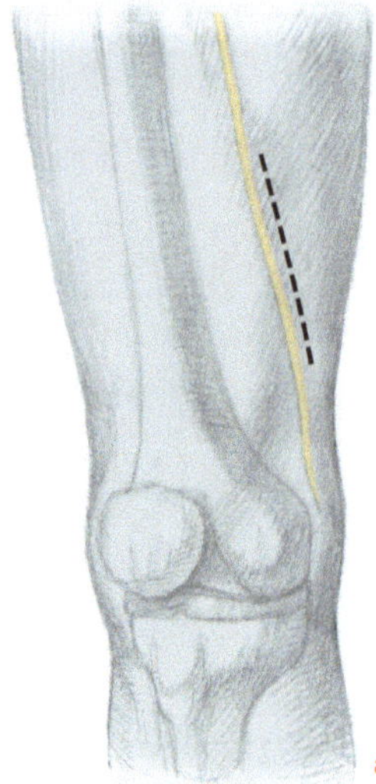
a

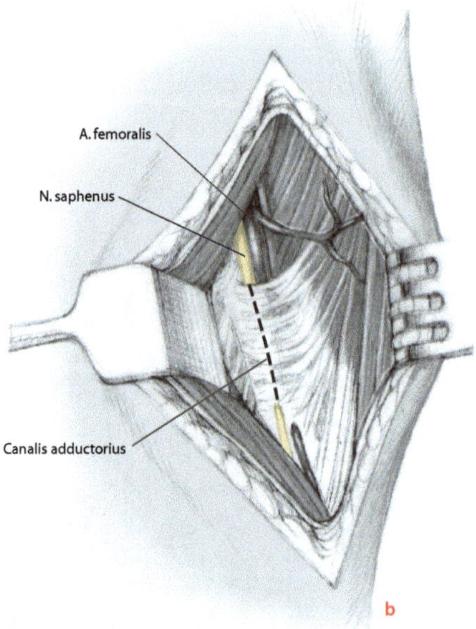

b

Figure 5.25a,b

Saphenous nerve entrapment (right leg). a Skin incision; b aponeurotic roof of the adductor tunnel is to be incised

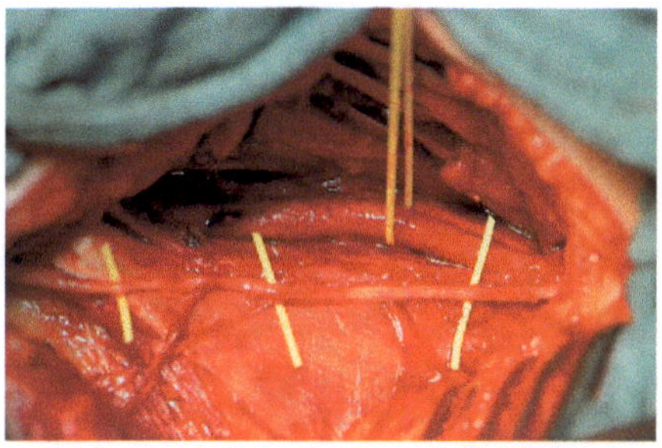

Figure 5.26

Saphenous nerve entrapment (right leg). View at its medial aspect, nerve underneath *yellow* loop pieces, femoral artery alongside

judged as the causative factor (▶ Fig. 5.26). Instead, the patients' histories frequently contain incidents such as bleeding after arterial punctures, bleeding after removal of the saphenous vein or comparable events as the possible origin of the symptoms. The surgeon never finds reasonably causative alterations within the channel.

After surgery, a suction drainage and a slight compression bandage including the lower limb and foot are required. There is no need for immobilization. General anesthesia works better than spinal anesthesia, because most cases requiring surgery involve elderly patients, who find it difficult to avoid body movements during the time-consuming surgery.

5.17 Common Peroneal Nerve Entrapment at the Knee

The common peroneal nerve enters the compartment of the peroneal muscles after turning around the fibular bone 2–3 cm below the tibiofibular joint. Two locations of compression neuropathy of the nerve are seen: first, the location between skin and bone beside the fibula, a location comparable to the situation of the ulnar nerve at the elbow level, which involves comparable risks of repeated crush traumas, for example, during operations; second, the entrance point into the muscle compartment, which is often surrounded by a fibrotic arch acting as the origin of the long peroneal muscle. Comparable to the arcade of Frohse with the posterior interosseous nerve, this arcade or the fibrotic arch often causes a compression syndrome, now rarely related to trauma, but instead mostly associated with spontaneous onset. Sometimes, activities requiring extremely flexed knee joints over a long period of time induce chronic entrapments. As expected, the point of the maximally elicitable Tinel sign is located over one of two entrapment points, so that the diagnosis and the indication for surgery depends on this clinical sign. The accompanying weakness and numbness stem from the distributions of the usually simultaneously affected superficial and deep branches of the peroneal nerve. The diagnosis may be completed by neurographic and electromyographic tests.

Of special interest are cases with subtotal or total lack of common peroneal nerve function following hip joint surgery. It is not fully understood why the peroneal part of the sciatic nerve is then affected at a much higher rate than the tibial part. We have mostly seen cases of severe sciatic nerve disturbances following surgery within the buttocks, for which the tibial nerve but not the peroneal nerve slowly recovered over a period of more than 12 months. The downward migrating Tinel sign over the sciatic nerve stopped in these cases at the above-mentioned entrapment points of the common peroneal nerve. Surgical release at the joint level was astonishingly followed by an additional partial recovery of the peroneal muscles some months later.

Surgery requires an incision using the skin crease of the knee joint, leading to the lateral aspect of the popliteal fossa, and finally turning around the region of the tibiofibular joint into a distal direction (▶ Fig. 5.27). With this method, a triangular skin flap is lifted up from the muscle fascia and fascia behind the knee. With this incision line, the final skin closure does not cross over the course of the common peroneal nerve so that irritations to the nerve due to hypertrophic skin scars are prevented (▶ Fig. 5.28 a). In contrast to the situation of the ulnar nerve at elbow level, it is not possible to transpose the nerve into a more fully supported area so that the skin incision must absolutely be influenced by the very superficial location of the nerve. In a word, the skin incision has to be chosen far from the course of the nerve. Dissecting the nerve starts with an incision of the fascia of the popliteal fossa parallel to the expected course of the nerve. The nerve is situated in very close connection to this fascia. Therefore, even the incision of this fascia should be done very gently. After identifying the nerve, its course leads further dissection around the fibular bone and into the entrance point of the peroneal compartment. As with the ulnar nerve dissection, the peroneal nerve has to be raised and should be completely freed of adhesions to the fibu-

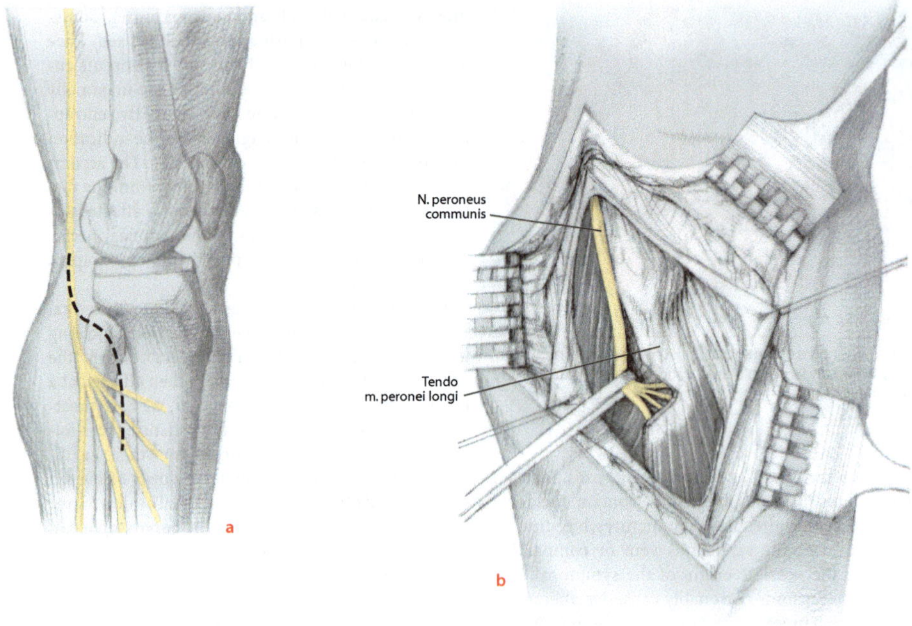

Figure 5.27 a, b

Common peroneal nerve entrapment at the knee (right leg). a Skin incision; b nerve release by incision of the aponeurotic peroneal muscle fascia

lar bone. After that, the main branches, the deep and the superficial branches are separated from each other, then as a final step, the above-mentioned fibrotic arch at the entrance point into the muscles should be incised so that the surgeon's finger can also enter the peroneal muscle compartment (▶ Fig. 5.28 b, c). Arising branches have to remain in view during the transsection of the fibrotic arch because they may be situated very superficially and are in danger of being damaged.

At the end of the operation, a closure of the fascia of the popliteal fossa is impossible because that would cause transverse strangulations at different levels, thus causing a new entrapment of the nerve. In order to prevent strangulation, we prefer a wound closure by skin stitches only after positioning a suction drain far from the nerve. A slight compression bandage is necessary, including the entire lower limb and foot. Mobilization can start the first day after surgery, the skin stitches should be removed after 14 days at the earliest.

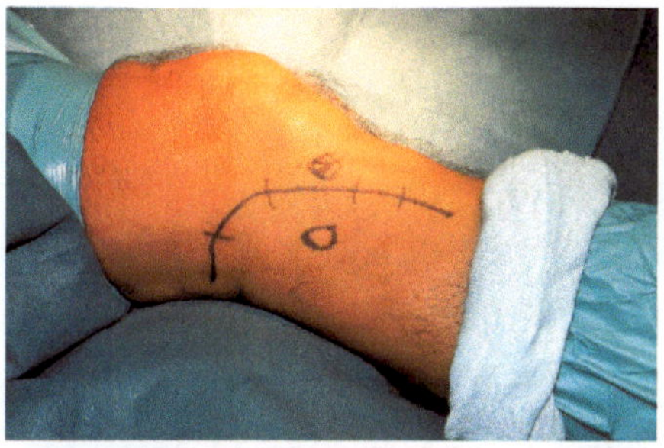

a

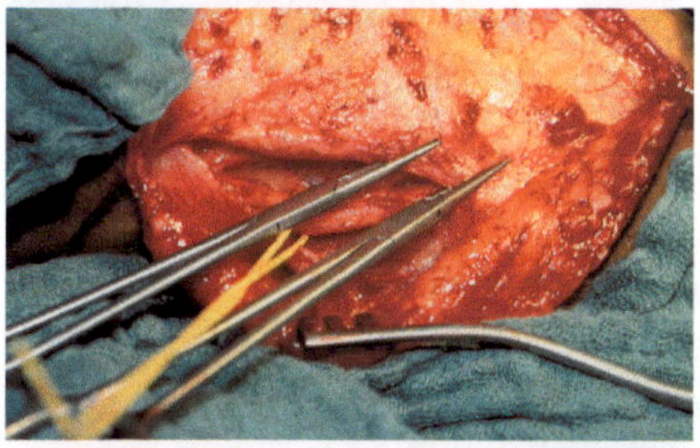

b

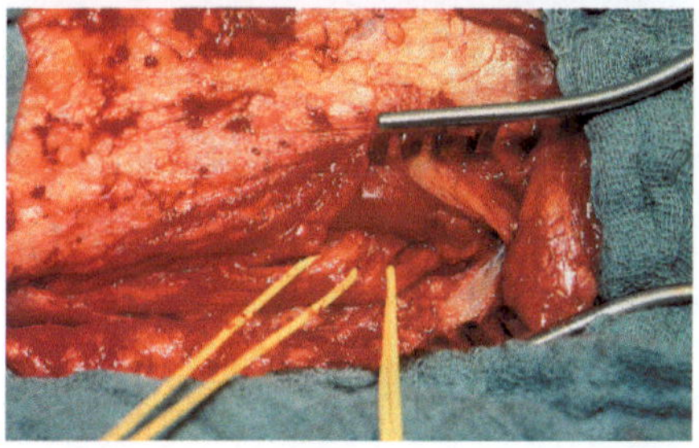

c

Figure 5.28a–c

Common peroneal nerve entrapment at the knee (right leg). a Skin incision; b identification of the nerve beside the tibial-fibular joint; c nerve release by incision of the peroneal muscle fascia

5.18 Tibial Nerve Entrapment at the Ankle

A few centimeters above the medial malleolus, the tibial nerve starts to divide into two main branches, the medial and the lateral plantar nerves. These two branches are covered by the flexor retinaculum, where they run along the posterior tibial artery through a channel identical to the carpal tunnel. When entering at the exit zone into the plantar region, the artery is situated between the two main branches of the tibial nerve, but it is important to know that the artery has variable branches intertwining the two nerves. The region under the flexor retinaculum (tarsal tunnel) contains not only the structures just mentioned, but also within a separated compartment and slightly nearer to the medial malleolus, the posterior tibial muscle tendon. As with the carpal tunnel, the tarsal tunnel is a pre-existing narrowed channel, with its entrapment syndrome (tarsal tunnel syndrome, according to Keck 1962) mostly presenting with spontaneous onset, possibly influenced by additional anomalies, as can be the case in other irritation zones. But if its symptoms are taken into consideration, the similarity between the carpal and tarsal tunnel syndromes deceives: the tarsal tunnel syndrome consists of a combination of entrapments of the median and ulnar nerves at the wrist level, in other words, an involvement of both the medial and lateral plantar nerves. Therefore, the associated symptoms are not so clearly separated and involve all the small muscles of the sole as well as the skin of the plantar surface of the foot. Patients come to the physician usually suffering from severe pain over the plantar skin, whereas an ongoing weakness or even atrophy of the muscles within the sole does not play an important role in the patient's history. Nevertheless, rare cases exist with isolated involvement of either the medial or lateral plantar nerves only.

The diagnosis includes determining the maximum point of the Tinel sign, which is usually located at the level of the medial malleolus or slightly proximal to it, as well as comparing the sensitivity over the plantar surfaces of both feet and testing the flexion forces of the toes on both feet. The diagnosis is finally completed by electroneurography and electromyography, particularly of the abductor hallucis muscle and abductor digiti V.

Although spontaneous onsets and slowly advancing and decreasing symptoms are the norm in the majority of cases, entrapments are also related to distortions involving the ankle joint. The symptoms usually start a few weeks subsequent to the distortion and decrease more rapidly. In these cases following a

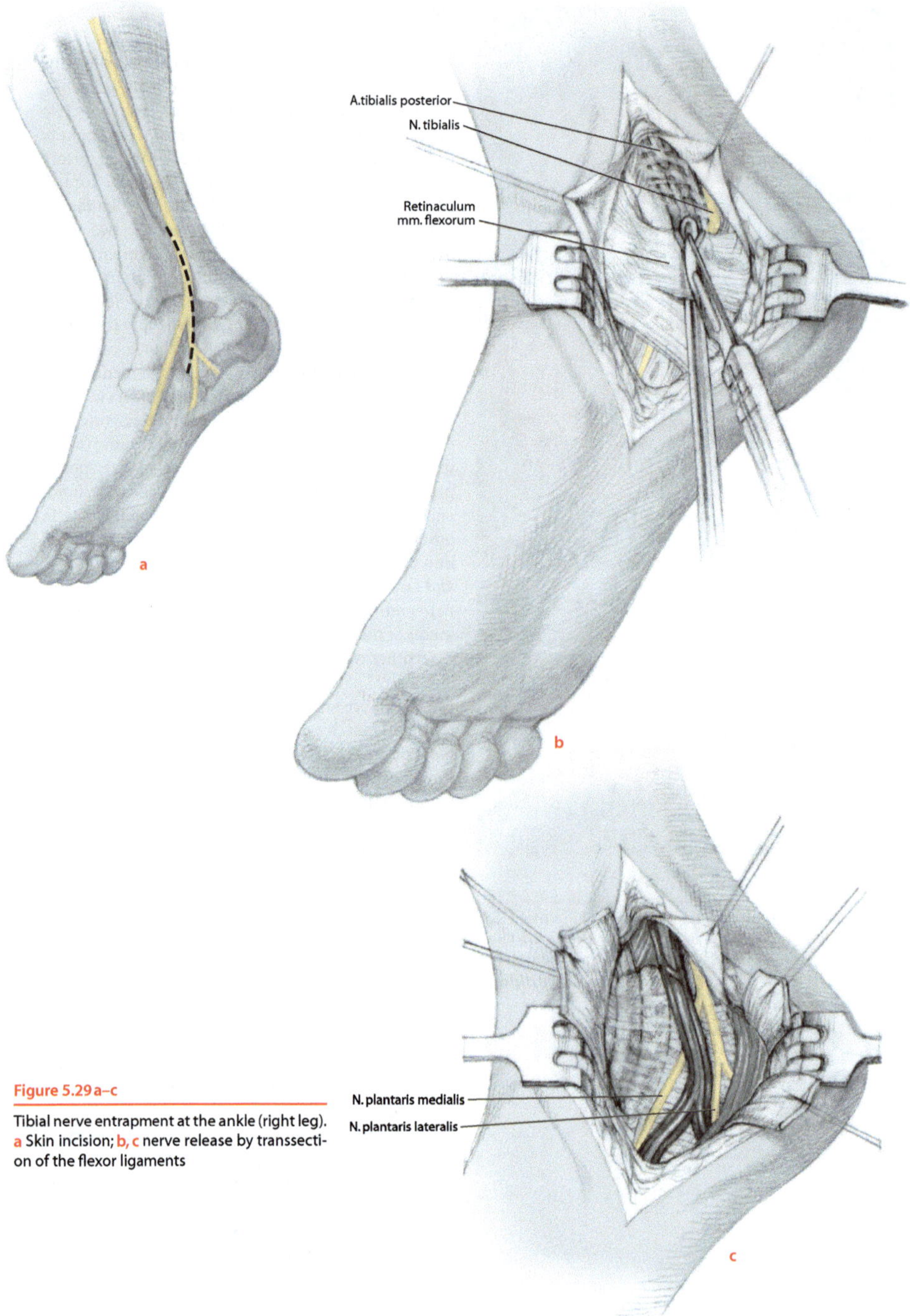

Figure 5.29 a–c

Tibial nerve entrapment at the ankle (right leg). a Skin incision; b, c nerve release by transsection of the flexor ligaments trauma, the plantar nerves need an earlier release than in pure spontaneous entrapments, because extensive extraneural and intraneural scar tissue will occur, endangering the nerves to irreversible damage. Nevertheless, despite a surgical release in time, long-lasting or even chronic pain syndromes of the tibial nerve can result, especially if related to trauma. Therefore, it must be pointed out that the prognosis decisively depends on the amount of intraneural damage due to scar tissue. This facts must be explained to the patient before surgery because they influence the decision and the patient's expectations of surgical success.

The operation starts with a slightly curved incision behind the medial malleolus, traveling upward 3–4 cm above the malleolus and about the same distance downward (▶ Fig. 5.29). At the distal level, incising the skin over the plantar surface, as is often described, should be avoided because the resulting skin scar would compress the plantar nerves just at their entrance point into the sole with each step. The dissection of the nerve and accompanying posterior tibial artery starts at the proximal level because identification is simple after a longitudinal incision of the fascia (▶ Fig. 5.30 a). The transsection of the flexor retinaculum still follows with the nerve or both branches in view. One should not start straight over the flexor retinaculum, which could lead to the wrong compartment and thus destroy the hypomochleon of the posterior tibial muscle tendon. The artery very frequently shows a serpentine course, and arterial and venous branches intertwine with the nerves (▶ Fig. 5.30 b). The small branching vessels should be identified before being disrupted, and they should be tied with bipolar forceps, keeping far from the nerves, and transected. Finishing the operation at that step, after the release under the flexor retinaculum might be unsuccessful because both nerves are also frequently compressed at the entrance to the sole. The abductor hallucis muscle is covered by a very strong fascia, which shapes two small holes, allowing the plantar nerves to pass under the plantar surface. These entrance points have to be enlarged by careful incisions, taking care not to harm the nerves themselves. This important part of the operation takes place at the distal part of the skin incision but it does not require a skin incision into the plantar surface.

At the end of the operation, we place a small suction drainage because rebleeding from the small intertwining arteries would cause an area of external scar tissue. We have unfortunately had the experience of unsuccessful reoperation after such developments.

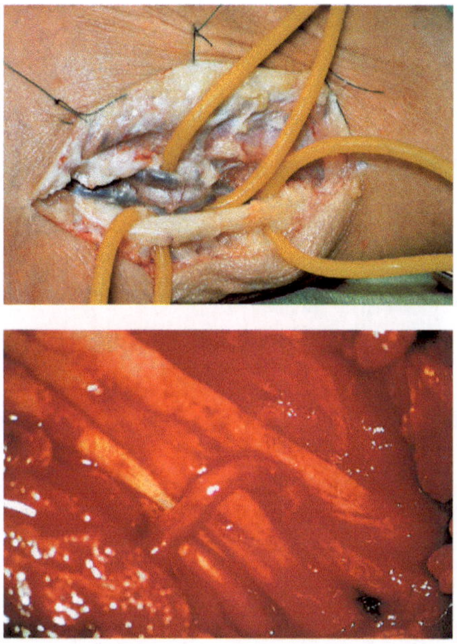

Figure 5.30 a, b

Tibial nerve entrapment at the ankle (right leg). a Exploration of nerve and vessels (in bloodless field); b another case, medial and lateral plantar nerves with intertwining vessels in between at the entrance of the sole of the foot

Depending on the operation field, which presents very little subcutaneous tissue, we usually avoid subcutaneous stitches so as not to produce transverse strangulations of the nerves. We only use skin stitches and leave them in place over a period of 14 days. Unfortunately, patients rarely follow instructions to remain inactive after surgery and we prefer to hospitalize the patient for a short time.

5.19 Deep Peroneal Nerve Entrapment at the Ankle

This very rare entrapment involves the final branch of the deep peroneal nerve, which runs along the anterior tibial artery at the level of the ankle joint between the extensor hallucis longus tendon and the extensor digitorum longus tendon. At this level, nerve and artery are covered by a retinaculum extensorum or, alternatively, by two of these structures. The nerve sup-

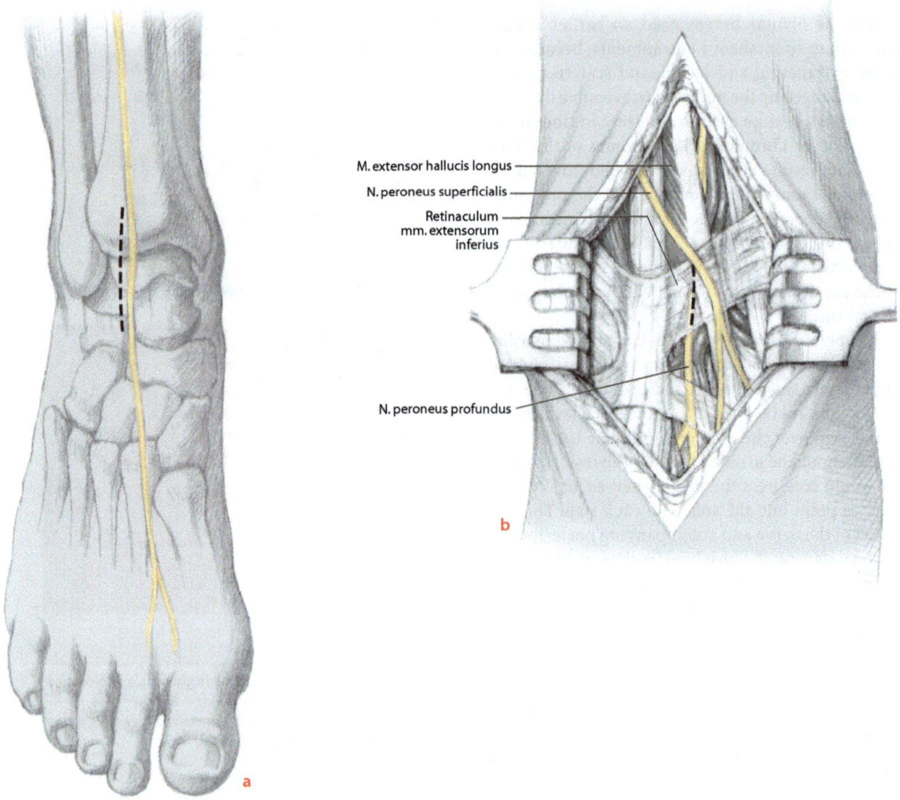

Figure 5.31 a, b

Deep peroneal nerve entrapment at the ankle (right leg). a Skin incision; b nerve release by transsection of the extensor ligaments

plies the extensor digitorum and extensor hallucis brevis muscles. The branches to these muscles arise just below the retinacula so that electromyographic tests can document denervation potentials in these small muscles. The sensory distribution of the nerve is represented by a small interdigital area between the first and second toes, comparable to the sensory distribution of the posterior interosseous nerve at the dorsal surface of the hand. This is the area where pain radiates in entrapment cases (anterior tarsal tunnel syndrome, according to Marinacci, 1968). The Tinel sign is to be elicited at a level where the 2.5-cm skin incision should be placed (▶ Fig. 5.31). The dissection of the nerve and the artery must pass between the extensor tendons and has finally to aim at a transsection of the disturbing parts of the extensor retinacula. Other parts aim at hypomochleon of the surrounding tendons The overlying superficial peroneal nerve leading to the medial aspect of the dorsal foot surface is situated subcutaneously, just above these retinacula. This nerve must be preserved, and much more important, it must not be mistaken with the deep peroneal nerve situated in a much deeper compartment (▶ Fig. 5.32).

We have treated two cases of anterior tarsal tunnel syndrome. The small nearly risk-free decompressive surgery unfortunately has two mitigating factors: ongoing compression forces due to shoes and a frequently rather late diagnosis compared to meralgia paresthetica.

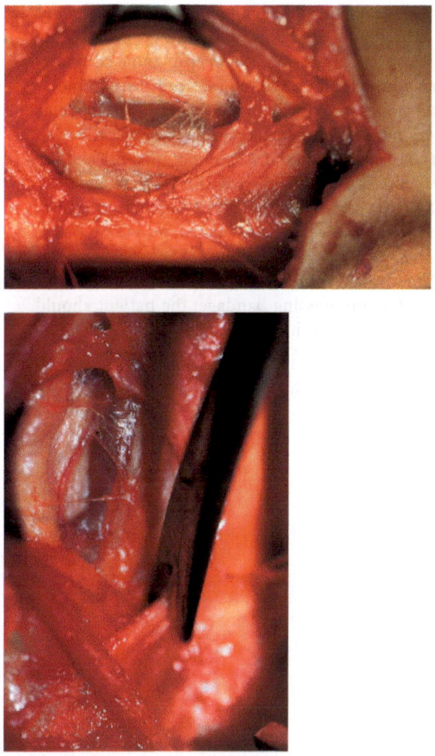

a

b

Figure 5.32 a, b

Deep peroneal nerve entrapment at the ankle (right leg). a Exploration of nerve and anterior tibial artery (superficial branch of the peroneal nerve below); b transsection of one of both extensor retinacula in order to release the deep branch

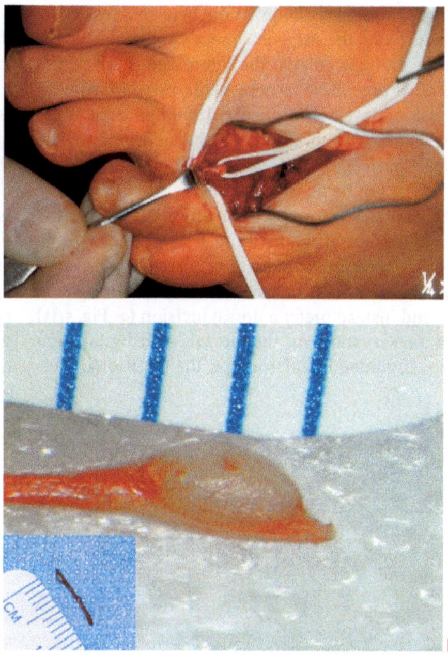

a

b

Figure 5.33 a, b

Plantar digital nerve entrapment (Morton). a Dorsal approach; b resected nerve with neuroma. (Courtesy of Prof. Tatagiba, Neurosurgical Department, University of Tübingen, Germany)

5.20 Plantar Digital Nerve Entrapment

The involvement of the common plantar digital nerves of the sole originates from a real compression between the heads of the metatarsal bones. The compression causes electric-current-like extensive pain radiating into the distribution of the affected plantar digital nerve, the space between two contiguous toes, mostly between the 3rd and 4th toes. Not rarely, neighboring interdigital spaces are alternatively or additionally involved. The syndrome is synonymously referred to as Morton's metatarsalgia, according to Morton's first description in 1876. Women are more affected than men. The pain is characteristically provoked by walking or manually pressing the toes against each other. On the other hand, it does not cease when the patient stops walking or removes his shoes. A detailed examination will show that the nerve damage is not caused by incidents called irritation or entrapment, but instead by compression between two heads of the metatarsal bones. Therefore, it should be understandable that the risk of developing a painful and irreversible neuroma is very high. Consequently, the chances of spontaneous relief of the radiating pain remain relatively low, even if the design of the shoes has been changed repeatedly.

The diagnosis consists of two tests: first, the physician should provoke the individually radiating pain by pressing the toes against each other by forced palpation within the interdigital space over the sole, and second, the pain should completely disappear after instillation of local anesthesia in the interdigital space for a period of 1–2 h.

If surgery is selected, the patient must understand that a procedure similar to neurolysis would be certainly unsuccessful because the nerve lesion originates from a real compression between two bony structures. As the surgeon cannot change this situation or perhaps enlarge the interosseous space, the operative procedure is necessarily neurotomy, with the risk of developing a new painful neuroma at the proximal nerve end. Of course, this neuroma will be located more proximal, within soft tissue with reduced risks of being irritated during walking.

Several authors incise the interdigital skin at the plantar surface of the foot and remove such neuromas. But because of frequent occurrences of hypersensitive scars at the sole, we never incise through the sole, and instead prefer a dorsal incision (▶ Fig. 5.33) with preservation of the dorsal interdigital skin nerve. If guided by microscope, the additional division of the metatarsal ligament advised by some authors to gain a better overview can be avoided. By means of magnification, the deep plantar compartment can be easily dissected between the two metatarsal bones proximal to their heads. The plantar nerve and the plantar artery have the same caliber, so that they must be identified and not mixed. Then the nerve is sectioned but the small artery preserved. A pathologist can examine a nerve segment to ensure that the right one has been treated, providing better arguments in case of recurrence.

The wound closure should include a small drainage and a compressing bandage; the patient should not put weight on the affected foot after the operation.

Trauma-Related Limb Nerve Lesions

The introductory review of types and degrees of nerve lesion, scar tissue reaction following nerve trauma, management of diagnosis, and timing of surgery subsequent to nerve injury (see Chaps. 2 and 3) applies to all trauma-related nerve lesions to be explored in the following chapters. These principles will therefore not be repeated here, other than several general remarks:

- During the operation, the surgeon should decide whether there is a chance of a spontaneous recovery when a nerve is in continuity or whether the nerve lesion needs nerve repair. If the affected nerve trunk is not disrupted and the surgeon remains unsure of whether to define the situation as pseudoneuroma or neuroma in continuity, a microsurgical procedure must be started, comparable to a stepwise neurolysis from above and below the affected nerve segment. By means of a longitudinally separating dissection between the fascicle groups, the lesion is approached and pseudoneuroma or neuroma can be better distinguished. The latter must be resected and reconstructed by grafts as described. Intraoperative nerve action potentials are helpful and therefore mandatory, particularly in this decisive operating step, as recently advised by Kline and Hudson (1995).
- A look at an anatomical atlas provides a three-dimensional picture before surgery on the affected nerve, with the vessels running alongside, and additional nerves that must be preserved, as well as the muscle borders that could lead to the surgical target. This will give an idea of the skin incision initially needed, where the only rule is "never cross over skin creases." No case resembles another in its details, one more reason that rules on how to explore injured nerves have not been assessed.
- Surgical explorations of the spinal accessory nerve, brachial plexus, circumflex (axillary) nerve, and facial nerve are the greatest challenge in peripheral nerve surgery. No surgeon should ingenuously start exploring lesions of these nerves located in extremely delicate locations without previous experience as an assistant to a highly skilled surgeon in this special field. Surgeons who take on surgical exploration must find a final solution to all intraoperative questions. Reoperations frequently fail because of the large amount of scar tissue. Nevertheless, the patient will recall the physician without fail 1 year later if surgery has not been successful.
- Each surgeon takes the responsibility for the primary intervention. We have encountered patients consulting us after an end-to-end epineural nerve suture. The only suitable advice must be to ask the primary surgeon if the suture is reliable. Any further decision will exclusively depend on this answer.
- A suction drainage is usually never allowed following nerve grafting, as its removal will most likely displace the transplants.

6.1 Accessory Nerve

The accessory nerve exits the skull base through the jugular foramen. Its course is situated lateral to the internal jugular vein. Its location is then variable: it may course either anterior or posterior to the internal jugular vein. Behind the digastric muscle, it turns a few degrees dorsal and leaves the jugular vein, then it runs parallel to and on fibers of the levator scapulae muscle, where the proximal third of the nerve is covered by the sternocleidomastoid muscle. The nerve exits into the posterior triangle of the neck beneath the posterior or lateral border of the sternocleidal muscle together with the occipital minor nerve, which wraps around the lateral border of the muscle. A few centimeters below these two nerves, the great auricular nerve wraps around the same muscle. Thus, the posterior sternocleidal border and the exit points of the occipital minor as well as the great auricular nerves form an important landmark leading to the accessory nerve or the proximal neuroma in case of

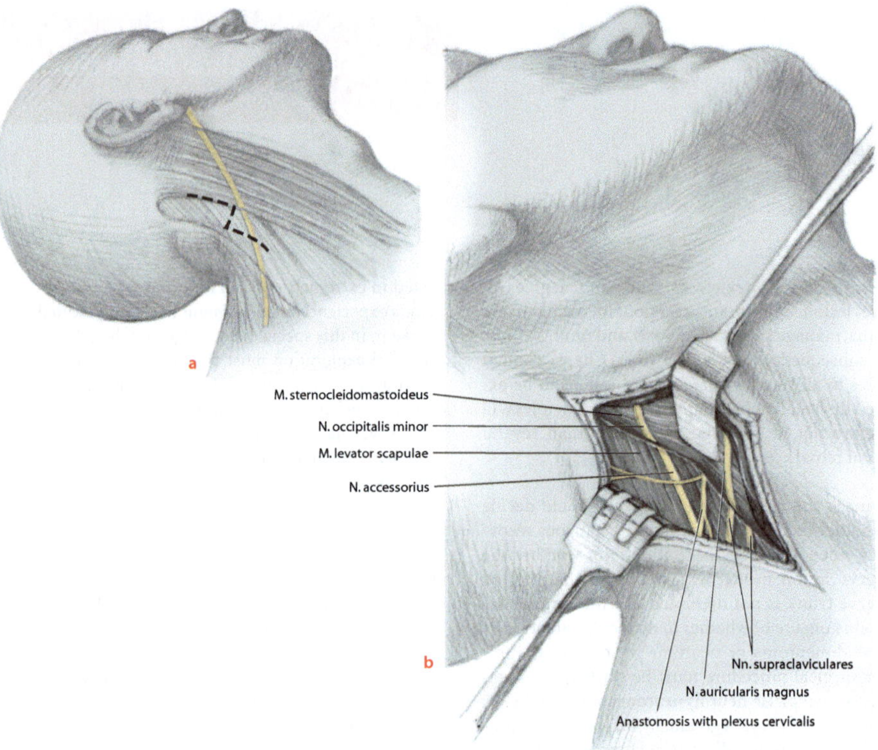

Figure 6.1 a, b

Accessory nerve lesion. a Skin incision; b nerve exploration started at the posterior border of the sternocleidomastoid muscle

discontinuity. The spinal portion of the nerve is then situated almost subcutaneously, and is therefore in danger during lymph node extirpations, unfortunately the most common origin of accessory nerve lesions. On reaching the anterior border of the trapezius muscle, the nerve divides into several branches, with the result that a more distal nerve lesion may make it very difficult to define an appropriate distal nerve stump.

The clinical findings after nerve lesion consist of a severe loss of trapezius muscle function. The supraspinatus and deltoid muscles abduct the humerus into a 90° position, but the further abduction requires the rotation of the scapula. This movement can be achieved by traction of fibers of the superior part of the trapezius muscle and additional fibers of the levator scapulae and rhomboid muscles. Meanwhile, the sternocleidal muscle remains intact because nerve branches to it leave the accessory nerve far proximal to its exit into the posterior triangle. In the case of a nerve lesion, a simple inspection already shows the atrophy of the superior portion of the trapezius muscle and a slight winging of the scapula, whereas a paralysis of the serratus anterior muscle causes a more severe winging of the scapula. Because branches of cervical plexus nerves also supply parts of the trapezius muscle, for example as described by Allieu et al. in 1982, we have never found a complete loss of function, making the diagnosis, the indication for surgical repair, and the timing of surgery unclear over a long period of time, all of which should be discussed with the patient.

This mixed innervation of the trapezius also leads to difficulties when trying to complete the diagnosis

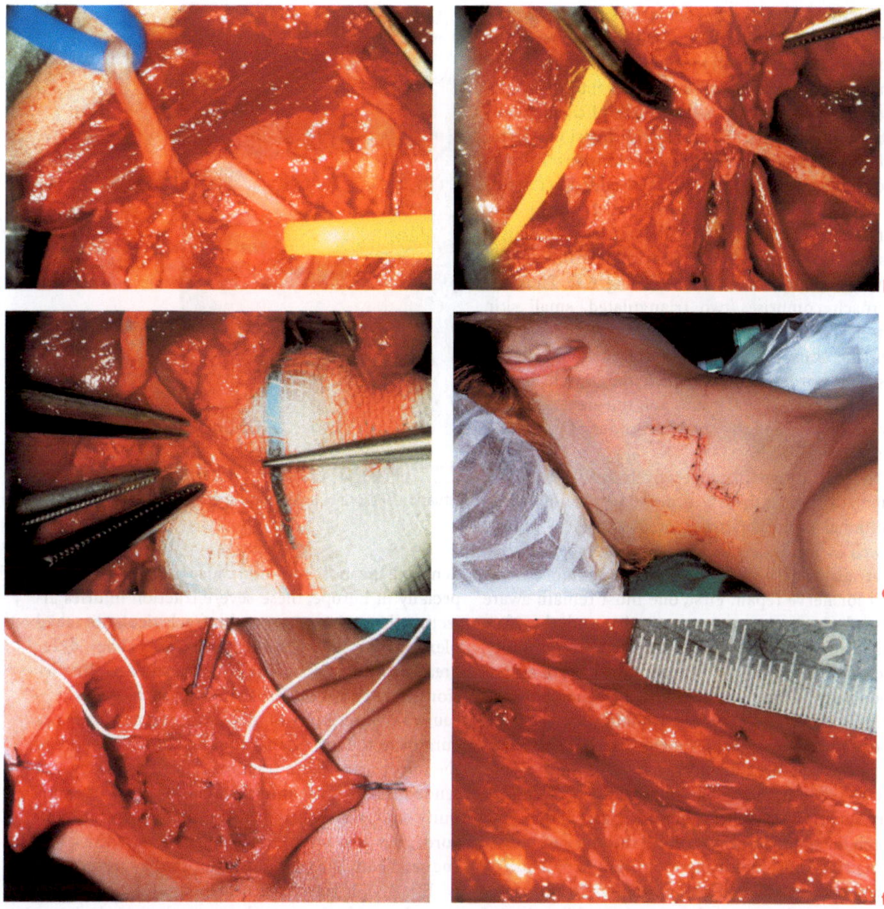

Figure 6.2 a–f

Accessory nerve lesions (right sided). a Exploration at punctum nervosum (accessory nerve, *yellow loop;* occipital minor nerve, *blue loop*); b neuroma in continuity; c epineurectomy; d situation after skin closure; e case with nerve discontinuity; f 18-mm nerve graft for repair

by means of electromyography. The test has to distinguish between voluntary potentials originating from preserved fibers of the cervical plexus and de-innervation or reinnervation potentials belonging to the distribution by accessory nerve fibers. Such electromyographic testing remains a great challenge to all electrophysiologists, often yielding misleading results.

Surgical exploration should be tried within the first 2 or 3 months. A remaining subtotal weakness would mean substantial functional loss and causes additional pain due to the permanently stretched soft tissue structures. On the other hand, surgical exploration is far more difficult, as can be expected with a first glance at an anatomical atlas. The mostly iatrogenic lesion leaves behind a subcutaneous field of scar tissue, and, more particularly, segments of the nerve may be completely avulsed together with the lymph node, resulting in the above-mentioned problems in identifying the motor entries into the trapezius. Nerve exploration is the source of cosmetically unfavorable results. The original incision, corresponding to skin creases situated transversely, must be extended: vertical limbs must be added to the primary small horizontal incision parallel to the posterior border of the sternocleidal muscle, making it possible to identify the nerve within healthy tissue above and below the scar area (▶ Fig. 6.1). Thus, the approach comprises two triangulated, small skin flaps. Nerve identification always succeeds at the level of the above-mentioned landmarks, beneath the posterior border of the sternocleidal muscle, beside the wrapping occipital minor and the great auricular nerves, and behind the anterior border of the trapezius muscle.

The use of an intraoperatively available nerve stimulator is mandatory to preserve the important additional motor branches of the cervical plexus, as well as to identify sensory nerves, especially the great auricular nerve, which can be removed and used for nerve repair. First, one must remain aware of exploring a nerve in continuity and therefore dissect very carefully. In case of preserved continuity, microsurgery as well as intraoperative nerve stimulation may distinguish between a pseudoneuroma (▶ Fig. 6.2 a–d) or a neuroma in continuity. The latter case requires nerve repair (▶ Fig. 6.2 e–f). The accessory nerve and the sural nerve as well as the great auricular nerve have comparable diameters. Extended nerve disruptions often require great patience to search for small branches behind the anterior border of the trapezius, indicating motor entry points. The interposed graft should be long enough to allow later movements of the neck because immobilization of the operating field is impossible. Wound closure must be undertaken with great care because the horizontal part of the skin incision crosses the graft and its suture lines.

Electromyographic follow-up again requires distinguishing between preserved voluntary potentials and special reinnervation potentials after nerve repair.

6.2 Brachial Plexus

Traumatic brachial plexus injuries are lesions affecting mainly young individuals. According to the major studies reported in the literature, motorcycle accidents are the most common cause of such lesions. Especially in Europe, these severe traction injuries affecting the entire supra- and infraclavicular brachial plexus bring in the majority of cases. They differ greatly from gunshot injuries, other penetrating lesions, or circumscript crush injuries to the plexus, because a discontinuity of all plexus nerves mostly occurs from the intraspinal root level to structures of the upper arm. These traction-related very long, extended lesions raise questions not only about continuity and scarring of the peripheral trunks and cords, but also on the continuity of the intraspinal rootlets and the roots within the neuroforamen (▶ Fig. 6.3). If intending nerve repair, a nerve graft should never be connected to roots that may be intraspinally avulsed or discontinued, because that would lead to a complete failure and also mean permanent loss of the grafts used. Our increasing experience has demonstrated that supraclavicular exploration was not sufficient to diagnose root avulsions, although this diagnosis remained fundamental to the decision about the type of nerve repair to consider.

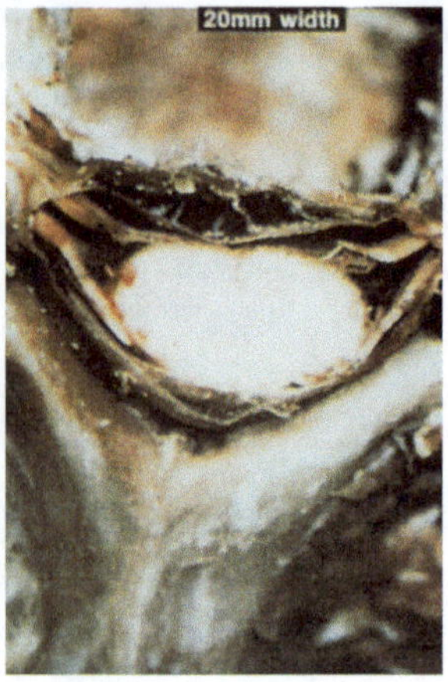

Figure 6.3

Situation of rootlets, anatomical specimen

Thus, one of the major issues, and generally the first step, during the management of a brachial plexus lesion that has to be addressed is whether the cervical rootlets C5–C8 are intact (Penkert et al. 1999). MRI studies with 1-mm C4–T1 axial slices should be acquired (▶ Fig. 6.4). If these studies do not sufficiently answer the question of continuity of the individual ventral and dorsal rootlets, CT myelography

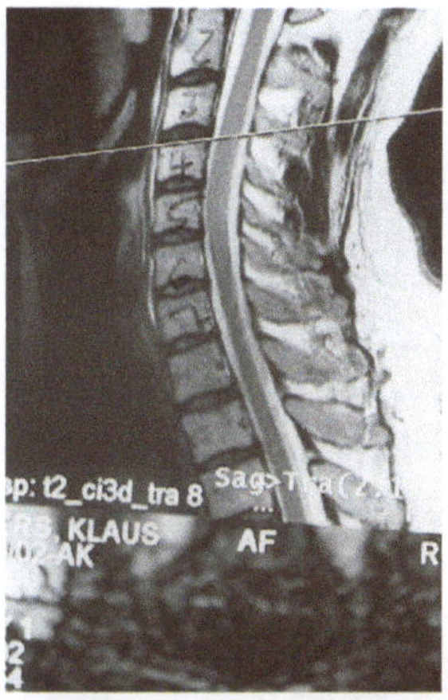

a

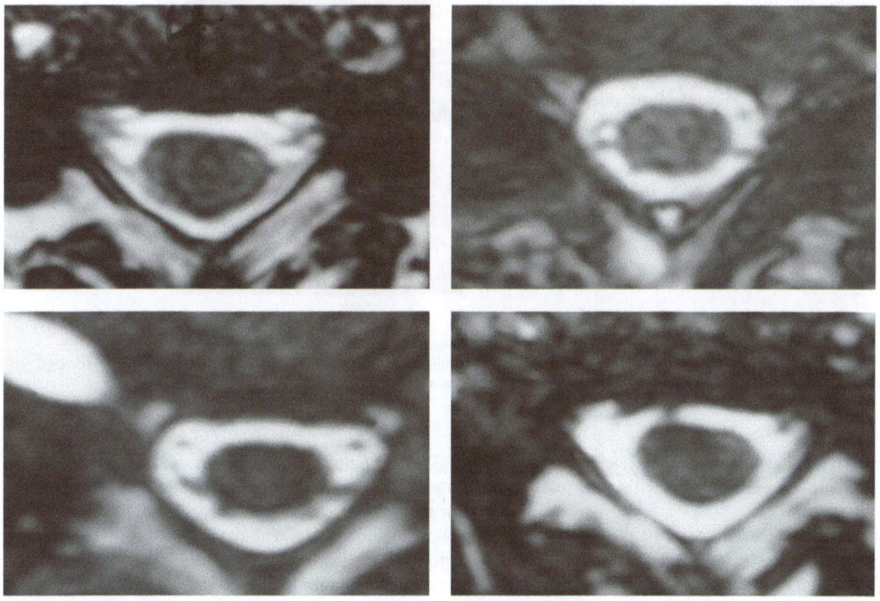

b c d e

Figure 6.4 a–e

MRI findings after brachial plexus lesion. a Scout, axial slices starting at C3–C4 level; b rootlets preserved; c discontinuity of both rootlets *on the left*; d preserved rootlets beside a pseudomeningocele (the rootlets will enter the next deeper neuroforamen); e both rootlets avulsed *on the left*

with 1-mm axial slices should be added. In special cases, intradural surgical exploration must be carried out via a hemi-laminectomy at the C5 and C7 levels, as described by Carvalho et al. in 1997 (▶ Fig. 6.5). Only the evidence of a ventral rootlet in continuity offers chances of axon sprouts with motor function. However, a Tinel sign that could be elicited in the supraclavicular area some weeks subsequent to a trauma only reveals the existence of sensory sprouts. With brachial plexus lesions, the Tinel sign consequently does not have the same importance as it has in the diagnosis of mixed nerve trunks in the periphery. The same holds true for somatosensory evoked potentials (SEP) before or during surgery, because they only show sensory fibers that may be in continuity. Of course, the opportunity to derive motor nerve action

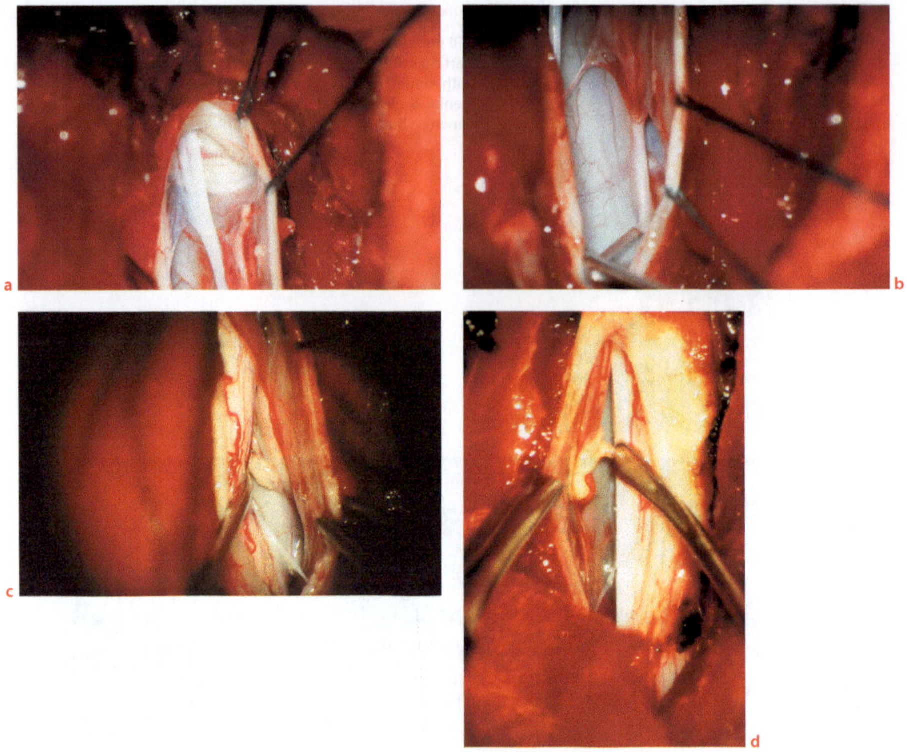

Figure 6.5 a–d

Intradural rootlet inspection. a Both rootlets preserved, denticulate ligament in between; b empty foramen, one level deeper; c intraforaminal disruption of the motor rootlet; d both rootlets avulsed

potentials (NAP) would intraoperatively offer a guarantee of sprouting motor fibers within the just-tested pathway.

Summarizing these factors, the diagnosis consists of the neurological investigation, an attempt to elicit the Tinel sign into a special dermatome, which answers the question on possible spontaneous recovery of sensory fibers, and finally an assessment of the intraspinal situation of the C5–C8 ventral and dorsal rootlets. A history of Horner's syndrome must be investigated, indicating a primary C8 avulsion. This sign often disappears before the lesion appears. Thus acquiring a view of the extent of the lesion, perhaps with a scheme of the principal plexus anatomy (▶ Fig. 6.6) and the number of available roots, the surgeon must decide to operate as early as possible.

The timing of the operation is extremely difficult to assess. Because of the initial ongoing scar tissue formation, we do not operate earlier than 2 months following the trauma. With the long distances that the sprouting axons need to overcome, the indication remains uncertain for a long time. On the other hand, the operative results substantially worsen if the time interval increases, as pointed out by Samii et al. (1997). In case of a complete root avulsion, there is no doubt about an immediate indication. But if roots present as preserved during the diagnostic assessment, the indication might remain questionable. If in doubt, we would advocate operating early rather than remaining reserved too long, so as not to waste recovery forces, at least 3–4 months after the injury. When operating at that time, reconstruction of the median

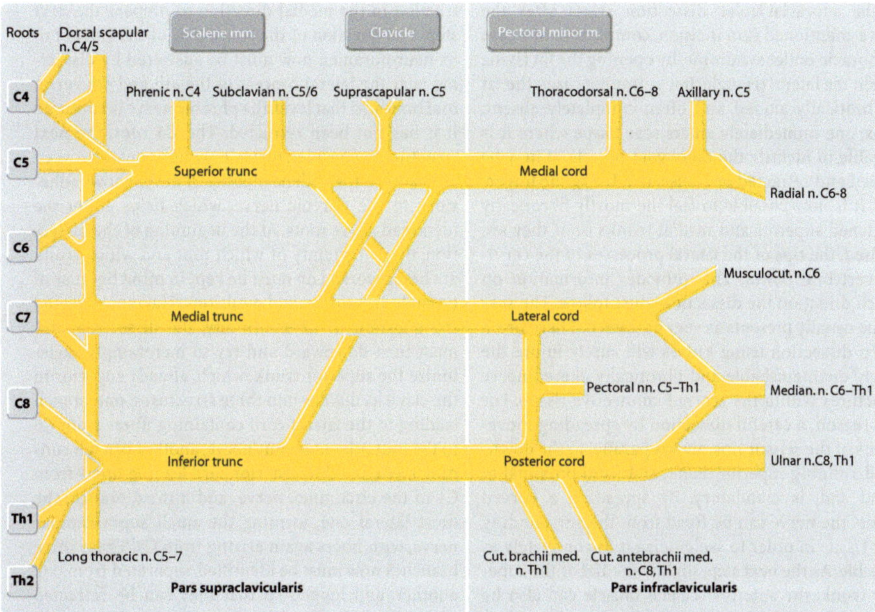

Figure 6.6

Scheme to demonstrate the principle of the brachial plexus anatomy at trunk and cord levels. (We owe the idea for this scheme to Dr. Schwandt, Neurological Department, Altona Hospital Hamburg, Germany)

nerve function can be targeted in order to achieve some wrist and finger flexion. This result would provide the opportunity for additional hand surgery efforts attempting to reconstruct a primitive grip function.

Without operation, more than 70 % of our brachial plexus patients would suffer from irreversible paralysis of the arm. If exclusively aiming at a stabilization of the shoulder and recovery of biceps function, our studies surprisingly revealed that late nerve reconstructions stand a good chance of reanimating the upper parts of the formerly paralyzed arm; therefore, we would advocate satisfying these patients if they ask for surgery even more than 6 months after the lesion (Penkert et al. 1999).

No case resembles another. Since different cases cannot be compared with one another, we can only assess principles: Different types of skin incisions were described, for instance, by Millesi in 1992. We use a combination of a transverse incision comparable to that used in the exploration of thoracic outlet syndromes, extended a few centimeters, for an incision parallel to the clavicle. This incision can be extended with no harm parallel to the lateral border of the sternocleidal muscle cranial, so that a triangulated skin flap can be turned aside. We then use a second incision leading downward from the clavicle to the axilla, comparable to an extended incision that we would choose to treat the hyperabduction syndrome. The skin over the clavicle is preserved, but the subclavian muscle below the clavicle must frequently be transected Thus, the clavicle is skeletonized with the exception of the skin bridge above it, and it is never transected. The continuity of the pectoral minor and major muscles and tendons is preserved. If necessary, clavicle and muscles must individually be looped and retracted in one or the other direction. The supraclavicular approach offers the exploration of the C5–C7 roots with their superior and medial trunks, whereas the infraclavicular exploration proximal to the pectoral minor muscle offers the approach to all cords and the inferior trunk with roots C8 and T1.

The supraclavicular dissection starts after the above-mentioned skin incision, comparable to a case of thoracic outlet syndrome, by opening the fat tissue within the lateral triangle. But in trauma cases, the fat is fibrotically altered and often completely absent. Thus, one immediately enters scar tissue where it is possible to identify the omohyoid muscle. It may be looped and retracted or transected. Using the fingertips, it is now possible to feel the mostly fibrotically hardened superior and medial trunks or, if they are avulsed, the tips of the lateral processes of the cervical vertebral bones. This provides information on which direction the dissection must follow. The scar tissue usually presents as very hardened. Therefore, a sharp dissection using knives will surely injure the barely distinguishable and fibrotically altered nerve structures within the scarred connective tissue. For this reason, a careful dissection by spreading movements of the scissor tips, always parallel to the downward-running superior trunk, and from proximal to distal end, is mandatory. By spreading a curved clamp, the nerve can be freed from the surrounding scar tissue in order to skeletonize it as completely as possible. As the next step, slightly medial of the superior trunk, the anterior scalene muscle can also be identified, which is also fibrotically altered. By carefully opening its scarred fascia, the more vertical downward-running phrenic nerve should be identified. If the C4 root was not avulsed, electrical stimulation of the nerve always helps identify it. This nerve serves as the borderline of the dissection. Running medial to the phrenic nerve is not advised because one could enter the internal jugular vein, which is also embedded within scar tissue. In our opinion, it is of great importance to preserve the phrenic nerve because its laceration would produce a significant reduction in lung volume, which would worsen later in life. One must be aware that the diaphragm presents no collateral innervation via the phrenic nerve of the contralateral side. The high position of one half of the paralyzed diaphragm remains irreversible for life. Consequently, we never use the phrenic nerve for a neurotization procedure (see Sect. 6.2).

After dissection and identification of the superior trunk, a further dissection in the proximal direction leads to the division into C5 and C6 roots if available and not avulsed. The phrenic nerve crosses over the C5 root at a very high level and at this spot, difficult adhesions can endanger the small nerve. On the one hand, this cross-point helps to anatomically identify the fifth root and phrenic nerve; on the other hand, separating the structures from each other seems necessary because the phrenic nerve requires careful retraction in the medial direction to prepare the next step. The question of the continuity of the C5 root to its neuroforamen now must be answered by dissecting near the lateral process of the 4th and 5th vertebral bones. At that level, the phrenic nerve is ruptured if it has not been retracted. The C6 root, the next structure to consider, turns more horizontal between the fibers of the scalene muscles. It never shows adhesions to the phrenic nerve, which helps count the identified nerve roots. At the beginning of the dissection, the uncertainty of which root and which trunk are being worked on must be kept in mind because of possible intraforaminal avulsions. Having answered the question of C6 continuity, the dissection now must turn downward and try to increasingly skeletonize the superior trunk, which, already superior to the clavicle, divides into three structures: one branch leading to the lateral cord containing fibers from C6 to the musculocutaneous nerve, another branch running medial to the posterior cord leading fibers from C5 to the circumflex nerve, and a third branch, the most lateral one, forming the small suprascapular nerve, with fibers again arising from C5. These three branches now must be identified, separated from one another, and looped so that they can be retracted slightly lateral.

The next step involves turning medial and identifying the C7 root and the medial trunk. In patients with a short neck, the cranial-convex curve of the subclavian artery may cover the 7th root. This is dissecting within scar tissue. Sharp dissection will surely harm the artery and cause a disaster. Spreading preparation using scissor tips parallel to the course of the clavicle helps find the subclavian artery. Very often, the arterial pulse can be felt by the fingertips, facilitating the preservation of the artery. The necessity of this preventive measure cannot be repeated often enough at this operating step. After that, the artery should be retracted downward under the clavicle, making it possible to now find the 7th root normally 1 cm caudal to the 6th root. Root and cord do not have proximal branches but, below the clavicle, the cord has a division into two main branches: one of them leads to the lateral cord-containing fibers running into the median nerve, and the second branch leads to the posterior cord-containing fibers running into the radial nerve. These distal branches must be identified and preserved if they have not been injured in the trauma.

Contrary to thoracic outlet syndromes, which show no fibrosis of the surrounding connective tissue, a dissection at this step to identify the inferior trunk with its C8 and T1 roots should not be tried from this approach, because, within the hardened scar tissue, these nerve structures can very easily be destroyed.

In order to solve this problematic situation, Kline and Hudson (1995) described an additional dorsal approach medial to the border of the scapula, which requires a transsection of fibers of the rhomboid, levator scapulae, and trapezoid muscles as well as the resection of a first rib segment. We think that the identification of the inferior trunk with both its roots always safely succeeds via the infraclavicular approach, which is anyhow necessary to answer questions on the continuity of all the secondary brachial plexus structures.

After the skin incision leading vertical to the clavicle to the axillary crease, as a first step, the cephalic vein must be identified over a long distance, particularly proximally within the scar tissue near the clavicle. The preservation of this vein provides some certainty of having collateral venous drainage in the event that the subclavian vein is injured, which cannot completely be avoided during infraclavicular exposure because this structure is the softest involved. The position of the cephalic vein leads into the area between the deltoid and the pectoral major muscle. Sometimes it is difficult to separate these muscle bellies because of scar tissue, especially if emergency surgeons had to reconstruct a ruptured subclavian or axillary artery. These preoperated cases present the greatest problems for entering the infraclavicular groove. If no former surgery has been done the space between the pectoral and deltoid muscles can be easily entered, and the muscles must be separated from each other completely. Next comes identification of the pectoral minor muscle fibers running transverse. These muscle fibers do not need to be transected, but instead, the muscle belly should be isolated and looped so that its retraction proximal or distal is permanently possible. One must be aware that great parts of the fat tissue within the infraclavicular groove are fibrotically altered or even completely lost. Under the pectoral minor muscle, a sharp dissection using a knife should therefore be completely avoided for the same reasons mentioned above. Spreading dissections parallel to the expected infraclavicular nerve and vessel structures and vertical to the clavicle will lead to the plexus structures, which often can be felt using the fingertips moved transverse to the nerves.

The most superficially located structure is the lateral cord. Its branches arise from the superior and medial trunks. First, the lateral cord proximal to the pectoral minor muscle must be identified; then the pectoral minor can be retracted rostrally and follow the lateral cord into the axilla where it divides into two branches: one leads laterally and forms the musculocutaneous nerve, the other leads medially and joins a branch from the medial cord forming the so-called median fork. Once the musculocutaneous nerve is reached, this is the most important target structure to be repaired.

Further and more difficult steps of the dissection will be the identification of the more deeply located structures. The posterior cord is the most laterally situated structure, and it is also located very deep. Nevertheless, as the next step, it has to be separated, skeletonized, and looped. The posterior cord receives branches from all three trunks, which, if they have not been destroyed following the trauma, are difficult to preserve, but they must still be identified, requiring a stepwise transsection of the subclavian muscle below the clavicle to gain the necessary overview. The transsection of the muscle fibers should be done piece by piece because the muscle belly contains an artery and vein whose injury can cause bleeding that is difficult to control. The transected parts of the muscle bellies can be pushed to both sides so that the clavicle is completely skeletonized and merely covered by the preserved skin bridge over it. Now all questions on preserved or destroyed nerve continuity within the most difficult area can be answered, one area under the clavicle, where true plexiform structures, macroscopically visible, are present.

When the posterior cord is followed distally, the axillary (circumflex) nerve is found, frequently arising from the cord, astonishingly at a rather proximal level (see Sect. 6.4). It turns lateral and deep. Distal to this important branch, the continuation of the cord forms the radial nerve leading to the axilla and upper arm region. This posterior cord, axillary and radial nerves should be regarded as the most laterally situated nerve structures in the infraclavicular region.

The next step should be the identification of the subclavian and axillary artery, which is to be felt with the fingertips. The artery must be skeletonized over a long distance. At distal levels, meaning distal to the pectoral minor muscle belly, it runs through the median fork. Identifying this region including the fork helps identify the median nerve as well as the musculocutaneous nerve.

The medial cord is situated under the subclavian artery and its identification requires a skeletonized and retractable artery. If trying to dissect the medial cord within scar tissue by spreading movements of an instrument, of course parallel to the expected nerve structure, one must now be aware of the above-mentioned subclavian vein, the most endangered structure. The vein shows close adhesions to the bony thorax. Contrary to the artery, it should not be skeletonized because it is surrounded by scar tissue and ruptures easily. Its location must be kept in view at all times when dissecting around the medial cord.

Identification of the inferior trunk with the C8 and T1 roots has remained unsolved until now. Following the medial cord proximal and using the infraclavicular and supraclavicular spaces together will lead to the inferior trunk, the deepest and most dangerous point of the surgeon's time-consuming efforts. The medial cord arises from the C8 and T1 roots. They join about 1–2 cm lateral to the spine and form in the inferior trunk. The medial cord receives an additional important branch from the medial trunk. Answering questions on the continuity of these nerve structures is one of the most difficult parts of neurolysis.

Far distal, the medial cord divides into one branch leading lateral, forming one part of the median fork, a second branch leading more medial, forming the ulnar nerve as well as one small additional branch forming the medial cutaneous antebrachial nerve, which often serves as an additional and easily available nerve graft. The median fork forms after the union of both of its branches in the median nerve trunk of the upper arm. The exploration has approached and ended at the pectoral major muscle tendon. But not rarely, the area of healthy nerve tissue has not been reached at this point, indicating a situation where injury proves far more extensive than expected. Particularly in cases of associated shoulder joint distortions or proximal humerus fractures, the nerve injury and tissue fibrosis also involve the upper third of the arm, sometimes also associated with a completely changed anatomy following vessel reconstruction.

The skin incision has to be extended over a long S-shaped distance to overcome the axillary crease and achieve the medial aspect of the upper arm. This makes it possible to enter the medial compartment containing the median nerve, brachial radial artery and vein, ulnar nerve, and more dorsally located, the radial nerve (for details of the approach, see Sect. 6.6). One must be particularly aware of the artery, which has to be skeletonized over the entire distance to have it safely under control, and of the vein, which cannot be isolated completely without rupturing it. Extremely difficult to manage in this operating step are cases of reoperations after primary vessel repair, not only caused by surgery but also by extensive scar tissue formations involving connective and muscle tissue itself. Vessel ruptures must be repaired at once using 6–0 or 5–0 stitches with a guarantee of sufficient preserved vessel diameter. The median nerve is the most superficially located structure seen when opening the vessel–nerve compartment. In the next step, both vessels must be identified and observed during all of the following steps: identifying and answering questions on fibrosis, continuity or discontinuity of the ulnar and radial nerve, the latter with its branches to the triceps muscle (see Sect. 6.6).

The pectoral major muscle and its tendon need no transsection; rerupture is a danger when they are reconstructed or reinserted. It is rather easy to isolate and mobilize parts of the peripheral muscle, including its tendon, and form a tunnel that joins the infraclavicular approach and that of the upper arm. All the nerves within this tunnel segment remain isolated structures and have no cross-connections; consequently, their dissection presents relatively few difficulties. Only the above-mentioned vessels require the greatest attention. With their previously identified location at the upper arm region in view, preserving and dissecting them over the complete distance from infraclavicular to the arm region can be successful. Vessel branches, of course, should be seen before rupture, tied and transected, to achieve an anatomically clear situation so that decisions on eventual nerve reconstruction can be made.

The dissection of all these structures sounds relatively easy and logical, keeping ▶ Fig. 6.6 and perhaps ▶ Fig. 6.7 in mind, but great patience is required. Our preliminary remarks on the importance of reliable preoperative assessments of the intraspinal root situation now seem reasonable, particularly because clearly defined extraspinal findings such as in ▶ Figs. 6.8–6.10 are far rarer than expected: structures that were proved as intra- or sometimes extraspinally avulsed do not require preservation or attention during dissection. Knowledge of structures to be preserved at all cost and structures that can be sacrificed facilitates and shortens the time-consuming neurolysis, an important factor, because a decision must be reached as to which structures need repair by grafting. Following this the grafts must be excised, a procedure requiring time and careful handling because each dissipation of grafts leads to a lack of grafts.

Now, the microsurgical part of the operation begins. Because plexus injury cases can never be compared, an assessment of decision-making rules depending on the intraoperative findings seems impossible. Instead, we limit ourselves to the vast field of nerve repair in plexus surgery discussed below. The

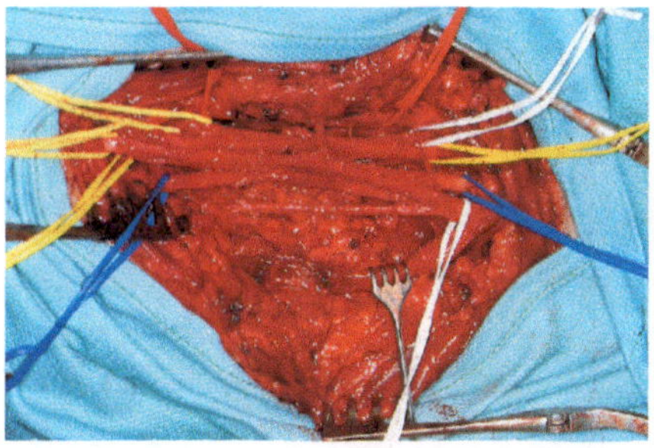

a

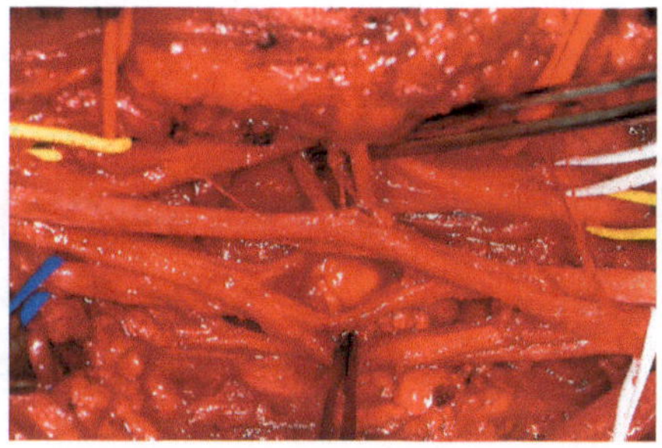

b

Figure 6.7 a, b

Brachial plexus anatomy, clavicula removed

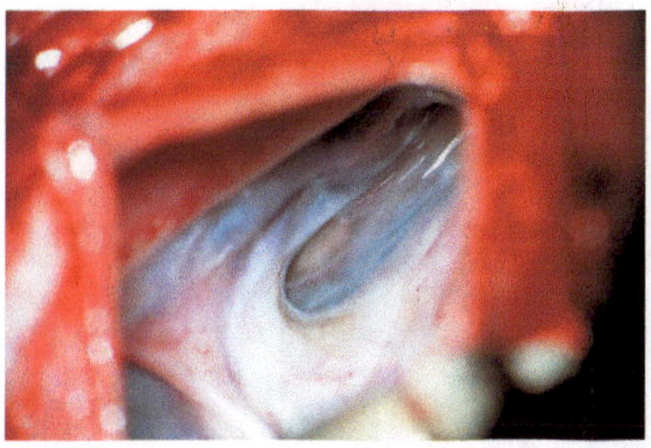

Figure 6.8

Extraspinal exploration: pseudomeningocele opened, empty neuroforamen

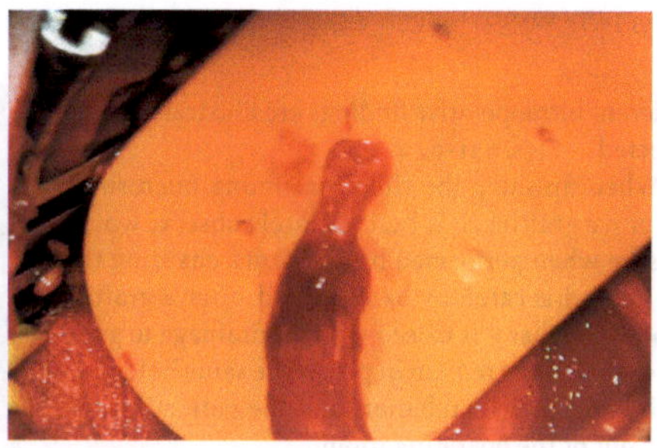

Figure 6.9

Extraspinal exploration: avulsed rootlets (C7) during extraspinal approach

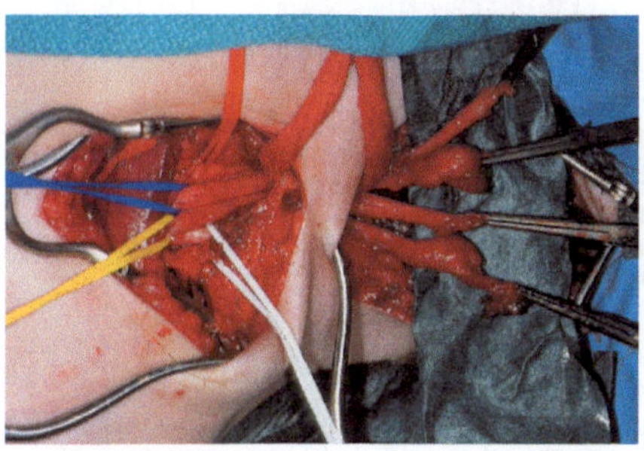

a

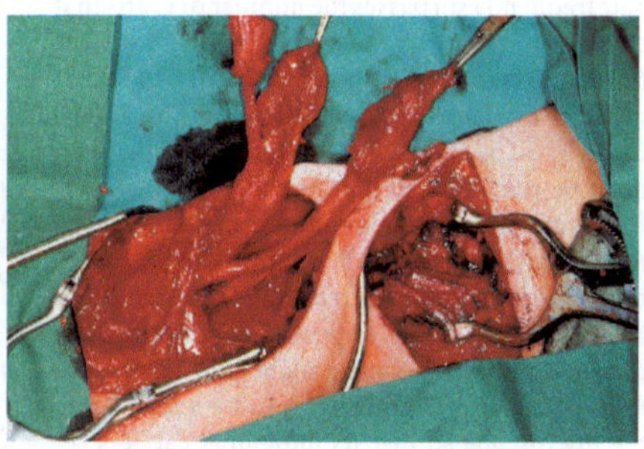

b

Figure 6.10 a, b

Two cases of two-portal brachial plexus exploration. a Complete trunk avulsion; b trunk avulsions, one root stump proximal

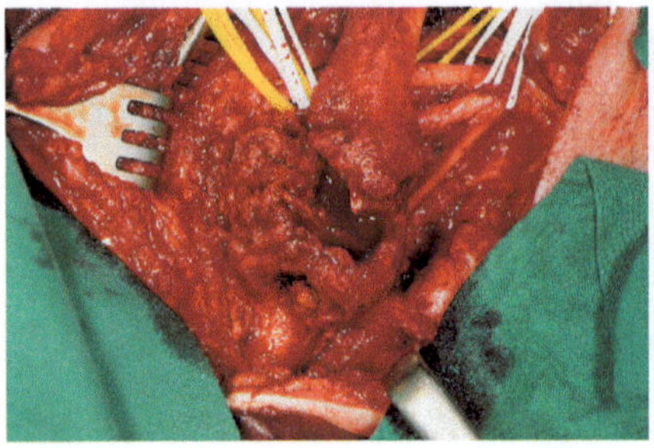

Figure 6.11

Preserved plexus anatomy including the suprascapular nerve underneath a pseudarthrosis of the clavicula (proximal on the right)

different intraoperative findings are illustrated by the selected ▶ Figs. 6.11–6.14.

When finishing the time-consuming microsurgical nerve grafting, it is best to closely observe wound closure when performed by assistants, ensuring that the wound is carefully handled and, after a grafting procedure, that it is closed without drainage to guarantee that grafts remain in place. The same holds true with bandaging, extubation, and the patient's transport out of the operating room.

A number of principles of plexus repair should be remembered:

- Because of the very long peripheral plexus nerve lesions, the number of grafts needed for nerve repair frequently surpasses the number of grafts that can be removed. If the preoperative diagnosis has revealed a certain avulsion of C8 and T1, the ulnar nerve is available as an additional graft (Millesi 1992). It can be removed over a long distance, but it must be remembered that its caliber, if used as a free graft, does not allow sufficient spontaneous revascularization out of the recipient bed. If the ulnar nerve is chosen as a free graft, the epineurium has to be longitudinally opened over the complete distance of the nerve, and a slight additional separation into fascicle groups has to be added using the microscope so that its individual calibers resemble that of the sural nerve caliber.
- Because of the relative lack of grafts, a frequent lack of donor nerves, as well as the rather long distance that has to be bridged by these grafts, priorities must be established as to the targeted nerves. In adults, the first priority is the restoration of the

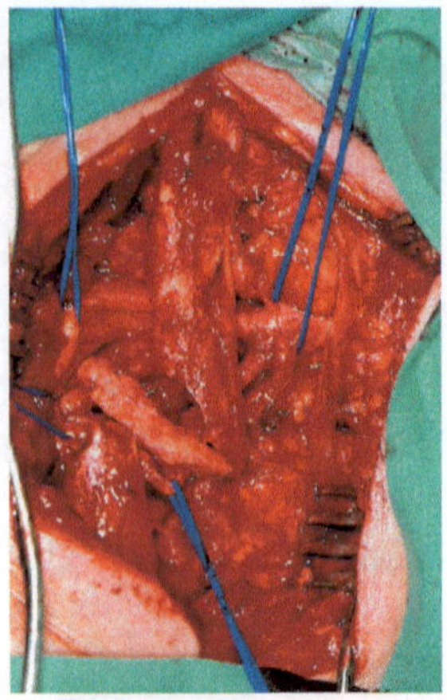

a

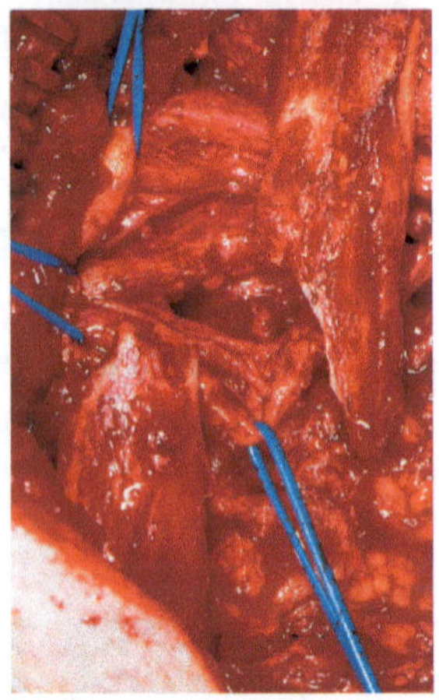

b

Figure 6.12a,b

Brachial plexus lesion due to clavicula fracture. a Fragment still in place; b fragment removed, laceration of cross-connections between superior and medial trunk to the posterior cord (proximal on the right)

Figure 6.13a–h

Brachial plexus repair. a Two-portal approach; b neuromas of all three trunks at the supraclavicular area; c nerve stumps after neuroma resection; d monofascicular structure at root level, greater magnification; e cord stumps at the infraclavicular area; f supraclavicular positioning of grafts; g infraclavicular positioning of grafts; h overview at the end

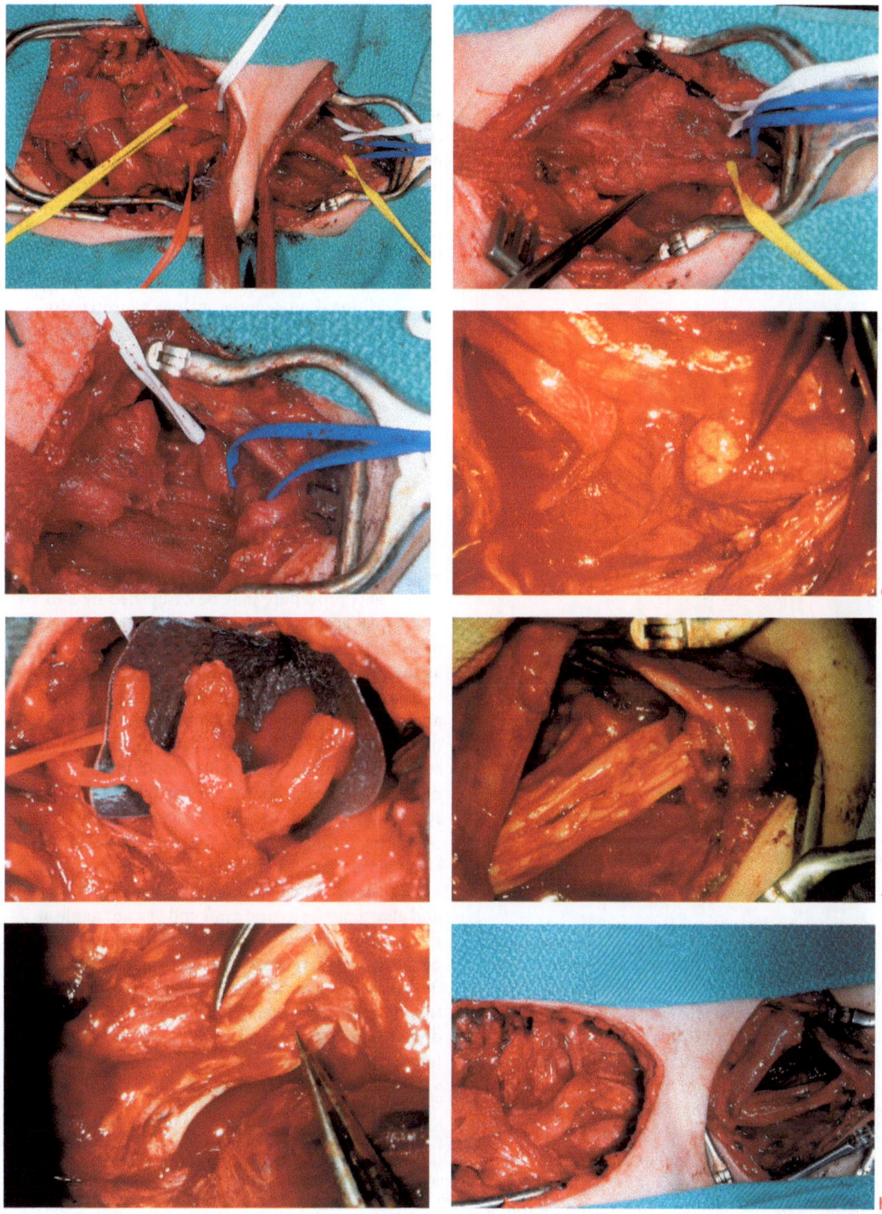

a
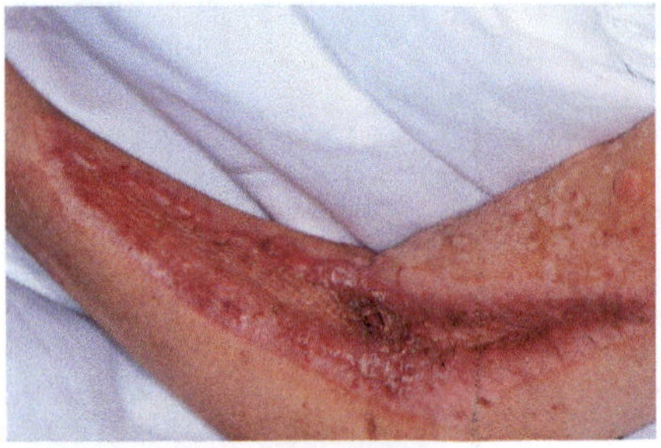

b
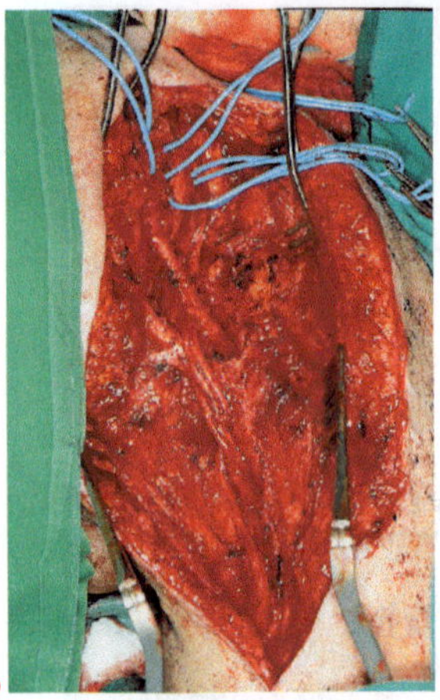

Figure 6.14 a, b

Unrepairable brachial plexus lesion. a Situation after additional extremity traumatization; b nerves and vessels torqued at the upper arm level (same case as a)

biceps function, then the shoulder abduction and external rotation via the suprascapular nerve, functions that remain rather insufficient if the scapula cannot be kept in place (long thoracic and dorsal scapular nerves), then the deltoid and the triceps muscles. The triceps can later be used as a synergist of the biceps by transposing its attachment at the biceps tendon. The median nerve may serve as a target only in cases operated on very early, and of course, if enough donor roots and their respective nerves are available.

- Depending on the number of donor nerve roots, the target structures are assigned a relative importance to achieve as many nerve adaptations as possible. On the other hand, the donor nerve root stump and the target nerve stump should be chosen at levels where scar tissue is completely absent (▶ Fig. 6.13). This frequently results in very long nerve gaps that must be bridged by grafts. One should interpose long nerve grafts because, according to our studies, the length of free nerve grafts and the number of nerve grafts chosen to bridge a particular pathway do not significantly influence the result (Penkert et al. 1988; Samii et al. 1997).
- If only a single nerve root is available as a donor nerve, or if all motor rootlets are lost due to avulsion, additional procedures such as neurotization (nerve transfer) should be primarily considered. The first priority is using the distal part of the spinal accessory nerve and/or intercostal nerves. The spinal accessory nerve is either directly connected to the suprascapular nerve or via the sural graft to the musculocutaneous nerve. Intercostal nerves serve better as sensory fiber donors and should be connected to the median nerve. If function of the so-called lower plexus is preserved, branches to the pectoral major muscle may be sacrificed and directly connected to the musculocutaneous nerve. This procedure may be completed by a direct spinal accessory to suprascapular nerve connection. The phrenic nerve, if transected and used as the donor nerve in a neurotization procedure, will probably cause later pulmonary restrictions and remains controversial in our opinion. The innervation of both halves of the diaphragm is strictly separated. We therefore avoid the phrenic nerve as the axon donor. On the other hand, in 1994, Viterbo et al. described experimentally encouraging results by testing the method of end-to-side neurorrhaphy. Using the phrenic nerve as donor, this procedure fenestrates its epineural sheath and anastomoses a sural graft end at a 90° angle at this window. Just recently, Millesi (2002) reported on attempts to reinnervate the long thoracic or dorsal scapular nerve distributions using an end-to-side graft connected to the phrenic nerve, also done to the conventional spinal accessory and intercostal nerve transfers.

Figure 6.15 a–h ▶

Neurotization procedure. a Accessory nerve as donor with its two branches; b, c one branch is transected; d connection of sural graft with the accessory branch; e a second graft connected with cervical plexus nerve; f connection of grafts with musculocutaneous nerve, infraclavicular area; g, h result 15 months later, no significant trapezoid palsy

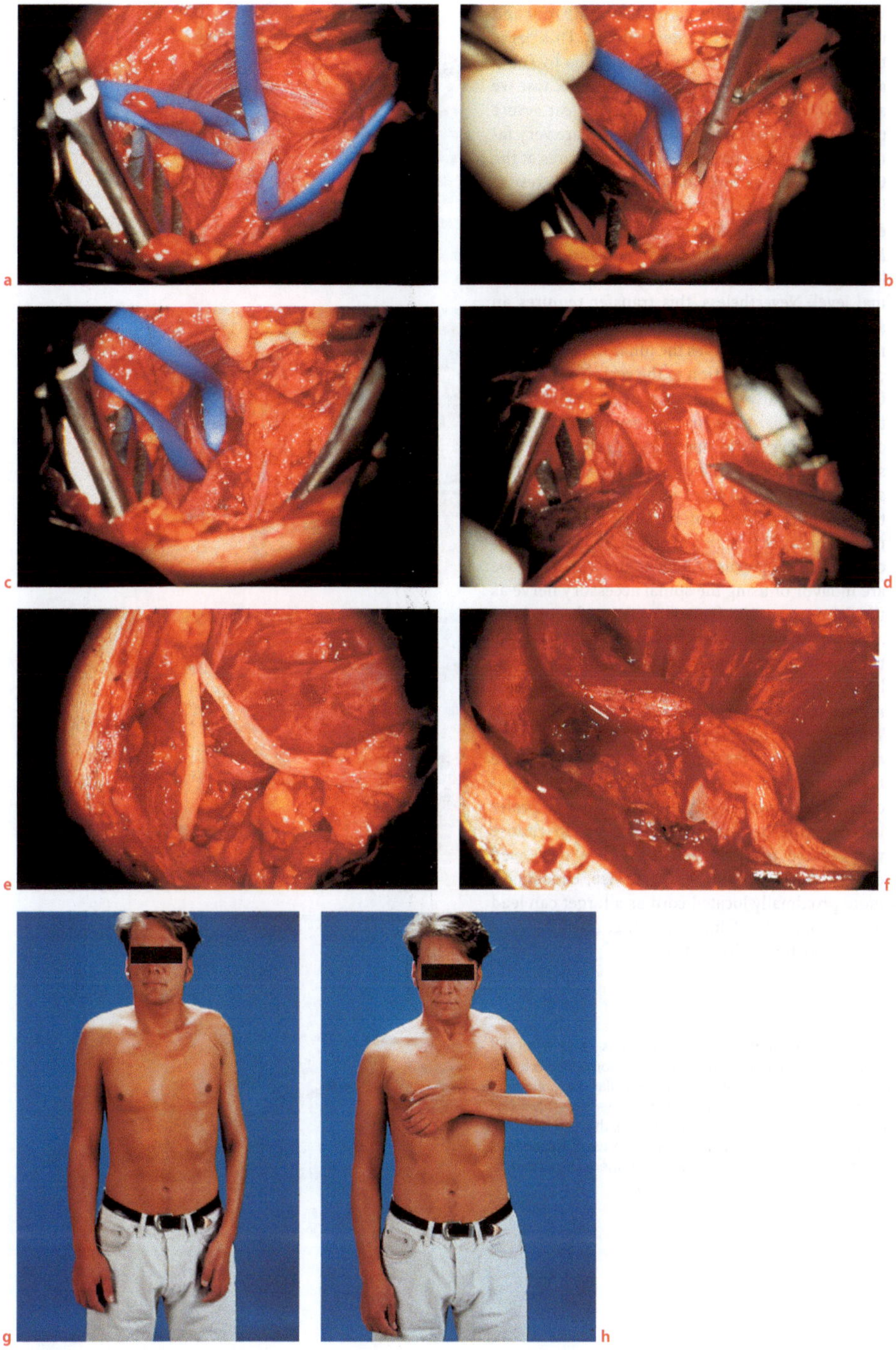
a
b
c
d
e
f
g
h

- We have not utilized the contralateral C7 root and its posterior division as a nerve donor. This nerve transfer was recently described in China by Gu et al. (1992). We do not favor this method because we agree with Birch and co-workers, who fear severe postoperative pain. We neurosurgeons are very familiar with severe pain due to disc ruptures at the C6–C7 level or, as Birch described in 1998, resulting from traumatic C7-root laceration. On the other hand, during recent personal communications, Millesi and Fansa reported that pain and palsy following C7-root sacrifice would remain at a minimal level. Nevertheless, this transfer requires an available long graft; some authors report that the most suitable graft serves the ulnar nerve with microvascular reconnection to the recipient bed.
- Our postoperative studies on neurotizations between the spinal accessory nerve and the musculocutaneous nerve via one nerve graft revealed a successful recovery rate of about 80 %. The transsection of the spinal accessory nerve far enough in the periphery does not paralyze the trapezoid muscle because it is also supplied by motor fibers of the cervical plexus (Allieu et al. 1982). Thus, we are in favor of using the spinal accessory nerve as the donor nerve if sufficient roots are absent. After accessory nerve transfer, the horizontal part of the trapezoid muscle in particular remains collaterally sufficiently supplied and can even later serve for muscle transfer (▶ Fig. 6.15a–f).
- The length of the grafts needed may only be taken as an indicator of the extent of the injury and of the fibrotic reaction within the plexus nerves. We occasionally encounter situations in which we prefer longer grafts because they enable us to choose well-defined target structures with a decreased danger of mis-sprouting. Otherwise, choosing a more proximally located cord as a target can lead to a higher rate of mis-sprouting, resulting in a greater postoperative deficit.

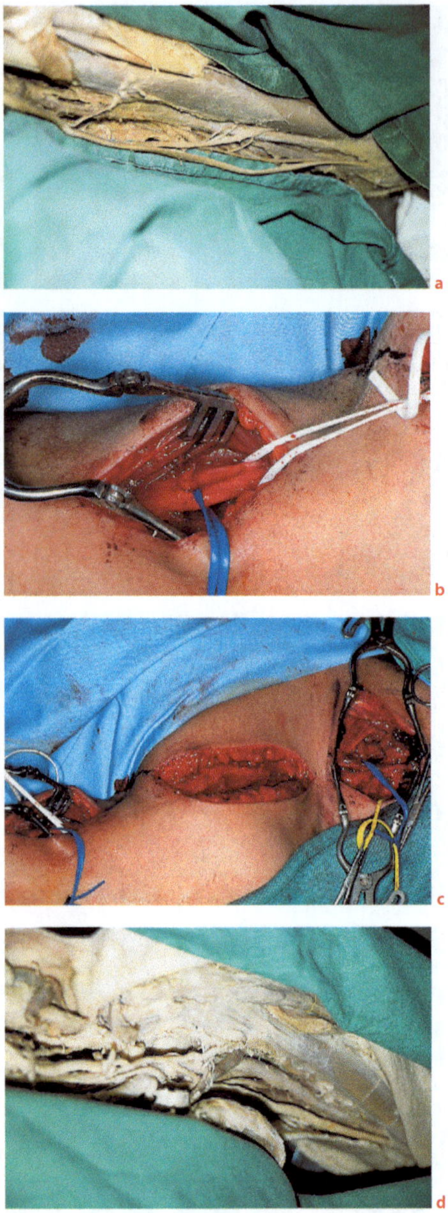

Figure 6.16 a–d

Anomalous origin of the musculocutaneous nerve from the median nerve at mid-upper arm level. a Anatomical specimen; b lateral cord at the peripheral infraclavicular area, ramification into median and musculocutaneous nerves visible, but both nerves remain together; c same case, the real ramification starts at the mid-upper arm level (musculocutaneous nerve at blue loop); d another anatomical specimen with normal origin of the musculocutaneous nerve

- The identification of the musculocutaneous nerve as the target of first priority may present problems: it is not rare that the ramification of the lateral cord into this nerve and the median nerve branch has been found absent. Instead, the musculocutaneous nerve then arose in the mid-upper-arm level from the median nerve, with a short transverse course into the biceps muscle (▶ Fig. 6.16). Of course, in such situations the grafts needed are quite long.

6.2.1 Addendum

Root reimplantation, as done several times by Carlstedt and colleagues, remains a challenge, as recently described in Birch et al. (1998). In humans, these operations lose any realistic chance of proper recovery if done later than 48 h after the trauma because after this time, the peripheral nerve structures irreversibly retract or become fixed within the neuroforamen. Opportunities to operate on these cases within the first 48 h seem to arise very rarely. Other technical considerations also stand out: the ventral root entry zone does not sufficiently come into view when accessed from the dorsal approach into the spinal canal. It becomes visible only if the cord is rotated, a dangerous procedure from a functional point of view. In our opinion, it must be pointed out that the sprouting forces of the far proximal motor axons are questionable if compared, for example, to that of the spinal accessory nerve. We know from experience with the facial nerve that sprouting forces decrease the nearer the proximal stump is situated to the facial nucleus. If this is as true for the anterior horn cell bodies and their root axons, it would be an argument against the reimplantation technique. Carlstedt himself points out that recovery seems to have a somewhat better chance if the rupture level of the root is situated peripheral to its transitional zone – meaning the zone where the matrix of the nerve changes from oligodendric or astrocytes to Schwann cell matrix. Thus, the procedure, according to Carstedt, should not consist of a reimplantation but instead of a readaptation to short anterior rootlet stumps. Further experiments, particularly cases of complete root avulsions and experiments on animals, are of course needed to advance this technique.

6.3 Long Thoracic, Suprascapular, Dorsal Scapular, Thoracodorsal Nerves

Isolated trauma-related lesions of the long thoracic, suprascapular, dorsal scapular, and thoracodorsal nerves are imaginable when resulting exclusively from penetrating injuries and therefore they rarely occur; questions about their repair remain of theoretical importance. However, their lesions are usual in association with brachial plexus stretch injuries. Paralysis of the supraspinatus, infraspinatus, serratus anterior, rhomboid, and latissimus dorsi muscles then indicates a brachial plexus lesion at a high level and therefore gains importance in clinical diagnosis of these complex lesions.

The suprascapular nerve takes high priority as a target in plexus nerve repair. Isolated lesions may quite rarely occur as a result of scapular fractures, which then involve not only the final ramification of its two main branches, but also the muscles themselves. Nerve reconstruction would theoretically succeed by combining a supraclavicular plexus approach with a posterior access, the latter comparable to that on the suprascapular nerve entrapment via an incision over the spina scapulae. But the supra- and infraspinatus muscle fibers are often fibrotically altered following such injuries, which is indicated by a loss of spontaneous muscle potentials in electromyography. Nerve reconstructions then would become questionable.

Lesions of the long thoracic nerve, which arises at root level from the brachial plexus, result in severe winging of the scapula. Very rarely, patients sustain sudden and spontaneous paralysis. An entrapment between portions of the scalene medial muscle, between the edge of the scapular bone and the chest, or sudden stretch injuries subsequent to heavy lifting is being debated as the origin. The nerve is deeply situated, and its course is covered by transverse fibers of the serratus, pectoral minor, and pectoral major muscles, so that a direct access without a mental picture of the lesion's location seems questionable in our opinion.

The dorsal scapular nerve takes a comparably deeply situated course. It arises at root level as well, runs more dorsal, and supplies the rhomboid muscles. We have not had a single patient requiring repair of the dorsal scapular nerve.

The same holds true with the thoracodorsal nerve. Its course is covered by the overlying scapular bone. Although this nerve is classically described as arising from the posterior cord of the brachial plexus, considerable variations are seen: it may arise from the axillary nerve or even from the radial nerve. A latissimus dorsi muscle palsy indicates a low-level brachial plexus lesion if, as is usual, it is associated with these injuries.

Comparably simple plastic or reconstructive surgical procedures must be considered in case one of the four nerves is completely injured. These procedures are more effective (see Chaps. 11 and 12).

6.4 Axillary (Circumflex) Nerve

The axillary nerve arises from the posterior plexus cord and occasionally branches as the thoracodorsal nerve. It supplies the deltoid muscle, which abducts the humerus between 15° and the horizontal. Further abduction is completed by rotating the scapula nearer to the spine by means of the trapezius, rhomboid and levator scapulae muscles. For deltoid muscle function to be effective, the suprascapular nerve, supraspinatus muscle, and rotator cuff must all be intact. In later axillary nerve repair, this is of great importance because the deltoid fibers will only be effective after the initial abduction done by the rotator cuff. From the opposite perspective, in case of associated suprascapular nerve lesion or rotator cuff rupture, axillary nerve repair would be worthless.

The axillary nerve consists of motor and sensory fibers of the 5th nerve root. After passing away from the posterior cord the nerve takes a short course running alongside the circumflex artery around the collum chirurgicum of the humerus into the posterior aspect of the shoulder. There, it appears within a triangle shaped by the posterior border of the deltoid muscle, the long head of the triceps muscle and the superior border of the teres major muscle. Several branches (some authors mention two main branches) disappear behind the deltoid muscle belly, where they also supply the teres minor muscle.

Patients suffer from a loss of effective abduction of the humerus and a small numb area over the cup of the shoulder, which often quite quickly disappears as this skin area has mixed innervation by cervical plexus fibers. Electromyography of all three portions of the deltoid muscle is mandatory as well as additional tests of the infraspinatus muscle, the latter ones for the above-mentioned reasons. The clinical investigation must preserve the intactness of the initial 15°–20° abduction to exclude the possible additional rotator cuff rupture before considering axillary nerve exploration.

Nonpenetrating and noniatrogenic injuries are the majority of the causes of axillary nerve palsies, in other words, typical trauma-related shoulder joint luxations. At exploration, neuromas in continuity near the posterior cord or complete disruptions are to be found following luxations.

The decision on eventual nerve repair is not easy in so far as spontaneous recovery of the nerve usually takes at least 9 months, or more in case of a degree II lesion or more according to Sunderland's classification. Unfortunately, most luxations cause such a lesion, making the period of spontaneous sprouting too long. Therefore, the decision must be made earlier and conclusively must be discussed thoroughly with the patient. Because of the deep location of the nerve, the Tinel sign unfortunately does not help at all.

The exploration is always composed of two combined approaches: one follows the typical infraclavicular access to the brachial plexus, the other accesses from posterior into the triangle between the deltoid, triceps, and teres major muscles (▶ Fig. 6.17). The patient must be turned about 30° on the healthy side and the arm must remain freely movable anterior or posterior to the body so that both approaches are available in one procedure. The operation starts with the infraclavicular approach, comparable to that in hyperabduction entrapment. All the brachial plexus structures must be dissected and identified stepwise, even and especially the subclavian artery and vein, in order to preserve both of them safely. During the entire exploration, it must be kept in mind that all nerve structures above the target nerve must remain preserved with absolutely no harm done to them. For this reason, we prefer not to loop the plexus nerves in these cases and to use only careful manual retraction. Identifying the axillary nerve requires primary identification of the posterior cord; the ramification between cord and nerve is usually found between the clavicle and the pectoral minor muscle, whereas the further nerve dissection needs to retract the pectoral minor muscle in the rostral direction. The nerve disappearing in the deepness of the axilla can be followed with the fingertips to ensure continuity or discontinuity, the latter eventually supported by evidence of a proximal neuroma (▶ Fig. 6.17 a, b). The posterior approach requires a vertical skin incision parallel to the posterior border of the deltoid muscle (▶ Fig. 6.18). The arm lies anterior rotated. Manuel retraction of the muscle bellies will aid in entering the posterior triangle. The nerve and the circumflex artery can be identified beside the collum chirurgicum, but with extended nerve branch avulsions, if the posterior nerve segments no longer exist, the identification of motor entry points may remain impossible in

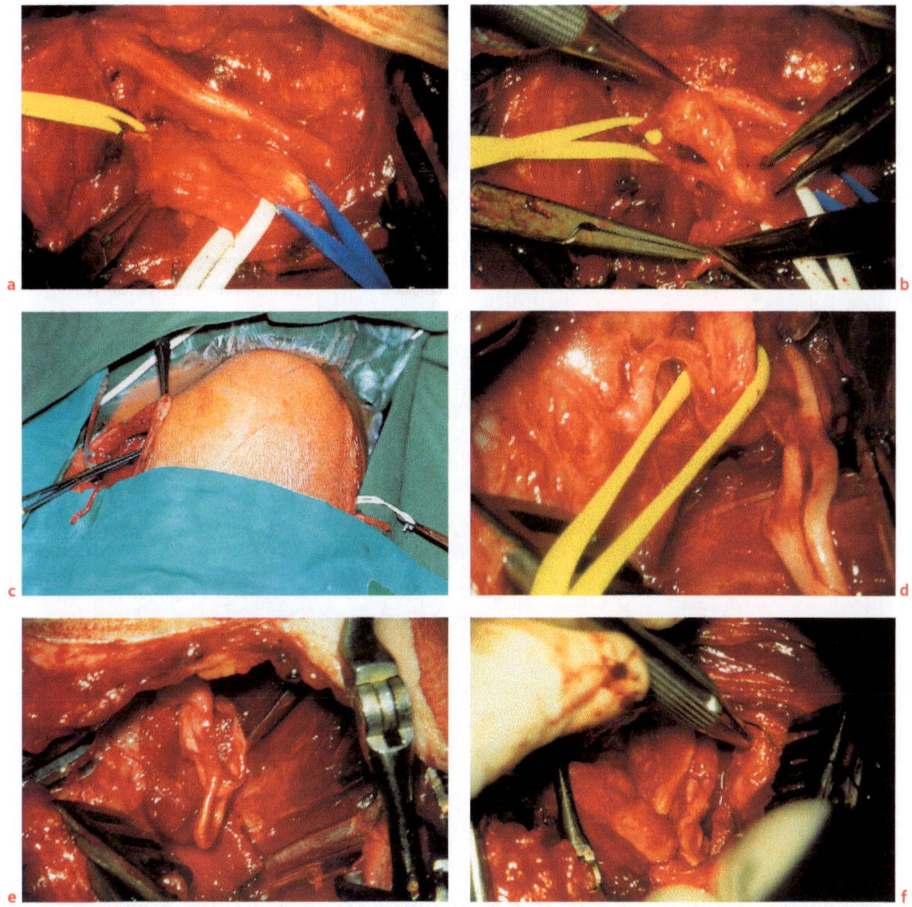

Figure 6.17 a–f

Axillary (circumflex) nerve repair, two-portal approach (left shoulder). **a, b** Infraclavicular approach, axillary nerve with neuroma (*white and yellow loops*), radial nerve side by side (*blue loop*); **c** positioning of sural graft from infraclavicular to dorsal; **d** peripheral axillary nerve branches and two grafts in position, view from dorsal; **e** dorsal anastomoses; **f** proximal anastomosis of grafts with the axillary nerve stump

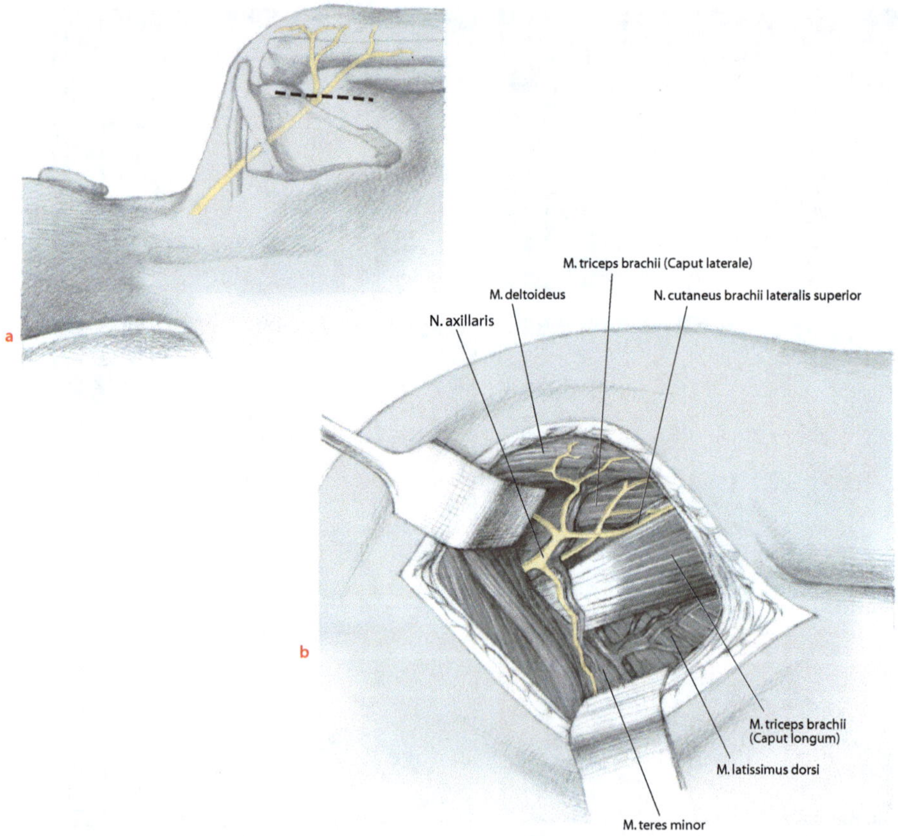

Figure 6.18 a, b

Approach to the axillary (circumflex) nerve from dorsal (right shoulder). a Skin incision; b exploration of nerve and its ramification between lower border of the deltoid muscle and both heads of the triceps; the teres major muscle body may be individually lifted up or held downward

certain cases. If a distal nerve segment is available, intraoperative nerve action potentials will help in deciding on nerve repair. If reconstruction becomes necessary, one sural nerve is usually sufficient to reconstruct the gap between the anterior and posterior stumps; two side-by-side grafts roughly 12 cm in length are pulled from infraclavicular to posterior (▶ Fig. 6.17c–f). Because of the reduced risks of missprouting (mainly motor fibers within the axillary nerve, no innervation of antagonists), chances for recovery are excellent following nerve repair.

6.5 Musculocutaneous Nerve

The musculocutaneous nerve mainly consists of fibers of the C6 root, which pass the superior trunk, change to the lateral cord, and leave the cord far distally in the lateral direction, whereas the median nerve shapes the continuation of the lateral cord into the periphery. Of great importance is that the musculocutaneous fibers occasionally do not separate from the lateral cord at this level, but instead arise from the median nerve at mid-upper arm level (▶ Fig. 6.16).

Clinical findings and the possibilities of nerve repair then differ radically from cases with normal anatomy. Isolated musculocutaneous nerve lesions occur very rarely, and if they do, either as result of a penetrating injury or associated with far proximal humerus fractures, they produce extended disruptions and additional difficulties if associated with brachial plexus lesions.

Eventual nerve repair requires a two-portal approach comparable to that of the axillary nerve: one aims at exploration of the lateral cord via an incision vertical to the clavicle to the axilla crease, a typical infraclavicular approach. Below the pectoral minor muscle, the lateral cord is the first structure to be found because it is situated the most superficially. Following the lateral cord, one passes the junction with fibers from the medial cord, the median fork. At this level, the lateral cord divides into the median nerve branch and the musculocutaneous nerve in the lateral direction. On entering the coracobrachial muscle, further dissection is often hindered by severe trauma-related fibrosis of all the soft tissue structures, including the pectoral major tendon. For this reason, we usually choose a second approach to identify the nerve below the lesion safely and then follow the nerve from distal to proximal. Via a longitudinal incision over the anterior aspect of the mid-upper arm, fibers of the biceps muscle can be separated and the nerve can be found within a layer between the biceps and brachial muscles. At this level, the ramification of the musculocutaneous has already started, which makes it necessary to dissect carefully enough to preserve all the small motor entry points. A neuroma in continuity or even discontinuity mainly involves the nerve segment that passes through the fibrotically altered coracobrachial muscle. Two relatively short sural nerve grafts must then be interposed between both the approaches for nerve repair, providing an excellent chance of recovery because the nerve contains mostly motor fibers.

If a mostly iatrogenic lesion exceptionally involves the ramification itself – frequently due to unusual ventral approaches on humerus dislocations – distal nerve connections may remain absent within the scar tissue. If the biceps muscle belly showed no sign of fibrotic alterations before operation, direct neurotization might succeed, as described by Millesi and Walzer (1981).

6.6 Radial Nerve

The components of the radial nerve consist of fibers of the spinal segments C6–T1. The nerve shapes the continuation of the posterior cord below the separation from the axillary nerve fibers. Occasionally, the thoracodorsal nerve arises at a distal level from the radial nerve. After its relatively deep course through the axilla, it traverses the spiral groove of the humerus, and then abruptly turns downward within the lateral aspect of the humerus, where it pierces the lateral intermuscular septum. At first it takes its course between the biceps and brachioradial muscles, then between the brachial and brachioradial muscles, where it divides into the superficial branch and the posterior interosseous nerve (deep branch). The latter branch passes the supinator channel supplying nearly all the extensor muscles of the forearm and, of course, the supinator muscle itself, whereas the superficial branch mostly contains sensory fibers. It is important to know that the superficial branch also leads some motor fibers supplying the short extensor carpi radial muscle (see Sect. 5.8). Trauma-related upper radial nerve lesions always result from humerus fractures causing dislocation or stretch forces at the bone fragments. Open and closed repositions and stabilizations create additional risks of crushing the nerve. The same risks are also present with the posterior interosseous nerve, which is then injured in radius fractures or radius stabilization. Upper arm lesions result in a complete hand drop, whereas lower arm lesions present preserved wrist extension associated with radial abduction via the short wrist extensor.

It is claimed that fracture-related palsies recover in 80% of cases, but a patient with radial nerve paralysis presents particular problems in case of upper arm lesions: the time it takes for spontaneous sprouting processes in case of preserved nerve continuity is too long. The most proximal muscle to be electromyographically tested is the brachioradial muscle, possibly indicating ongoing de-innervation or starting re-innervation. In contrast, the triceps function usually remains preserved because its supplying branches separate from the radial nerve at a very high level, far proximal to the spiral groove. Nevertheless, the decision on nerve exploration has to be made earlier than spontaneous recovery would have been expected. The decision in case of posterior interosseous lesions is easier for three reasons: spontaneous nerve sprouting requires less time; fractures and stabilizations at the radius mostly cause a severe lesion if the nerve is involved; opening the trauma-related narrowed supinator channel is mandatory and might be valued as an

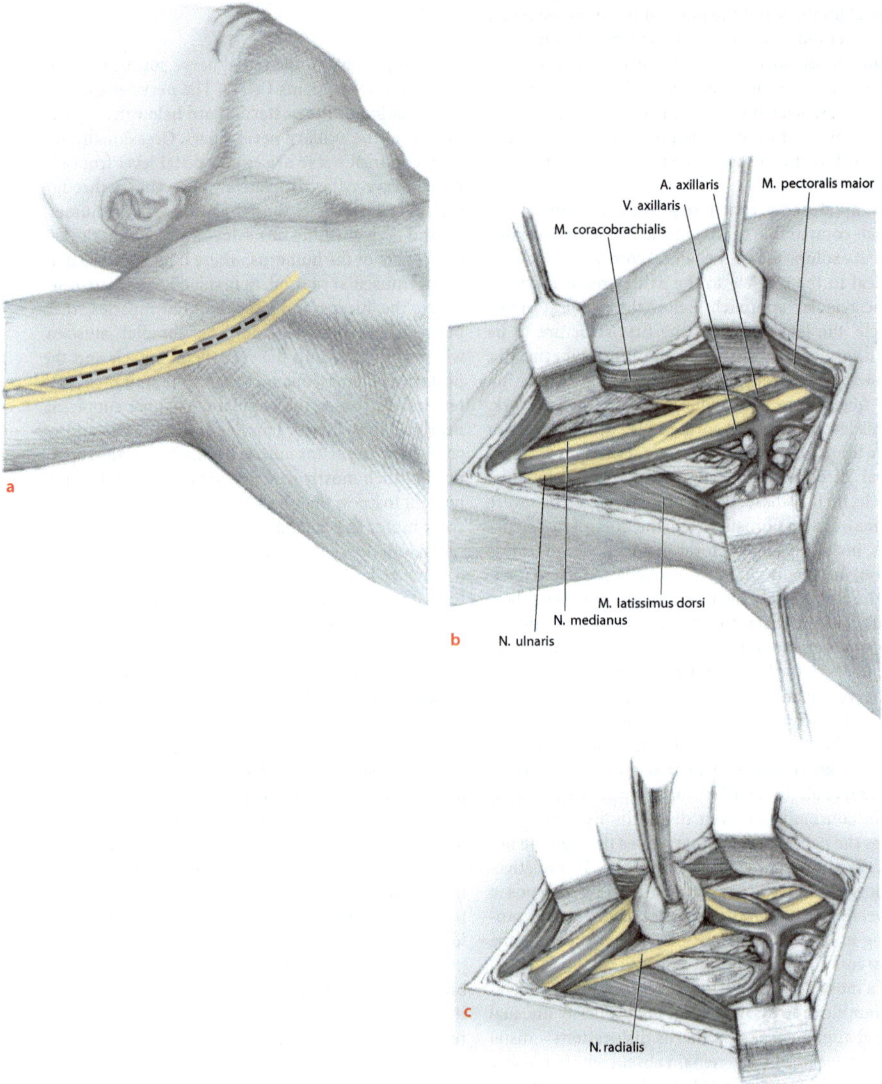

Figure 6.19 a–c

Principle of the radial nerve exploration distal to the axilla. a Skin incision; b nerve exploration after gently lifting up median nerve and brachial artery, then the brachial vein and ulnar nerve, motor branches to the triceps muscle have absolutely to be identified and preserved if preoperatively functional; c radial nerve and its triceps branch in detail

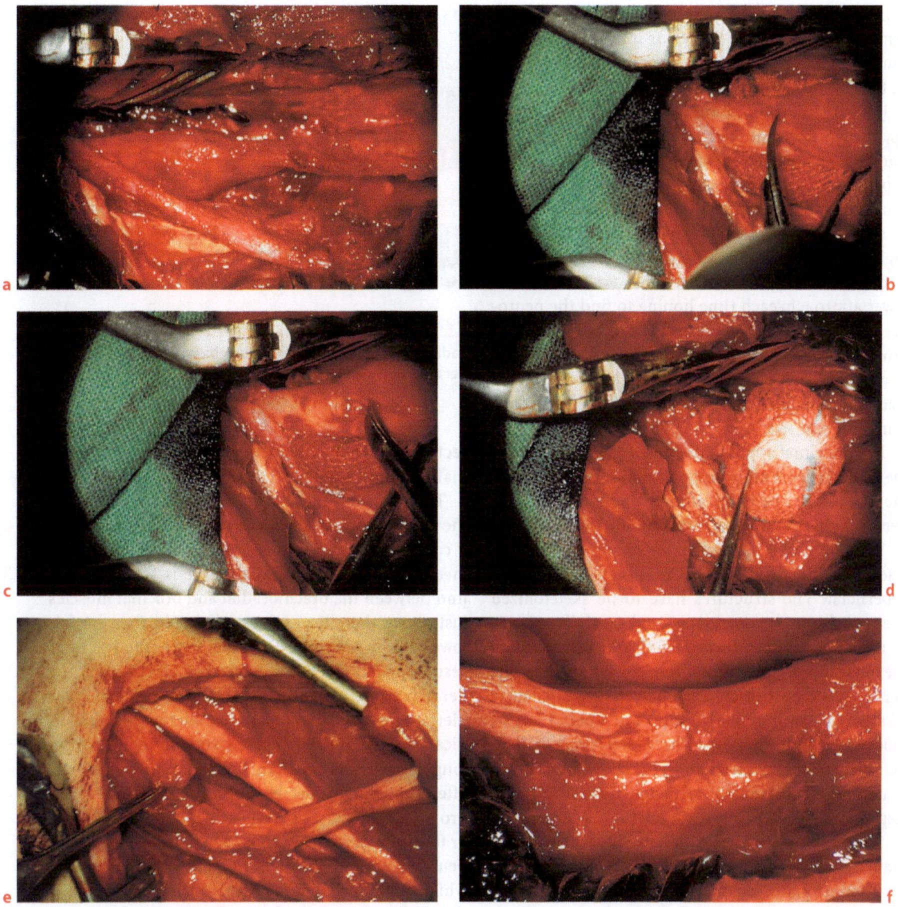

Figure 6.20 a–f

Radial nerve repair (upper left arm), two-portal approach. a Proximomedial approach (view at the arm's medial side), neuroma of the main nerve, branch to the triceps side by side preserved; b, c nerve transsection; d monofascicular nerve stump; e connection of grafts to the proximal stump, grafts ventrally positioned and crossing over the median nerve; f connection of grafts to the distal nerve stump via a second approach from lateral, a few centimeters above the elbow level (view at the arm's lateral side) emergency. The Tinel sign is helpful only at the upper arm level, whereas the posterior interosseous rarely contains sensory elements and consequently cannot be triggered.

If a surgical exploration of the radial nerve at the upper arm is considered we prefer the supine position and do not split or even transect the functionally preserved triceps muscle; a two-portal approach is usually sufficient to manage all intraoperative issues. In case of fractures involving the mid-humerus or higher structures, we start via the proximal approach; in case of fractures at lower levels, we start via the lower approach, each time hoping to find the neuroma and the two nerve stumps via one of the two approaches. However, in the majority of cases, the two-portal approach unfortunately cannot be avoided in fracture-associated cases because of the extended intraneural scar tissue covering long distances.

The proximal approach requires a skin incision at the medial aspect of the upper third of the upper arm; the fascia must be longitudinally incised to feel the nerves and the brachial artery with the fingertips (▶ Fig. 6.19 a–c). The median nerve and the brachial artery are identified first because they are the most superficial. The structures have to be skeletonized over roughly 10–12 cm, looped and carefully retracted upward so that by turning in the dorsal direction, the ulnar nerve and brachial vein come into view. The nerve should be dissected again over a long distance, whereas the vein easily ruptures and should not be touched if at all possible. The radial nerve is then found deep and dorsal when all the above-mentioned structures are manually retracted upward. At that step, intraoperative nerve stimulation is mandatory to identify and preserve the two or three nerve branches supplying the triceps muscle, which are always functionally intact and are still surrounded by an outer layer of epineural sheath of the radial trunk at that level. This epineurium should be incised longitudinally so that the triceps branches can be mobilized in the proximal direction and increasingly separated from the possibly nonfunctioning radial nerve trunk, which does not react on stimulation. The nerve trunk may be followed with the fingertips around the spiral groove making it possible to identify or exclude a proximal neuroma. If a neuroma is found, the radial nerve trunk must be transected so far proximal that the cross-section is reliably free of intraneural fibrosis to guarantee unhindered axon sprouting following repair. The cross-section shows a rather variable fascicular pattern at this proximal level, sometimes more or less monofascicular (▶ Fig. 6.20 a–d), but also a polyfascicular aspect. During nerve transection, the triceps branches must permanently remain in mind and in view.

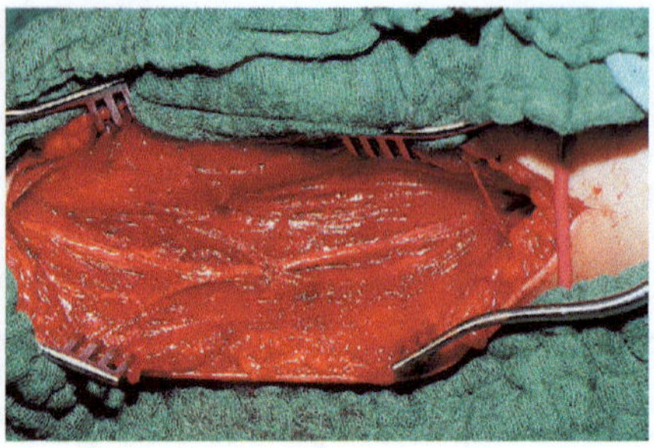

Figure 6.21

Radial nerve with branch to the brachioradial muscle (left upper arm, view from lateral side)

The distal approach requires a skin incision over the lateral aspect of the lower third of the upper arm; it can easily be extended using the elbow crease in a medial direction. The radial nerve is the easiest to find between the brachioradial and brachial muscles just above the elbow joint and should then be followed in the proximal direction, where the fracture-associated scar is quickly reached. Frequently, the nerve is strongly attached to the bone here and completely fibrotic. This typical situation rather surely indicates nerve grafting. Reconstruction requires very long nerve grafts, meaning both sural nerves, which, after tunneling, must be pulled side by side from proximal to distal; the grafts may be situated posterior to the humerus or anterior to it (▶ Fig. 6.20 e). Depending on the position of the main scar and plates, which will be secondarily removed, the opposite side should be chosen for the grafts. Grafts of approximately 30 cm in length should be imposed as often as necessary because of extended intraneural fibrosis (▶ Fig. 6.20 e, f); the outgrowing axon sprouts only require that Schwann cells be alive and nerve tissue revascularized in time. In 1978, Sunderland even suggested excluding the superior branch of the radial nerve as a target of repair in order to ensure ingrowth of axons into the motor pathways of the deep branch exclusively, a method he termed funicular exclusion. In case of preserved brachioradial muscle function, the relatively proximal arising branch to this muscle must be identified and preserved (▶ Fig. 6.21). On the other hand, if the damage to the radial nerve occurred proximal to this branch, it should serve as a target for one graft.

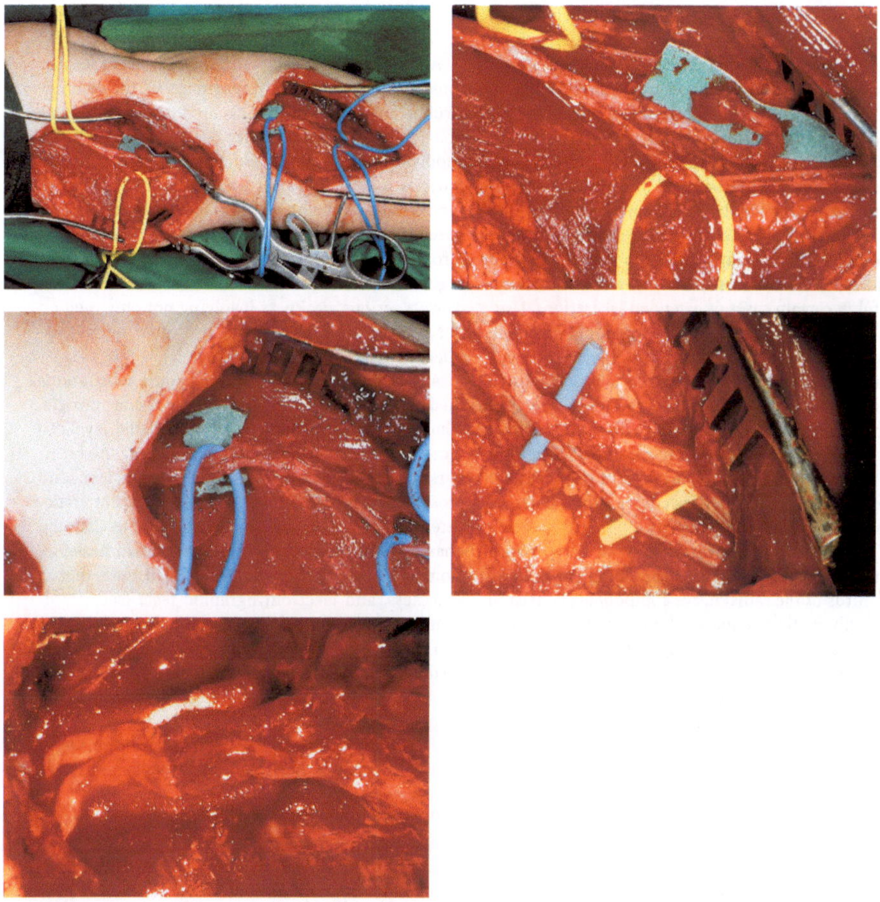

a b c d e

Figure 6.22 a–e

Radial nerve repair at right forearm level. a Two-portal approach; b proximal situation, neuroma of the deep branch, superficial branch and branch to the short wrist extensor (*yellow loops*) preserved; c ramification of the deep branch distal to the supinator muscle; d grafts positioned through the supinator channel, proximal anastomosis; e distal anastomosis

Lesions at the forearm level also require a two-portal approach (▶ Fig. 6.22 a–e), in which the two incisions and approaches on the supinator channel entrapment are used (see Chap. 5), thus preserving the supinator muscle and minimizing any intraoperative soft tissue harm. The lower approach between the extensor muscles of the forearm leads toward the interosseous membrane between the forearm bones where the posterior interosseous nerve divides into several small branches. All these branches must be dissected very carefully within the fracture-related scar tissue; their identification may remain unsuccessful in certain cases of extended lacerations. Usually, however, two sural nerve grafts should be pulled through the supinator channel and interposed, even if distal nerve stumps are only available as small branches. If not available, the graft ends are split slightly and placed between muscle fibers only (direct neurotization according to Millesi and Walzer 1981 and Millesi 1992). A later removal of a primarily inserted radius plate clearly becomes impossible because it endangers graft integrity.

The chances for recovery following nerve repair even over long distances are again excellent because two-thirds of the radial nerve components consist of motor fibers, thus reducing the amount of possible mis-sprouting (Mirzai et al. 1993). The postoperative use of splints prevents overstretching the extensor tendons and should therefore always be used until voluntary muscle contractions reappear.

6.7 Median and Ulnar Nerves

The median nerve originates with two branches from both the lateral and medial cords; their junction shapes the median fork with the axillary artery between them. For the motor pathways, the median and inferior trunks and their respective C7–T1 roots contain nerve fibers to the median nerve. The artery may hide the medial cord so that careful and extended dissection may be necessary to bring all structures into view. The ulnar nerve is only supplied by fibers from the medial cord and the C8 and T1 roots. It is located more medial to the median nerve, and an additional small branch arises just beside it, the medial cutaneous antebrachii nerve, which can be used as another nerve graft. Both main nerve trunks pass the upper arm at its medial aspect quite superficially; their individual courses at elbow level have been described in the discussion on the pronator teres, interosseous anterior, and cubital tunnel entrapments (see Chap. 5). They pass the forearm again superficially enough so that detailed descriptions on the necessary approaches are not of great importance.

All physicians dealing with median nerve lesions must bear in mind the importance of the Martin-Gruber anastomosis existing in 15% of individuals according to Sunderland (see Sect. 2.1). Motor fibers supplying some of the ulnar innervated intrinsic muscles may at first pass within the median nerve, then cross over at elbow level to the ulnar nerve using special branches or even sometimes the anterior interosseous nerve. Injuries to proximal median nerve segments or to the anterior interosseous nerve then cause a serious weakness involving not only median nerve innervated muscles but also ulnar nerve-supplied intrinsics.

Another variation in such anastomoses contains median nerve fibers destined for the thenar muscle, which leave the median nerve at variable levels to cross over and join the ulnar nerve. These thenar fibers then leave the ulnar nerve at the palm level and cross over all longitudinally orientated palm structures to enter the thenar muscle (Riche-Cannieu anastomosis). In these cases, lower median nerve lesions are astonishingly not associated with thenar weakness, and electromyographic tests lead physicians to reject the need for nerve repair at all.

The particular skin incisions must be chosen at the medial aspect of the upper arm: at elbow level including the S-shaped elbow joint crease, at the forearm longitudinally, and at wrist level with the wrist crease (▶ Fig. 6.23). Incision lines that cross transverse creases over joints must be avoided so as not to induce irreversibly constricting scars.

Fracture-related lesions of the median nerve sometimes occur following very low forearm fractures, resulting in a trauma-induced carpal tunnel entrapment. Nerve explorations or repairs then need to open the carpal tunnel to improve chances of recovery by facilitating the eventual resprouting processes. After tunnel release, the situation then makes it possible to identify the fascicle group containing fibers to the thenar muscle by microdissecting from distal to proximal. The thenar branch group can be carefully separated by following it to the cross-section of the prepared distal stump so that, in case of nerve grafting, this individual group receives sufficient supply by axon sprouts, guaranteeing thenar muscle reinnervation.

Fracture-related ulnar nerve lesions mostly occur at elbow level, almost always requiring neurolysis and transposition to the ventral aspect of the elbow region. In our opinion, it would be a mistake to avoid the transposition because elbow fractures induce ex-

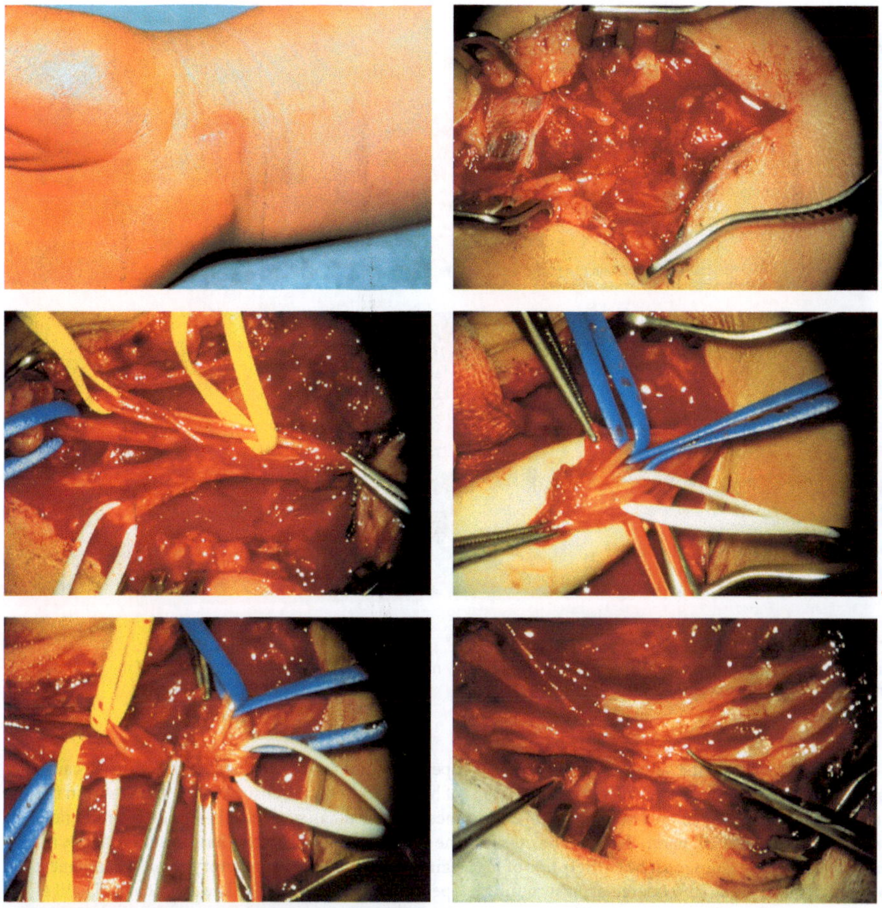

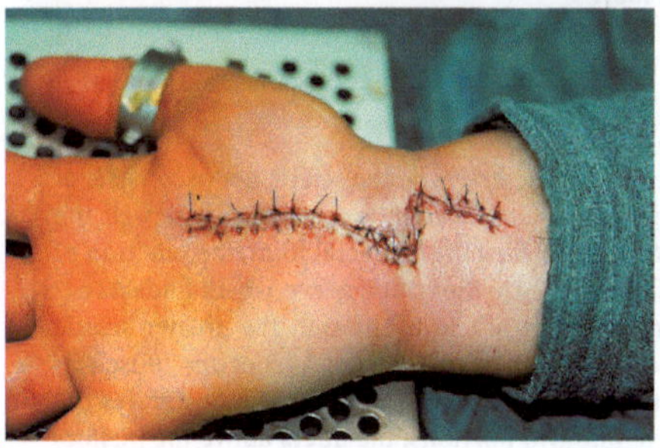

Figure 6.23a–g

Median nerve repair after endoscopic CTS release (right hand). a Neuroma at wrist; b exploration of the carpal tunnel; c identification of the median nerve branches (thenar branch, *yellow loops*); d separation of proximal fascicle groups; e both the nerve ends torn end to end, situation ready for interfascicular grafting; f positioning of grafts; g skin incision used

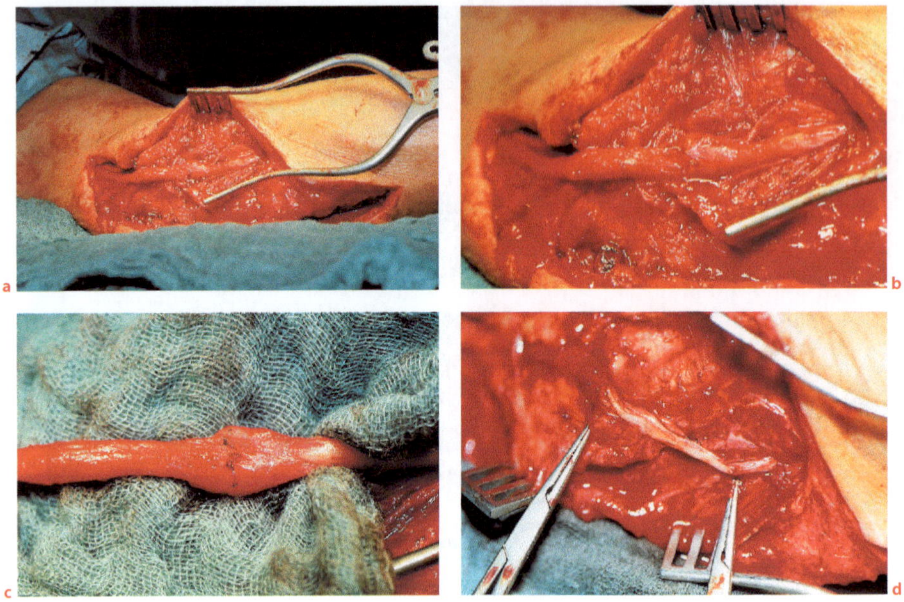

Figure 6.24 a–d

Ulnar nerve repair at elbow level subsequent to previous primary nerve suture (right arm). a–c Exploration of the neuroma; d repair by means of three grafts

tended scar tissue within the sulcus region. By transposing the nerve, roughly 1.5 cm of nerve length is gained, making it possible to try a microsurgical end-to-end suture in case of nerve repair. The nerve stumps and fascicle groups must be entirely free of fibrosis and tension for an unhindered axon sprouting process. In case of insufficient transposition, tension forces during elbow flexion will undoubtedly induce a new suture neuroma, as illustrated in ▶ Fig. 6.24.

Ulnar nerve lesions at wrist level always require the additional opening of the distal ulnar tunnel comparable to the above-mentioned low-level median nerve lesion, again allowing an unhindered outsprouting of axons. At wrist level, the deep ulnar nerve branch of the palm can be dissected and followed by separating microdissection to the distal nerve stump, again ensuring that, in case of nerve repair, this important branch gets enough axon supply to re-innervate the intrinsic muscles.

All nerve grafting procedures require postoperative immobilization while still in the operating room, especially when joint regions are involved and postoperative movements can displace the grafts. Because of higher numbers of sensory components within the median and ulnar nerves, mis-sprouting influences the results more negatively than in radial nerve repair, but the chances for recovery remain excellent if operated early secondary or late secondary (Khalil et al. 1986).

6.8 Sciatic Nerve

The intrapelvic origin of the sciatic nerve consists of a division of the L4 root, then of the L5 as well the S1–S3 roots. Below the iliosacral joint, the junction of all five roots form the sciatic nerve, which finds its exit into the buttock level through the greater sciatic notch. The transverse-running piriformis muscle is either located above the sciatic nerve or divides the nerve into two portions; the fibers above the piriformis then contain the peroneal division, whereas the fibers below are comprised of the tibial contribution. The inferior gluteal nerve runs side by side with the sciatic nerve arising from it still at intrapelvic level and supplying the gluteus maximus muscle. The superior gluteal nerve exits above the piriformis muscle and turns upward, there supplying the medial and inferior gluteal muscles. Its ramification starts immediately after the exit so that eventual nerve reconstruction frequently fails because of the destroyed small motor entries into the muscle substance.

After the exit, the sciatic nerve turns downward and is situated on the two obturator muscles, the gemelli and quadratus femoris muscles when seen during operation from a conventional posterior route. Just below the hip joint, several branches arise and supply above all the biceps femoris muscle, which is important to remember for clinical and electromyographic diagnosis and eventual exploration. At the posterior side of the thigh, the sciatic nerve is surgically found between the semitendinous and semimembranous muscles at the medial side and the biceps femoris muscle at the lateral side. The separation between the tibial and peroneal nerve portions becomes more visible the lower the approach leads.

The clinical findings are obvious and severe but especially critical when superior and inferior gluteal nerves are also involved. Penetrating nerve lesions such as impalements or gunshot wounds are not frequently observed in Europe; the majority of high-level sciatic nerve lesions unfortunately occur with hip joint surgery, but particularly as failures of acetabulum reconstructions. We have seen long, extended nerve tractions, severe scarring following injury to the inferior gluteal artery and its emergency management, sometimes associated with nerve strangulations, as well as intrapelvic lesions due to reconstruction instruments.

When in doubt on the degree of nerve lesion, exploration is indicated and advised rather early because the outgrowing of nerve axons in this context requires the most time of all the extremity nerves. Paralysis of the gluteus maximus muscle in electromyography indicates a lesion at a very high level; on the contrary, a preserved biceps femoris function indicates a rather low lesion at the buttocks level. On the other hand, both muscles are the most proximally located ones to be tested, and they re-innervate comparably quickly. Therefore, they help in surgical timing. If signs of re-innervation of both remain absent, a late secondary exploration should be advised, as clearly defined: 3 months at the latest subsequent to the nerve injury. Many physicians unfortunately require waiting 1 year for surgery, when spontaneous recovery is expected in during this period. This is a mistake, as results after nerve repair decisively worsen following these waiting periods. Overweight and older patients do not easily decide for reoperation; nevertheless, chances of recovery rapidly decrease without early reoperation.

We prefer a two-portal approach into the buttocks and avoid large curved skin incisions with transverse transsection of the gluteal muscles described elsewhere, because these muscles may be functionally preserved, and the patient will permanently sit on scar tissue formations. We therefore take one approach, identical to that on the sciatic nerve entrapment syndrome (see Sect. 5.14), with the difference that we directly attack the nerve, the inferior gluteal branch and artery in an area where all structures are surrounded by scar tissue. Thus the principle of identifying nerves within healthy tissue only is abandoned. But contrary to other extremity nerves, the sciatic nerve has the caliber of a thumb, which reduces the danger of harming the nerve iatrogenically. Special care must still be taken on all the surrounding vessels because injuries of this nature are difficult to control when their stumps retract through the sciatic notch. If the nerve lesion and fibrosis extend into the pelvis the necessary parts of the sciatic foramen can easily be enlarged by means of a punch after transecting the always fibrotic piriformis muscle. Thus, an overview is gained on a few additional proximal centimeters of the sciatic nerve.

Lumbar plexus lesions will also involve the femoral nerve divisions, and these severe lesions only exceptionally come into question with a combination of these injuries. The retroperitoneal approach requires turning the patient onto the healthy side so that a second approach through the gluteal muscles remains available in case nerve reconstruction is necessary. Intrapelvic/extrapelvic nerve reconstructions remain single cases in the literature and in conference communications, as reported by Birch et al. (1998), and they should be attempted only if surgery has been done very early. Reinnervation periods of about 3 years were observed and described. All the details and risks of flank or abdominal wall incisions and approaches are not described in this context because general surgeons, who are more familiar with abdominal approaches, can assist. This also avoids postoperative complications from abdominal hernias following an eventually insufficient closure. The surgeon must remain retroperitoneal because intraoperative herniations and movements of the abdominal contents make microsurgery and the maintenance of microsutures impossible.

Sciatic nerve lesions below the sciatic notch are far easier to solve: an additional long transverse incision

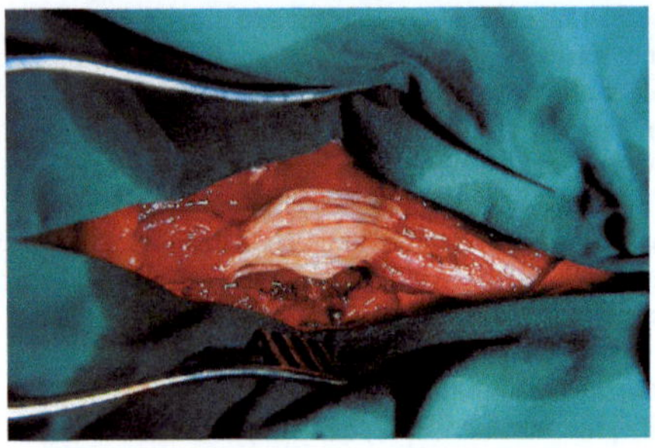

Figure 6.25

Interfascicular repair of a short distant sciatic nerve lesion

uses the buttock crease, which indicates the lower border of the gluteal muscles. It provides access between the biceps and semitendinosus muscles from below. The branches to these muscles must of course be preserved. Again by means of a two-portal approach, a tunnel can be formed between the sciatic notch access and this second lower access. The gluteal muscle fibers and the overlying intact skin are looped as a whole, and thus they can be lifted up by the assistant during the exploration part of the procedure. In special situations, these two approaches then extend the openings to the large approach with one skin incision and transsection of gluteal muscle fibers, as described by Kline and Hudson (1995), large approaches with one curved skin incision and transsection of the gluteal muscle fibers. If a sciatic nerve reconstruction is considered, a lack of available nerve grafts is an unresolved problem because of the nerve diameter, which would require extending the approach as mentioned above: the better overview will make it possible not to dissipate intact nerve segments and to end at nerve gaps not larger than needed in order to ensure that there is a maximum of transplant material. When nerve grafts are lacking, the reconstruction of the tibial nerve part is be preferred because recovery of the peroneal nerve part is often disappointing. The patient thus recovers sufficient foot flexion, and extension can subsequently be reconstructed via a tibial posterior muscle transfer.

Injuries to the sciatic nerve at the thigh level are mostly observed as a result of typical penetrating injuries (▶ Fig. 6.25); the longitudinal or S-shaped skin incisions needed depend on the lesion level. The approach uses the space between the biceps femoris and the semitendinosus as well as semimembranous muscle bellies. The nerve branches leading to these muscles already separate from the main nerve trunk at the lower buttock level so that they no longer come into view in lower-level explorations.

The postoperative plaster bandage presents difficulties but should nevertheless be used without exception.

6.9 Femoral Nerve

The femoral nerve originates from the roots and their anterior divisions L2, L3, and L4. Then it takes a relatively long retroperitoneal course, first on top of the psoas muscle, then at lower levels, along the medial border of this muscle. Branches supplying it and additionally supplying the iliac muscle arise very early, whereas branches to the sartorius muscle arise near the inguinal ligament. It then runs downward under the inguinal ligament, there located lateral to the femoral artery and vein so that it can be identified by palpating the femoral pulse. Nerve and vessels are situated within their own fascial compartments, separated from each other. About 3 cm below the inguinal ligament, the nerve divides into several motor branches to the quadriceps muscles and one main sensory branch, the saphenous nerve. The femoral nerve remains covered by the relatively thick iliac fascia, whereas the medially located artery and vein pierce this fascia and are only then covered by the superficial fascia of the thigh.

Injuries to the nerve at high intrapelvic levels hinder patients severely, given that walking and even standing without the psoas is impossible. Similarly, lesions at lower levels are problematic because the loss of the quadriceps muscle function makes walking or standing aids necessary. Early nerve explorations and eventual reconstructions are therefore of great importance because residual defects can lead to complete social isolation.

In our experience, lesions mostly result from penetrating injuries, more rarely and then at higher levels, from hip joint surgery or acetabulum reconstructions; we have seen one lesion resulting from a transvaginal hysterectomy. Unfortunately, although nerve axon regrowth has to overcome only a relatively short distance, recovery time is often long. We would therefore advocate early exploration if the patient decides that everything possible has to be done soon.

Because of the relatively short extrapelvic course, the surgeon has to be aware that a retroperitoneal approach will probably be needed even if a penetrating injury just below the inguinal ligament has occurred; the proximal stump will always retract a few centime-

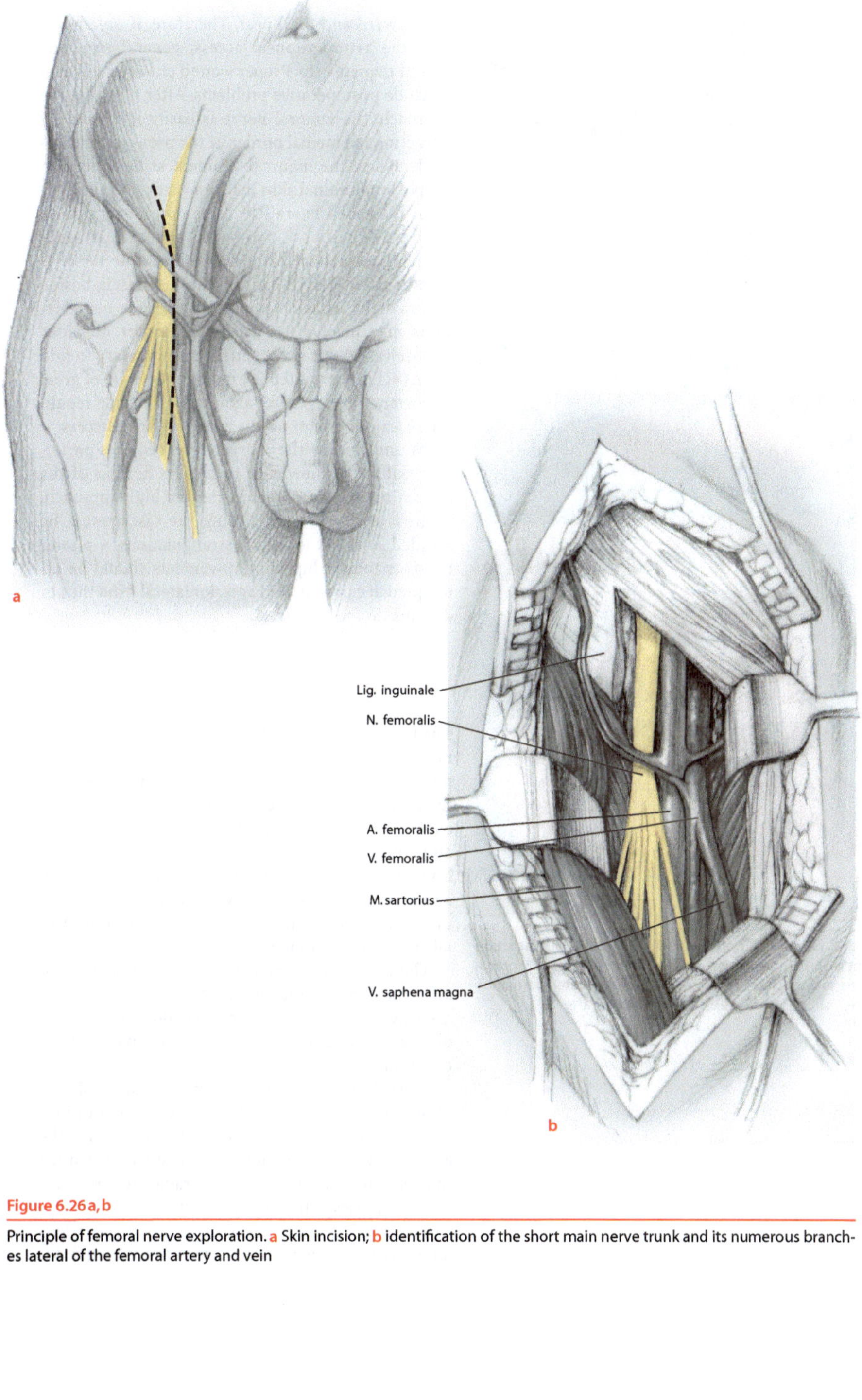

Figure 6.26 a, b

Principle of femoral nerve exploration. a Skin incision; b identification of the short main nerve trunk and its numerous branches lateral of the femoral artery and vein

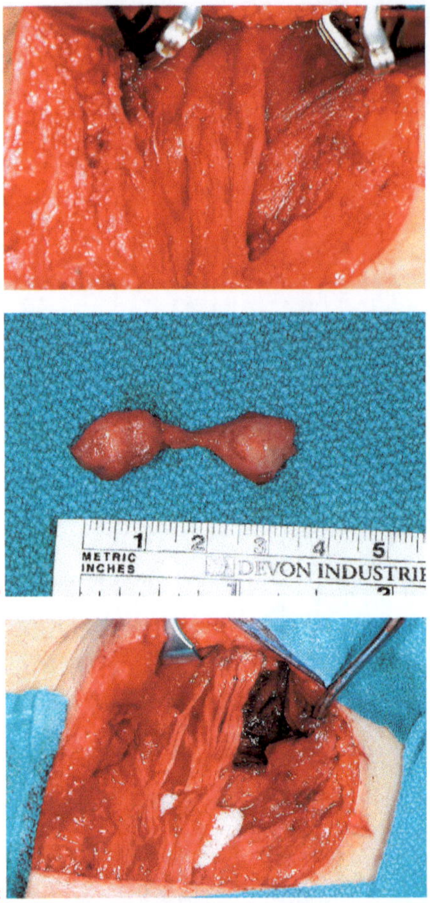

a b c

Figure 6.27 a–c

Femoral nerve repair after harmful neurofibroma resection (right leg). a Situation after re-exploration below the inguinal ligament, single fascicles preserved; b one resected part of the nerve; c situation after repair by means of grafts

ters upward and disappear. Therefore, if unfamiliar with the retroperitoneal access, general surgeons should request help. Proper wound closures will also preclude postoperative problems. After finishing the approach, the femoral nerve is easily identified by retracting the medial border of the psoas muscle laterally. Below the inguinal ligament at thigh level, a simple longitudinal skin incision vertical to the ligament is needed lateral to the femoral artery pulse (▶ Fig. 6.26). Thus, a two-portal approach is again available to manage extensive lesions. The nerve is identified not before incising the iliac fascia beside the medially located femoral artery. Low nerve lesions may involve the five or six motor divisions themselves so that great patience is necessary to find them (▶ Fig. 6.27). All these motor entries are of great importance as targets for axon sprouts during repair. These lesions do not need a retroperitoneal access.

Wound closure after nerve repair requires particular skills and knowledge to prevent hernias of the abdominal contents when using the high approach, whereas at thigh level, closing the fascia must be avoided so as not to induce strangulations. A plaster bandage to stop hip joint movements should be attempted. It can be placed anterior lateral from the abdominal to the knee level.

6.10 Tibial Nerve

The tibial nerve forms the continuation of the sciatic nerve. In the popliteal fossa, it is deeply located and pierces the origin of the soleus muscle together with the popliteal artery and vein, then nerve and vessels course downward, sheltered by the gastrocnemius and soleus muscles. At the lower third of the lower limb, it runs more medial toward the tarsal tunnel, and several centimeters above it divides into the medial and lateral plantar nerves with the posterior tibial artery between them.

The clinical findings depend on the level of lesion affecting either all the muscles of the calf and sole or exclusively the muscles of the sole. Both lesions hinder walking and therefore need nerve repair without question.

Most lesions result from penetrating injuries (▶ Fig. 6.28 a, b); lesions at lower levels may additionally result from fractures or distortions involving the ankle joints. They are then associated with extended intraneural scar tissue comparable to peroneal stretch injuries at the knee joint level.

The skin incisions needed depend on the particular level of the lesion: incisions over the popliteal fos-

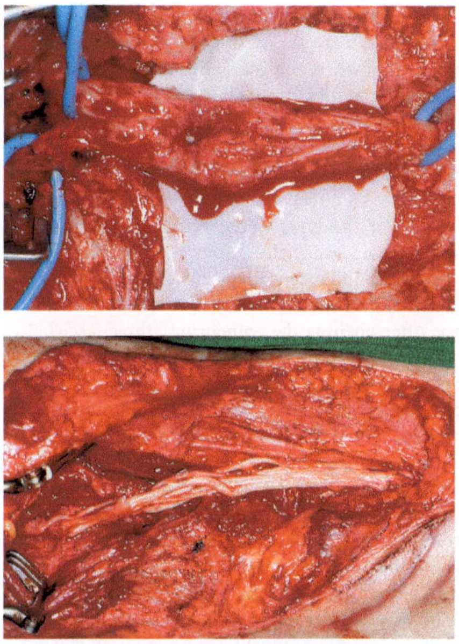

a

b

Figure 6.28 a, b

Tibial nerve repair after knee joint arthroscopy, patient in prone position. a Nerve laceration; b repair by grafts, proximal on the right

sa should be S-shaped to the popliteal crease, over the calf longitudinally downward, and lesions involving the ankle level require incisions described in Sect. 5.18 on the tarsal tunnel. Muscle fibers at mid-calf levels should be split and never transected. Combined or the typical two-portal approaches are possible .The surgeon must always be aware of the important tibial artery running alongside, which must be preserved. In contrast, reconstruction of the artery are never indicated if it has been damaged at the time of the primary injury; the development of sufficient collateral vessels can be expected, starting with secondary surgery. In case microneurolysis within the tarsal tunnel is needed, it must be pointed out that especially at ankle level, many interfascicular cross-connections are present, forming an intensive plexiform structure, according to Sunderland's studies. Thus, interfascicular separating dissections may cause small neuromas, resulting in disabling pain syndromes. The situation at that level is comparable to the one of the ulnar nerve at elbow level. Low-situated trauma-related nerve lesions always require a complete tarsal tunnel release to allow unhindered outgrowth of axons.

A postoperative plaster bandage for 10 days and immobilization are of course mandatory.

6.11 Medial and Lateral Plantar Nerves

Nerve lesions and the subsequent need for repair surgery on both the plantar nerves occur very rarely. We have seen only two cases caused by sharply penetrating injuries. In one case, both nerves were reconstructed using the old skin scars at the sole. Paresthesias such as a Tinel sign at each step before and unfortunately long after the operation made walking almost impossible; in our opinion, the nerve reconstruction remained questionable. The patient should be prepared preoperatively for these subsisting paresthesias. The only acceptable reason for nerve reconstruction should be avoiding muscle atrophy of the sole, which can cause severe problems for the patient.

Whenever possible, incisions into the skin of the sole must be avoided at all costs because the subsequent scar tissue will trigger the nerves for the rest of the patient's life. Skin incisions over the medial aspect of the abductor hallucis muscle are preferred, allowing approaches that lift up this muscle (patient lying supine). Both plantar nerves can easily be identified within the tarsal tunnel and then followed distally from that point into the plantar region. We chose this approach in one procedure to remove a neurofibroma from the lateral plantar nerve in which no injury had previously occurred.

6.12 Peroneal Nerve

The peroneal nerve divides from the sciatic nerve at variable levels and separates more and more as it turns lateral. In the popliteal fossa, it becomes more superficial as the nerve approaches the head of the fibula. Just at that level, the nerve is overlain by ligaments and a very thick fascia, an area where the nerve is mostly in danger of being crashed. Entering the peroneal muscles, it divides into the superficial and deep branches. Contrary to the anatomically comparable situation of the radial nerve at elbow level, both branches supply important muscles so that both of them should serve as target in case of nerve repair. The deep branch curves slightly anterior supplying the anterior tibialis, extensor hallucis and extensor muscles of the toes. The superficial branch takes a relatively straight course downward and supplies the peroneus longus and brevis muscles. Its sensory branch leads to the dorsum of the foot to supply the entire skin surface, with the exception of a small area between the first and second toes, which instead belongs to the only sensitive distribution of the deep branch. The situation is identical to that of the superficial and deep branches of the radial nerve.

Lesions of the deep branch cause a foot extension palsy, whereas the superficial branch is responsible for everting the foot; isolated lesions of one of the two branches occur very rarely and present sometimes unresolvable difficulties if nerve repair has been required, particularly because of the early ramification of the deep branch.

Most peroneal nerve lesions result from injuries to the knee joint, mostly severe injuries causing distortions and ruptures of the lateral and crucial ligaments. The virtual nerve injury then consists of a nerve traction in the longitudinal direction. Unfortunately, the peroneal nerve is relatively fixed in length between the division of the sciatic nerve and the fibula joint level, providing little elasticity when stretched.

In our experience, these injuries do not have a reliable spontaneous chance of recovery and therefore require exploration. Nevertheless, it should be pointed out to the patient before operation that these long extended stretch injuries have a poor prognosis in terms of either spontaneous recovery or nerve repair. This should be explained with the following arguments: first, this type of lesion causes long, extended intraneural severe scar tissue so that sometimes after the resection of the scarred nerve segments, gaps of 25 cm or more result; second, for unknown reasons, the regenerating forces of the peroneal nerve remain unsatisfactory and they present the worst regenerating forces if compared to the outgrowing forces in other extremity nerves in humans (see also Chap. 5).

In lesions involving the popliteal fossa and fibula joint region, the patient lies prone. Both legs are prepared for eventual sural nerve removal. The contralateral sural nerve has priority, so as not to cause an additional loss of sensitivity in the affected limb, but very frequently, the sural nerve of the affected side must also be removed to overcome the above-mentioned long nerve gaps. The incision starts S-shaped over the popliteal fossa to the popliteal crease but rather frequently must be extended proximal in order to identify the sciatic nerve and the arising peroneal nerve (▶ Fig. 6.29). Then at the distal level, the surgeon must identify the deep and superficial nerve branches within the muscles far enough below the fibula joint within healthy tissue. The dissection then follows the nerve from proximal and distal. The main trauma-related scar tissue is to be found proximal to the fibula joint where the lateral ligaments have ruptured and sometimes, in case of other open injuries, wounds have been débrided. Following such injuries and secondary operations requires safe identification of the peroneal nerve, successful only within healthy tissue, whereas a direct attack to the nerve at the lateral aspect of the knee would result in iatrogenic nerve damage. Nevertheless, after skeletonizing the nerve only, the full extension of the lesion cannot be estimated with the naked eye: a microscope is mandatory. After opening the epineurium, three fascicle groups become visible, frequently giving the impression of a neuroma in continuity over quite a long distance (▶ Fig. 6.29b). In such situations, intraoperative nerve action potentials can be helpful. It is astonishing that the neuroma frequently becomes thicker the more proximal the dissection of the intraneural nerve structures is. After transsection of such a high nerve segment, its cross-section then shows a neuromatous mass with no interfascicular pattern. These unexpected situations require resecting more and more of the proximal stump so that even the skin incision itself sometimes must be extended proximal a few times. A proximal stump with a very soft fascicular structure at its cross-section is often to be found not before the mid-thigh level, where the peroneal nerve and tibial nerve already have a common epineural sheath. These typical situations explain why such long nerve gaps emerge and why nerve repair may even lead to a relative lack of nerve grafts. Defects of 25 cm or more can only be reconstructed by two grafts (▶ Fig. 6.29f). At the end of exploration and eventual nerve repair, the fascia of the popliteal fossa and over the peroneal muscles remains open to prevent strangulations. A postoperative posterior plaster bandage is of course necessary. It should not only immobilize the knee joint but also the ankle joint to avoid foot flexion contractures. Ten days later, a peroneal splint should be applied.

Further difficulties emerge when the lesion affects the lower limb. Tibia fractures and their reconstructions leave behind severe scars and extended fibrosis of the peroneal muscles. Nerve reconstructions at this levels are a challenge; nevertheless, they may completely fail when the small branches of the deep peroneal nerve are involved. The situation is again comparable to lesions of the posterior interosseous nerve. A fibrosis of the peroneal muscles must be excluded by electromyographic tests before operation. A precondition of successful nerve repair is that the muscle fibers remained alive, which must be proven by ev-

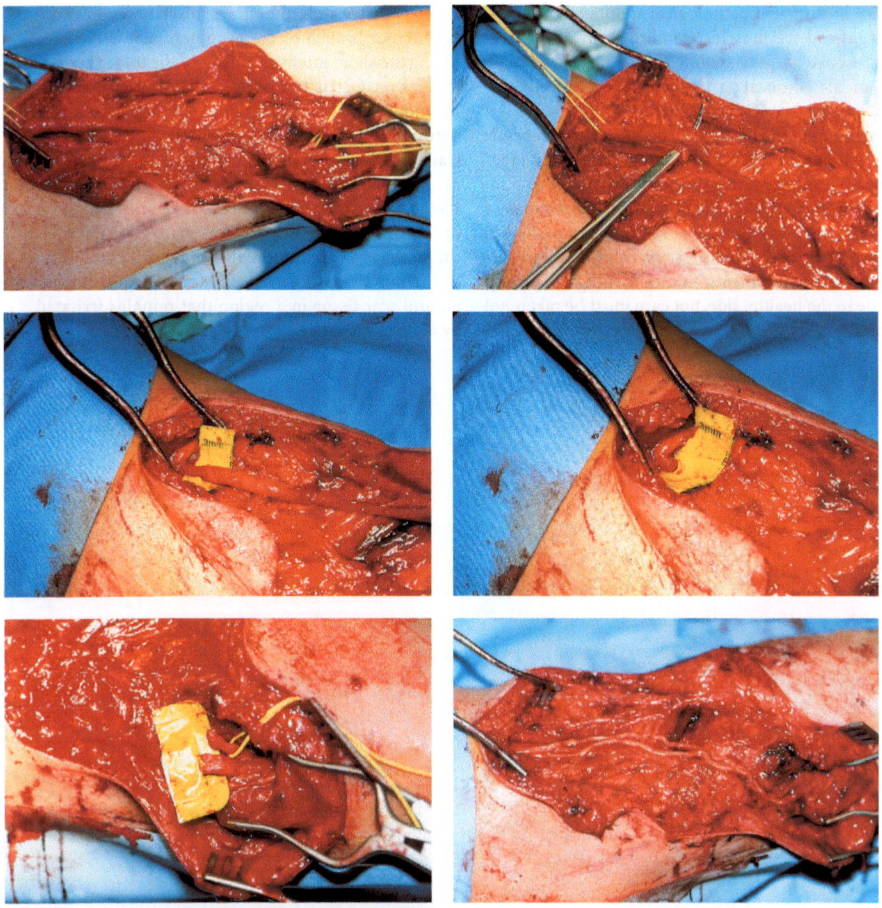

a b c d e f

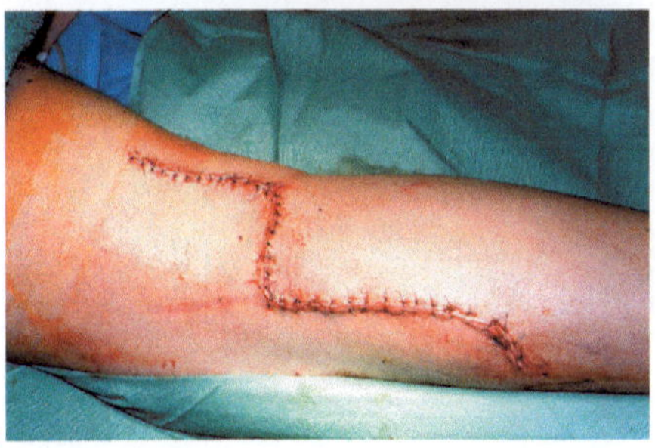

g

Figure 6.29a–g

Peroneal nerve repair after knee injury, patient in prone position (left leg). a Nerve continuity preserved, but fibrosis over 25 cm present (superficial and deep branches, *yellow loops*); b proximal neuroma 5 cm in length; c, d proximal nerve transsection above the neuroma; e distal nerve stumps below the tibial–fibular joint; f both the sural nerves as grafts 30 cm in length; g skin incision used idence of sufficient pathological spontaneous activity. If instead the muscles are fibrotically altered, reconstructive surgery should be done at once, as in case of late peroneal paralysis, a tibial posterior tendon transfer (see Chap. 11).

Positioning the patient during operation depends on the level of the lesion expected. As already mentioned, a lesion affecting the popliteal fossa and fibula joint region requires the prone position, whereas a lesion at the lower limb level requires the patient in the supine position. Nerve lesions comparable to peroneal nerve entrapments require turning the patient a little to the healthy side, but care must be taken not to cause pressure sores if eventual nerve repair takes a few hours.

Special issues are sometimes raised in repair of the final motor branch of the deep peroneal nerve supplying the short extensor muscle of the toes. Theoretically, a reconstruction should technically succeed if the motor entries are identified. But these lesions are naturally associated with transsection of the superficial final sensory branch resulting in a neuroma and causing disturbing electrical-current-like pain over the dorsum of the foot. If the patient still complains of this pain before surgery, we remain restrictive because a nerve exploration always requires extension of the initial wound, eventually resulting in further painful scar tissue in a region that remains irritated by the patient's shoes.

Facial Nerve

Peripheral nerve repair on facial nerve injuries of the face is indicated if the nerve lesion involves the nerve peripheral to the stylomastoid foramen. Lesions caused by cerebellopontine angle tumor surgery, Bell's palsies, or fractures of the temporal bone are therefore not discussed in this chapter.

If the facial nerve was removed for reasons of radical parotid gland tumor surgery, nerves must be repaired in the same session for the best results. Immediate restoration of nerve continuity seems to be the best logical consequence in that situation. Of course, the indication to do so depends on the prognosis and the dignity of the tumor. If palliative radiation is indicated after surgery, the recipient bed for eventual nerve grafts would become fibrotic to the point that the outgrowth of axon sprouts would be blocked completely.

Alternative facial nerve lesions, unrelated to tumor, are caused by penetrating injuries of the face, mostly a matter of secondary nerve exposure and restoration of continuity.

In contrast to muscles of the extremity, which undergo irreversible atrophy starting a few months after the lesion, it is often surprising how long muscles of the face can reassume function with nerve repair. Their potentially contractile ability often remains preserved for a period of a few years due to cross-innervation, meaning that nerve fibers supply some muscles from the contralateral facial nerve. Before treatment of a facial nerve lesion, the existence of pathologically spontaneous activity of the involved and noninnervated muscles of the face must be proved by electromyographic studies. The electromyography must also distinguish between voluntary potentials coming from the contralateral side and voluntary potentials coming from the affected side; the latter would indicate spontaneous nerve recovery. The distinction can additionally be made by stimulating the affected nerve at the level of the stylomastoid foramen. The presence of potentials after stimulation at the affected side would indicate preserved peripheral nerve continuity.

In summary, an attempt to restore facial nerve function depends on electromyography, and repair should not generally be denied even if the injury occurred a long time ago.

7.1 Macroscopic Anatomy

After its exit from the stylomastoid foramen, the nerve usually divides into two first-order branches just after penetrating the parotid gland. These two branches divide again after a short distance into second-order branches. Within the gland, a great variation in anastomoses between these branches is present, forming the so-called parotid plexus. More peripherally, there are further divisions that form three groups of peripheral branches, which are referred to as zygomatic, buccal, and mandibular branches. With a certain selective frequency, six main types of ramification have been published in the literature (cited in Millesi 1979).

The existence of this great variability in nerve ramification explains why surgery on these nerves remains a great challenge and why success in nerve repair still depends mainly on immediately and exact nerve identification.

7.2 Microscopic Anatomy

Meissl published studies on ten facial nerves in human cadavers performed in the mid-1970s (cited in Millesi 1979): at the level of the primary trunk, all nerves primarily consist of three major fascicles and several much smaller ones at the medial side; coming more peripherally, the three major fascicles fuse together and then subdivide into three fascicle groups again. There was some functional grouping to be observed in so far as upper portions of the nerve proved responsible for zygomatic fibers, middle portions for buccal fibers and lower portions for mandibular fibers.

The type of microsurgery that should be used in nerve anastomosis depends on the intraneural structure of the terminal nerve segment. In the monofascicular or polyfascicular nerve stump, small nerve grafts should cover the entire cross-section, whereas when there are fascicle groups, an interfascicular adaptation should be attempted. This differentiation reduces nerve fiber aberration at suture lines as far as possible and prevents neuromas.

7.3 Facial Reanimation

7.3.1 Facial Nerve Repair

The proximal nerve trunk, its intraparotid plexiform ramification, and its peripheral varying branches can be exposed at three levels: beyond the stylomastoid foramen, between the major superficial part of the parotid gland and its minor deep part, and at the level where the different nerve branches leave the parotid gland.

Because of the danger of damaging the parotid gland and its duct, a surgeon without experience in ENT surgery should not explore the plexus part of the facial nerve completely. Instead, nerve reconstruction should lead from a proximal nerve stump just beyond the stylomastoid foramen to peripheral branches beyond the lateral border of the parotid gland.

For surgery, the patient's head is turned to the contralateral side. Exposure at the stylomastoid foramen segment requires a skin incision posterior to the auricle, then curving around anterior and again turning downward, following the anterior border of the sternocleidomastoid muscle. The leading structure is the anterior border of the mastoid bone. It remains difficult, but of great importance, to find the connective tissue compartment between the anterior border of the sternocleidomastoid muscle and the posterior border of the parotid gland, because injury to the gland leads to fistulas. In any case, the great auricular nerve running transverse and superficially to this compartment should be identified at once, isolated over about 5 cm proximal and distal, and preserved during the entire surgery. It runs a little upward and behind the auricle to supply a large skin area, causing complaints from the patient if damaged. After identification of the two borderlines between the muscle belly and the gland, the anterior aspect of the mastoid bone must be followed about 1.5 cm or more in depth until the fingertip is able to feel the stylomastoid process. On reaching this structure, the attaching anterior parts of the sternocleidomastoid muscle must be carefully sectioned and isolated from the mastoid bone. Doing this carelessly may result in immediate injury to the small facial nerve and drilling the mastoid is required to find a nerve stump.

The nerve can be found slightly posterior to the process running downward and slightly anterior over fibers of the digastric muscle. The access is astonishingly facilitated when the microscope is used, particularly at the region of the stylomastoid process. There is an artery running alongside the nerve of the same caliber, which, in case of injury, leads to bleeding that is difficult to control without harming the nerve. Damage to the nerve stump by the surgeon may lead to a situation in which the mastoid bone must be drilled in order to find it within its intramastoidal course. Care must then be taken not to injure the chorda tympani, which leaves the facial nerve on its lateral aspect in the retrograde direction.

Further important structures, the internal carotid artery, internal jugular vein, external carotid artery and the spinal accessory, hypoglossal, vagus, and glossopharyngeal nerves are more deeply situated than the digastric muscle. The proximal access now aims at identifying the facial nerve or its stump, which then serves for connection with grafts if needed or anastomosis after nerve transfer.

The peripheral exploration of facial nerve branches beyond the parotid gland should be done using the injury-associated skin scar and, eventually, also limited vertical skin incisions situated over the expected course of the zygomatic, buccal, and mandibular branches. These incisions, if needed in the particular case, must be placed about 3 cm lateral to the lateral eyelid angle, 5 cm lateral to the nose wing, and about 3 cm lateral to the mouth angle. It is very helpful to take the microscope from the very beginning because the small and highly variably located facial nerve branches are rather superficial. The best way not to damage them is to spread the tissue from the beginning transverse to the skin incision by means of small scissors under magnification. A number of small arteries cross the operating fields; they should be identified, coagulated, and transected. Stopping diffuse bleeding without previous identification of the injured small vessel will destroy the small nerve branches before they have all been viewed. By manual retraction of the underlying skin, the operating approaches are enlarged as expected so that large curved skin incisions over the entire face should no longer be necessary. Roughly six small transverse-running nerves of zygomatic, buccal, and mandibular branches can be identified and looped; they will serve as targets for restoration of nerve continuity.

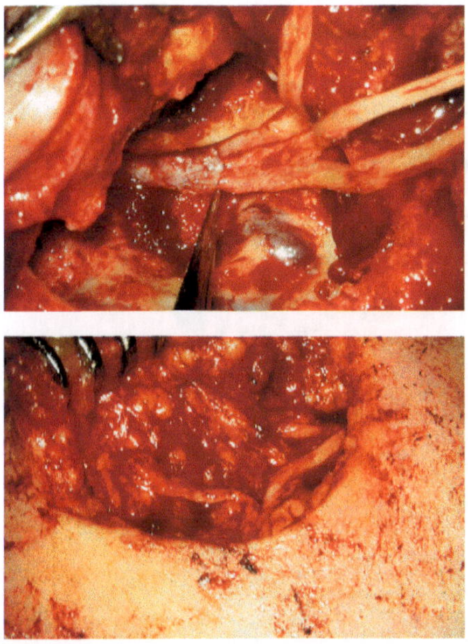

Figure 7.1 a, b

Direct facial nerve repair, two-portal approach. a Grafts connected with facial nerve fascicles proximal to the parotid gland; b distal nerve connections with zygomatic and buccal branches

After removing the sural nerve as graft, we are always confronted with great differences in nerve stump caliber: the caliber of the sural nerve is much larger than that of the peripheral facial branches, a situation we rarely see in other contexts. In this situation, the microscope must be used to separate a few fascicle groups within the graft so that nerves of smaller diameter appear. Interfascicular surrounding tissue should be removed slightly so that really naked small nerve stumps are available. The grafts are subcutaneously placed between the proximal approach at the stylomastoid level and the three approaches in the periphery (▶ Fig. 7.1).

The peripheral nerve coaptation is difficult to perform because of small diameters. Depending on the surgeon's experience, fibrin glue may be a consideration. The central anastomosis must have a view of the particular nerve structure of the facial nerve stump (see Sect. 7.2).

The wound must be closed without a suction drain, as always in nerve grafting, and extreme care must be taken not to displace the new nerve adaptations; postoperative immobilization is impossible. A loose bandage must cover as much as half of the affected face.

7.3.2 Nerve Transfer (Hypoglosso-Facial Nerve Anastomosis)

If a proximal stump of the facial nerve is not available, nerve transfer or neurotization is indicated and has proved to be very effective in the last decades. This procedure has been well known since Balance's reports on his experiences in 1909 as well as alternative nerve transfers which recruited the spinal accessory (Cushing 1903), glossopharyngeal (Balance 1924), or phrenic nerves (Hardy 1957) as the motor fiber donor. In the latter cases, results were disappointing. We saw patients after nerve transfer using the spinal accessory nerve, who developed dreadful voluntary mass movements of the entire face without achieving satisfying symmetry at rest. In order to avoid the sacrifice of a donor nerve, cross-face grafting was attempted: several grafts were connected with facial nerve branches as far peripheral as possible at the healthy side and with more centrally located branches of the facial nerve at the affected side, as Anderl reported in detail in 1973. One graft crossed over the face through the forehead, two of them through the upper lip, and one of them through the lower lip. The procedure was time-consuming and done in two sessions. A special challenge was to identify several peripheral branches on the healthy side, stimulate each individual branch, and decide, depending on the stimulation results, which branch could be sacrificed as the donor nerve.

Because of its difficulties and expenditure, we now prefer the hypoglosso-facial anastomosis, which includes the sacrifice of one hypoglossal nerve. It is interesting that patients do not sustain the atrophy of one half of the tongue and do not present the changed speech articulation we would normally expect.

Unavailable proximal facial nerve stumps may stem from temporal bone fractures, cholesteatoma surgery procedures, and other intratemporal tumor treatments as well as cerebellopontine angle tumors. With the first, direct nerve reconstructions from intracranial to intratemporal or even extratemporal must be considered. But the patient's situation or risks from a secondary intracranial approach may favor a simple nerve transfer.

For surgery, the patient's head is turned to the contralateral side, far enough to allow access under the

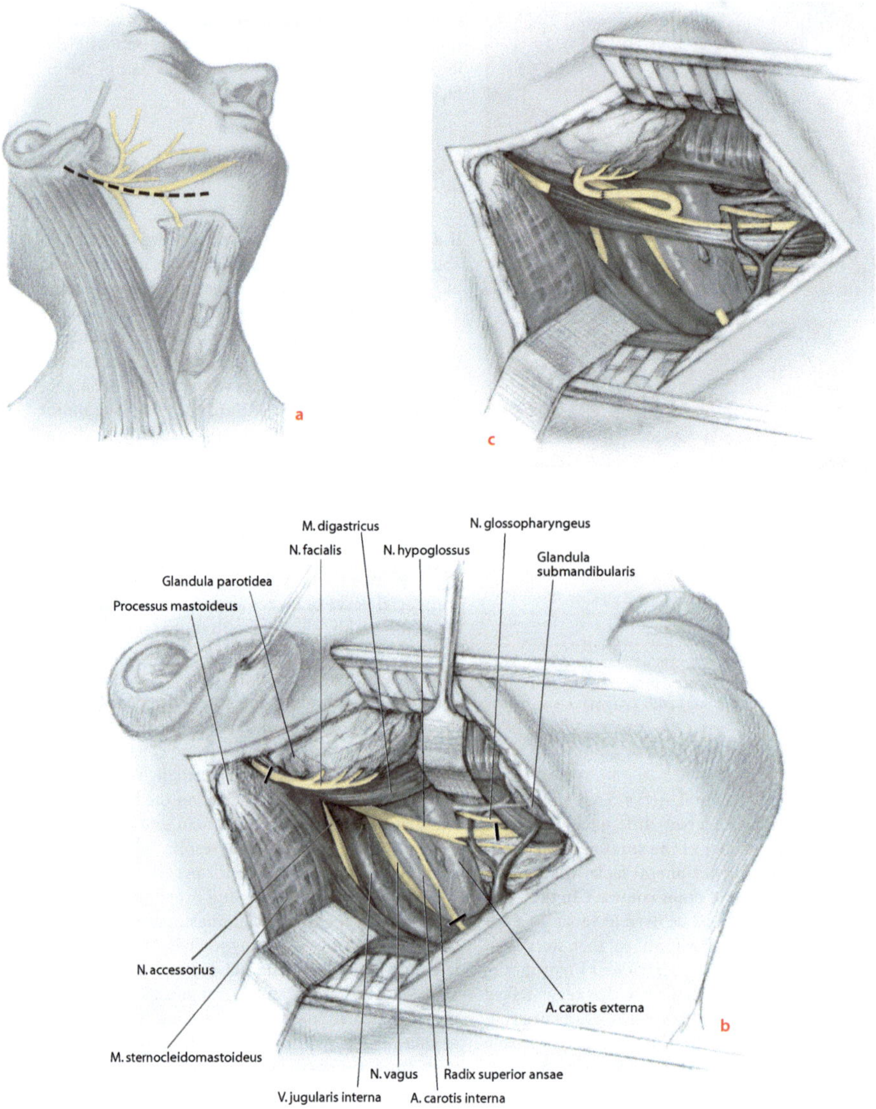

Figure 7.2a–c

Nerve transfer (right side). a Skin incision 1.5 cm behind the ear; b exploration between anterior border of the sternocleidal muscle and the posterior border of the parotid gland; transsection of the facial nerve as proximal as possible as well as of the hypoglossal nerve 1.5 cm distal to the external carotid artery; the digastric muscle is lifted up at the beginning; c anastomosis between facial and hypoglossal nerves; the digastric muscle is now situated below the nerve anastomosis; the cervical ansa may be secondarily connected to the distal stump of the hypoglossal nerve lower mandible. Surgery starts with the same skin incision and approach as described in the previous chapter concerning exposure of the central part of the facial nerve beyond the stylomastoid foramen (▶ Fig. 7.2). A microscope is used for nerve identification. The facial nerve transsection must be done as far proximal as possible, in other words, near the stylomastoid foramen, to receive a sufficient distal stump as the target. This is contrary to what was said in the previous chapter where we needed a sufficient proximal stump. If the facial nerve is transected near the parotid gland by mistake, its peripheral stump will disappear within the gland.

Exposure of the hypoglossal nerve requires extending the skin incision between the lower mandible and the anterior border of the sternocleidomastoid muscle. The bellies of the digastric muscle must be identified. This muscle should be isolated completely to allow retraction. Deep to the digastric muscle especially the external carotid artery should be identified using the fingertip. Care should be taken on branching intertwining arteries and veins because damage to them leads to diffuse bleeding. The surgeon must not get nervous in this situation, but try to identify the origin of the bleeding with careful suction, and use bipolar forceps only when the bleeding vessel stump is identified and visible. Careful maneuvers are also essential on the external jugular vein for the same reasons. The hypoglossal nerve crosses over the external carotid artery, turning anterior and parallel to the lower mandibula, and there it can be followed as far peripheral as possible, where it must be transected. The nerve is identified with nerve stimulation and by viewing the tongue, which should move during stimulation. After transecting the nerve, its central stump is turned and taken back; this procedure causes slight bleeding from the above-mentioned small branching vessels. Then the nerve stump is led under the lifted bellies of the digastric muscle and finally anastomosed to the already prepared peripheral stump of the facial nerve beside the stylomastoid process. The anastomosis is again done using the microscope, and it should be performed like an end-to-end suture (▶ Fig. 7.3). We place two 10-0 stitches to avoid rotation of the stumps against each other during wound closure.

To avoid atrophy of the homolateral half of the tongue, the descending small branch of the hypoglossal nerve can be transected as far peripheral as possible, turned upward and united with the peripheral stump of the main hypoglossal trunk.

During wound closure particular attention should be paid to the end-to-end anastomosis in front of the mastoid bone. It has proved suitable to place a small drain without suction far from the suture line but near the posterior border of the parotid gland, and to lead the drain outside through the lower edge of the skin incision. It can be removed 1 or 2 days later without harming the suture and avoids postoperative hematomas, because a compression bandage is impossible dealing with this type of surgery.

In contrast to all the alternative nerve transfers and cross-face grafting, sufficient symmetry at rest and sufficient voluntary face movements can be achieved. Even sufficient closure of the eyelids, the most important and the most difficult aim of facial nerve surgery, is often achieved. In our opinion, the hypoglosso-facial transfer is a relatively simple and effective method for facial nerve reanimation.

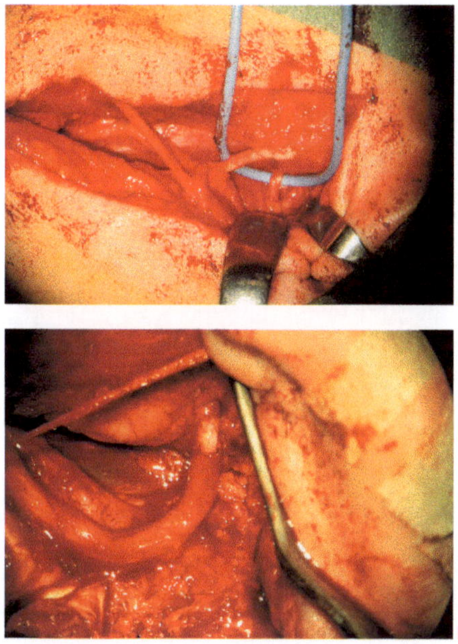
a
b

Figure 7.3 a, b.

Nerve transfer (left side). a Hypoglossal nerve beside the stylomastoid foramen, facial nerve at the *blue loop*, great auricular nerve preserved; b after transsection of the facial nerve and nerve anastomosis

[illegible]

lower mandible. Surgery starts with the same skin incision and approach as described in the previous chapter concerning exposure of the central part of the facial nerve beyond the stylomastoid foramen [illegible]

[illegible]

Nerve Tumors

The introduction of microsurgery and the associated encouraging reports over the last 40 years have extended the indications for its use and improved our results in tumor cases. Nevertheless, we have often received patients in whom a palpable tumor mass had been removed with the end result of nerve paralysis. As to be expected, secondary nerve repair procedures then achieved a lower functional level than a microsurgical primary procedure during tumor removal would have produced. For that reason, it must be pointed out that a primary microsurgical access to tumor-affected nerves should be deemed absolutely necessary. The inadvertent removal of nerves can no longer be accepted.

8.1 Symptoms and Diagnosis

Each space-occupying lesion involving nerve tissue, either extra- or intraneurally located, leads to an irritation of nerve axons causing the typical electric-current-like paresthesias and pain, comparable to symptoms of entrapment syndromes, and indicates degenerating and regenerating sprouts. The maximum point where these Tinel sign-like sensations can be elicited safely directs the location of the possibly growing tumor mass. If this mass is situated superficially it can be easily palpated, and then it usually proves as movable transverse to the nerve course and not in the longitudinal direction.

A growing mass within a nerve trunk first leads to degeneration of the myelin sheath, which can be measured by decreased conduction velocity in electroneurographic tests. Increased intraneural pressure causes the process referred to as Wallerian degeneration, which can be visualized by electromyographic tests: the investigation then reveals larger polyphasic and simultaneously longer potentials.

In advanced cases, neurological deficits also appear. If still in doubt as to the type of lesion, magnetic resonance imaging (MRI) should be performed to prove the existence of the tumor.

In conclusion, diagnosis involves:

- Palpation of tumor mass
- Assessment of special nerve-related deficits
- Evidence of a Tinel sign with maximum point at a special location
- Magnetic resonance imaging as an optional investigation

8.2 Therapy and Prognosis

Without operative exploration and tumor removal, the patient's disease will result in nerve paralysis. Therefore, surgery is mandatory, particularly in cases of benign histology. Since we do not know the histology before surgery, it is also required in order to answer the question concerning tumor dignity. However, when a general surgeon is unexpectedly confronted with a tumor traversed by a nerve, complete familiarity with microsurgical techniques is necessary if the intention is to intervene. If not, the operation should be stopped and more experienced surgeons called in; a macrosurgical technique will damage nerve axons and nerve function. Even a diagnostic biopsy endangers nerve axons and leaves behind scar tissue involving the outer layers of the tumor sheath. Thus, the situation usually encountered during secondary microsurgical tumor removal will result in a poorer prognosis.

The exploration first requires soft tissue separation, generally large enough to identify the involved nerve above and below the tumor. There should be 2–3 cm of the entering and exiting nerve segments visible, because the microsurgical procedure then starts at these healthy nerve segments. Skin incisions to be chosen follow the same principles that we developed to explore entrapment and trauma-related lesions: incisions should never run transverse over skin creases; two-portal approaches save soft tissue structures and avoid transsection of muscles. Patient and limb positions are always very similar to those chosen for entrapment surgery.

If the tumor is not simply attached to the nerve, like a solitary lipoma, but originates from the nerve, the epineurium of one of its two entering segments is longitudinally incised and partially removed so that a careful separation of fascicle groups is possible; the same procedure is repeated on the opposite nerve segment.

In case of benign tumors such as neurinomas, neurofibromas, intraneural ganglion cysts and quite rare cavernomas as well as hemangiomas, most of the fascicles and fascicle groups divide slightly and seem to disappear between outer layers of the particular tumor sheath or under a thin and widened layer of the nerve epineurium.

By gently incising these outer layers along nerve fibers, in cases of benign, solid neural sheath tumors, for example, many of these fibers can be identified as widespread over the tumor surface; under the microscope, they can be separated even more from inner tumor sheath layers. Returning to the entering and exiting nerve segments, the situation of neural sheath tumors finally makes it possible to identify the real microstructure from which the tumor originates. This small fascicle or fascicle group must be transected above and below the tumor. After ensuring that further adhesions between tumor and fascicles on its surface are excluded, the tumor itself can be easily removed as a whole mass. Very rarely, decreasing the tumor mass in order to facilitate the microsurgical separation of all the fascicles is necessary. If available, an ultrasound aspirator is helpful here.

As the anatomically visible fascicular nerve pattern does not simultaneously correspond to a functional grouping, the sacrifice of the involved fascicle or fascicle group does not automatically result in a substantial or measurable neurological deficit. Instead, a slight and diffuse functional loss emerges, and it is easily compensated during postoperative training.

The surgery of tumor-related nerve lesions presents particular dangers if structures of the brachial plexus, especially at the trunk level, are involved. On the one hand, its macro- and microanatomy is the most complex: within the junction between the C5 and C6 roots, we find an extremely plexiform microstructure over a short distance, which, after 1 cm, divides into one branch leading to the posterior cord, one to the lateral cord, a third one to the suprascapular nerve, and one more to the dorsal scapular nerve. Tumors involving this superior trunk area cause far more complex neurological deficits before and after operation. On the other hand, the plexus tissue also differs from more peripheral nerves in so far as an interfascicular pattern is absent in favor of a mono- or bifascicular structure (▶ Fig. 2.3 a). We find fewer collagen fibers within this large fascicle, and a perineurium is practically nonexistent. Therefore, the nerve structure has less resistance against manipulation, and the more sensitive the nerve structure is, the more necessary microsurgical techniques are. This makes macrosurgical removal of solitary tumors involving nerves in the lateral cervical triangle unacceptable.

Quite another comment on surgical prognosis has to be made concerning plexiform neurofibromas (see Sect. 8.3.3). They always originate from more than one fascicle group, and at the plexus level, they unfortunately tend to involve several trunks and perhaps grow into the neuroforamina. Such tumors can no longer be managed microsurgically, but instead, they need an en-bloc resection if possible at all, and if the patient accepts the subsequent sacrifice.

Tumors that are not solid also require an interfascicular preparatory dissection above and below the actual mass so as to visualize the number of structures that can be preserved. The following steps then need to be adapted to the different qualities of tumor growth: for example, one may unexpectedly run into a solitary or even multicystic intraneural ganglion, a vessel tumor, or even an infiltrating mass. Prognosis depends on the number of fibers preserved under the microscope.

8.3 Special Comments on Histology

8.3.1 Schwannomas (Neurinomas)

Schwannomas originate from Schwann cells of one nerve fascicle. Two series published by Kline and coworkers showed that the most common age is about 40, and that proximal locations are more frequent; consequently, plexus involvement occurs rather more frequently than believed (Donner et al. 1994; Lusk et al. 1987). In our comparably smaller experiments, these results were confirmed.

Brain nerves, with the exception of the first two, and peripheral nerves have a typical transitional zone where astrocytes stop and Schwann cells and collagen fibers start. Only the latter peripheral nerve segments can serve as the origin of a schwannoma. Tumor removal need sacrifice only one fascicle, as described above in detail (▶ Figs. 8.1, 8.2). The postoperative deficit remains insignificant. If operated early enough, the prognosis is conclusively excellent. Demyelinated axons caused by tumor pressure or surgical manipulation recover within 4–5 weeks. Axons suffering from axonotmesis recover within months by outgrowing. All the former targets can be finally achieved by nerve sprouts. There is no mis-sprouting to be expected.

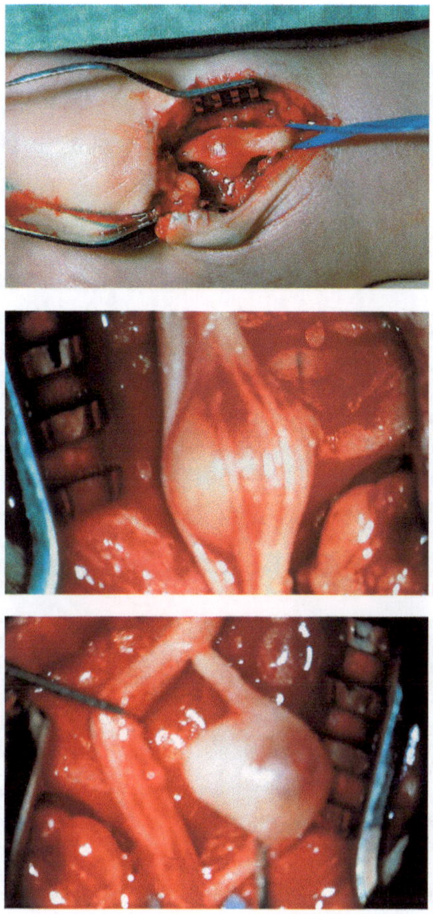

a b c

Figure 8.1 a–c

Digital nerve schwannoma. a Tumor exploration; b, c tumor originating from a single fascicle

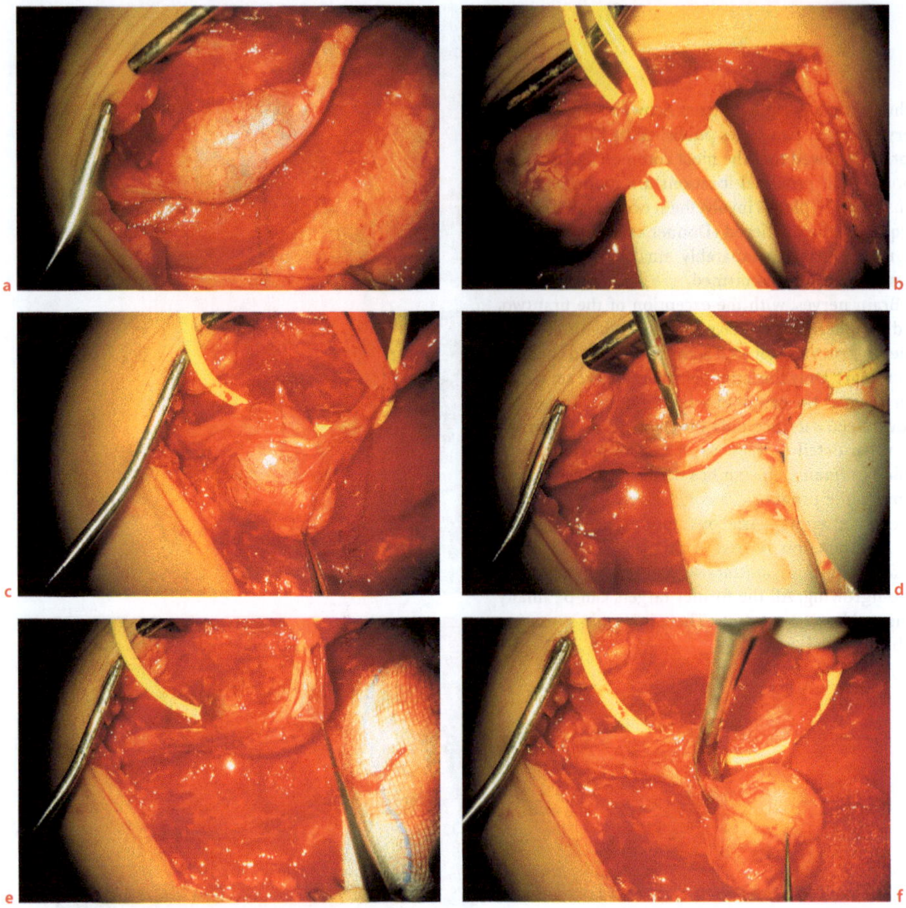

Figure 8.2 a–f

Ulnar nerve schwannoma of the upper arm. a Macroscopic view; b interfascicular separation above the tumor; c–e separation of noninvolved fascicles at tumor level; f transsection of the one involved fascicle

8.3.2 Neurofibromas

In 1987, Lusk and co-workers commented that epineurial fibrocytes should be the origin of neurofibromas, whereas Schwann cells should develop in the comparatively more benign neurinomas. The epineurial fibrocytes are more primitive cells, and they are therefore said to give rise to the more invasive neurofibromas. We have evidence that neurofibromas used to grow faster, involve not only one small fascicle, but very frequently at least one fascicle group or even a few fascicle groups, and we remember a higher rate of neurofibromas becoming malignant.

The principal surgery does not differ from surgical removal of schwannomas, but the structure the tumor is originating from presents larger, and therefore the particular preoperative deficit becomes more obvious. During microsurgery, intraoperative nerve stimulation mostly shows a complete functional loss in the involved fascicle group; consequently, its transsection and sacrifice are not yet a plausible explanation for additional deficits, but the separation and preservation of the remaining fascicles proves more difficult in detail because of severe adhesions to the tumor capsule.

Not rarely, multiple neurofibromas occur within one extremity simultaneously involving one or even several nerve trunks. All these tumors must theoretically be removed, using the above-mentioned technique. The patient must be aware that the tendency of neurofibromas to reoccur at other locations is higher if there are multiple tumor manifestations, thus requiring more frequent follow-up.

Neurofibromas in association with von Recklinghausen's disease (VRD) bear an even higher risk of secondary malignancy than tumors not associated with the disease. Therefore, if solitary and not plexiform (see the next section), its microsurgical removal should be the treatment of choice.

8.3.3 Plexiform Neurofibromas

Plexiform neurofibromas mean the manifestation of numerous neurofibromas originating from each fascicle group of one nerve trunk. These tumors may be located over a short or even a longer nerve distance. All tumors are together surrounded by a thin epineurial sheath. The entire mass is more likely to be painful than solitary schwannomas or neurofibromas. Besides an extremely intense Tinel sign, the tumor mass can be displaced only transverse to the expected course of the nerve trunk. As the tumor can originate in each fascicle group, complete removal would require sacrificing all fascicles and would lead to nerve paralysis (► Fig. 8.3a,b). Nerve repair by grafting should theoretically follow, but several arguments favor a conservative view in this situation: first of all, the number of available nerve grafts is limited, whereas the risk of tumor reccurrence at different nerve locations cannot be neglected, which would then need further resection and repair; secondly, it is never certain whether the nerve graft itself is free of tumor manifestation at the time of grafting (there is a higher risk of multiple occurrence in plexiform neurofibromas); thirdly, most patients are not ready to decide for a complete sacrifice of the preserved part of nerve function without guarantee of sufficient nerve recovery.

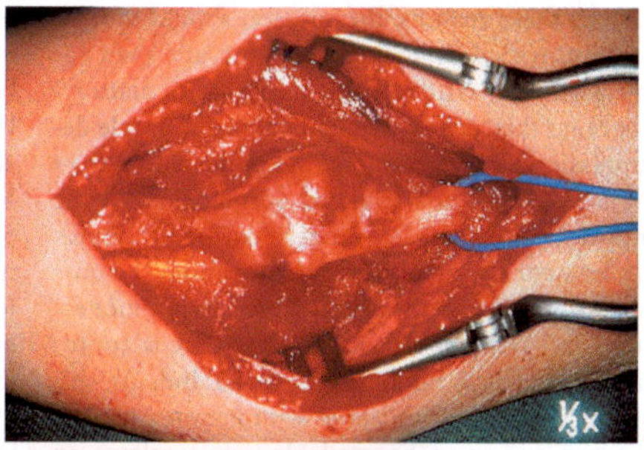

a

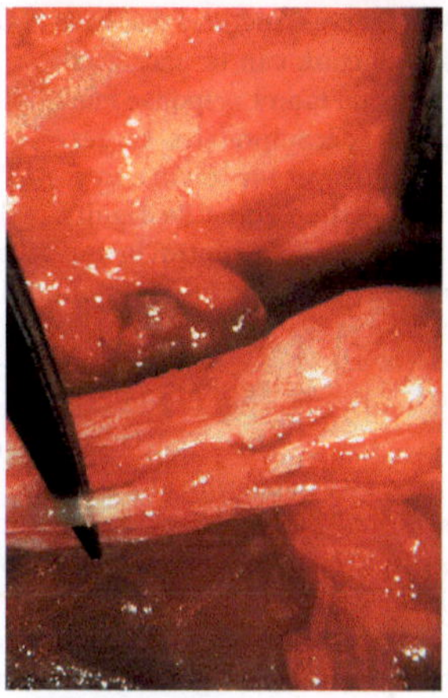
b

Figure 8.3a,b

Plexiform neurofibromas. a, b Tumors originating from each single fascicle

For all these reasons, the surgeon should discuss all options with the patient thoroughly, and then advise exploration at first, followed by careful neurolysis, because this technique should aim at a simple decompression. The circumferential epineurium must be removed, and the individual perineurium of the tumor-damaged fascicle groups must be longitudinally incised. Under higher magnification, the surgeon must now make the decision on which tumor resection and simultaneous fascicle sacrifice is appropriate, and which tumor to leave behind. At this moment, intraoperative nerve stimulation provides assistance and must be available, while relaxation must be ended. Tumor-like nerve structures that have lost their former motor function can be sacrificed, structures with preserved vital motor response must remain in continuity. Such decompressive surgery will reduce the triggered pain over the lesion and simultaneously answer the question about its dignity. Tumors to be left must be held under control by further manual palpation and eventual MRI.

8.3.4 Malignant Neural Sheath Tumors

A fast-growing tumor mass associated with an extensively positive Tinel sign and acute radiating pain when gently touched is suspicious of malignancy and simultaneous nerve involvement. Nevertheless, in surgical routine, most of these rare malignant neural sheath tumors are not suspected of being malignant at first, and therefore they frequently are blamed on biopsies or attempted tumor removal. However, a malignant histology after such attempts calls for muted action under any circumstances. The differential diagnosis between benign and malignant in cases of neural sheath tumors was reported as being not quite error-free. But a malignant histology indeed calls for en-bloc resection associated with complete nerve sacrifice. If preoperative investigations revealed no evidence of metastases, even the amputation of the involved extremity must be taken into consideration; if not, a higher risk of malignant reccurrence affecting the nerve stumps remains. A small remaining risk must be expected with the proximal nerve stump following amputation, because malignancy in the peripheral nervous system may be comprehended in terms of proceeding transformations of genes comparable to the situation of untreatable gliomas of the central nervous system. The value of adjuvant chemotherapy and radiation is still under debate, as recently pointed out by Ferner and Gutmann in 2002, who are investigating the issue with a multicenter study.

8.3.5 Ganglion Cysts

In terms of the rate of occurrence, ganglion cysts should be mentioned in third position in nerve-related tumors, after neurinomas and neurofibromas. Many of these ganglion cysts arise from joints or synovial sheaths. Several of these cysts compress nerves from outside, such as the Baker cyst of the popliteal fossa. These sometimes large solitary cysts are frequently connected with joints. Nevertheless, some of these cysts are not truly connected to joints. Their removal requires exploration of the affected nerve, followed by microsurgical separation of nerve tissue and cyst capsule.

Not quite comparable to these cysts causing an external nerve compression, similar cysts may alternatively occur within the interfascicular nerve tissue. Therefore, they remain surrounded by the epineurial sheath. These cysts require greater microsurgical efforts. They are completely attached to the perineural tissue of one fascicle, making its sacrifice reasonable. It is not known why intraneural cysts prefer to occur in the neighborhood of joints. We observed a predilection for occurrence near the wrist and elbow joints and within the tarsal tunnel.

Comparable to plexiform neurofibromas, multiple intraneural cysts over nerve distances of 10–15 cm were observed; therapy modalities are being debated (▶ Fig. 8.4). In our experience, removal of the affected nerve segments with nerve repair should no longer be considered; a microsurgical access following the above-mentioned principles should be the treatment of choice instead. As the multiple cysts originate from the perineurium of multiple fascicles, microsurgical removal of all the cyst walls must be avoided. Instead, each individual cyst must be opened only and evacuated. It is important to incise the epineurium of the nerve trunk far enough proximal and distal to ensure that none of these cysts are left behind. After cyst evacuation, the capsules may be dissected and only partially removed. The individual fascicles must be preserved to guarantee preserved postoperative nerve function. All our cases remained free of recurrence despite leaving parts of the tumor capsules behind (Tatagiba and Penkert 1992).

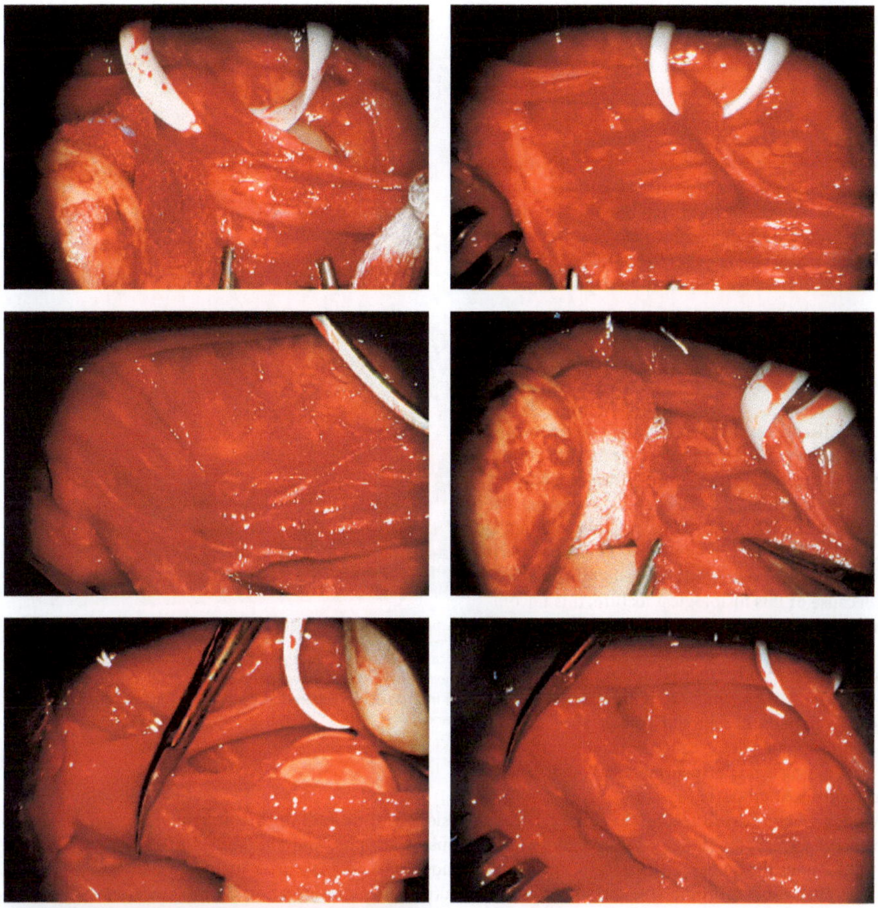

a b c d e f

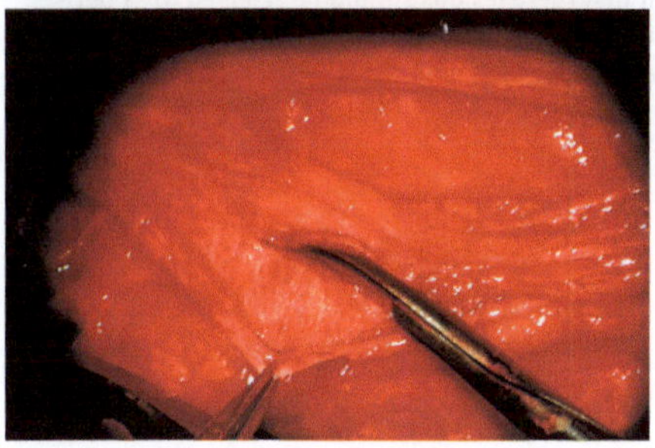

g

Figure 8.4 a–g

Multicystic intraneural ganglions, peroneal nerve beside the tibial–fibular joint. a Presentation after epineurotomy; b–e interfascicular separation, at the end one fascicle involved; f, g cysts opened, cyst walls remain in place

8.3.6 Glomus Tumors

The small glomus tumors arise from sympathetic fibers of final nerve branches and are situated under nail beds or in the subungual area of digits and toes. These tumors are much less common elsewhere on the extremity. They usually cause extremely sharp, nonradiating pain. Sometimes a dark point under the nail can be seen and should facilitate the diagnosis. The extirpation of these small tumors requires knowing how to incise beside or through a nail. Hand surgeons may be more familiar with these procedures.

8.3.7 Local Hypertrophic Neuropathy – Perineurioma

This rare disease results in hardening and thickening of a short nerve segment. Several case reports present only a few cases; the true nature of this disorder remains unclear. In 1995, Kline and co-workers described a proliferation of perineural cells surrounding each individual myelinated fiber. Fibrous tissue is said to tend to whorl around each individual nerve fiber. Because of this histological feature, this uncommon disease is referred to as "onion whorl disease." The origin of these lesions, which would provide a distinction between trauma-related or more tumor-like lesions, is not known, nor are treatment modalities clearly defined. Recently, Schröder (2001) ranked these lesions with what is called perineurioma, a tumor originating from perineurial cells, which usually develops from fibroblasts.

We have had one case affecting the peroneal nerve in the popliteal fossa (▶ Fig. 8.5). A skiing injury a few years before was the only trauma in the patient's history and, after a slowly progressive and finally subtotal peroneal palsy, a circumscribed neuroma was suspected and revealed by a highly dissolvable MRI study. The only option was to explore the nerve. A local hypertrophic nerve segment was found within the popliteal fossa and treated by internal neurolysis. At the end of the procedure, each fascicle group could be separated from the others but was left behind as a progressively hardening structure. Experience with similar cases described by Kline and Hudson led to their advice to resect these lesions and repair them by grafting. Similar small experiences are described in Birch (1998). Unfortunately, the diagnosis of these lesions is made over a long period of time, perhaps several years, propitious for advanced and irreversible atrophy of muscles. Predicting the prognosis following either neurolysis or grafting on these uncommon lesions will depend on the amount of preoperative muscle atrophy, and the still limited but growing knowledge on their true histological presentation. Taking into consideration Schröder's recent statement that these lesions should be referred to as perineurioma, better results can perhaps be expected from grafting than neurolysis.

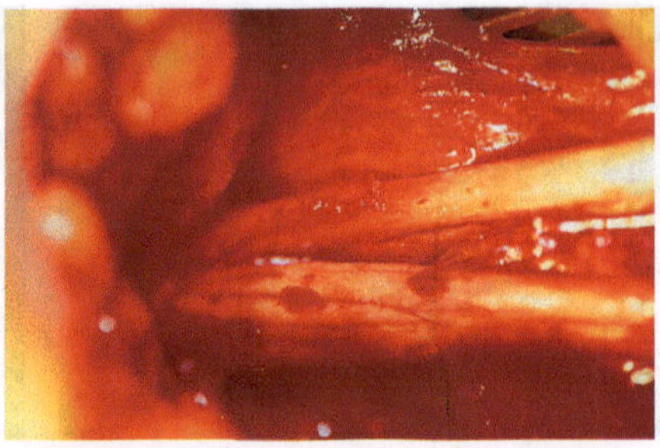
a

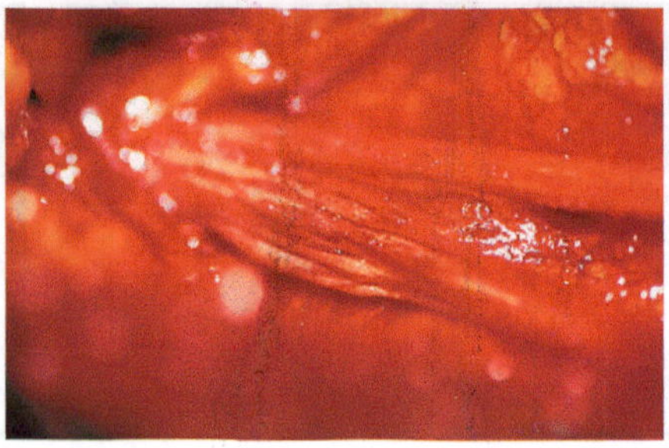
b

Figure 8.5 a, b

Local hypertrophic neuropathia (perineurioma). **a** Tibial nerve *above*, thickened peroneal nerve *below*, tibial fossa area; **b** after interfascicular separation, pathological fascicles remain in place

Pain Related to Nerve Trauma

9.1 Definition of Types of Pain

Untreatable pain related to a peripheral nerve trauma often results in complete social isolation of the patient. Many physicians tend to attach the label "psychologically peculiar" to persons with chronic pain that is more or less resistant to treatment. But what kind of treatment is really available if a nerve lesion causes more severe pain than first expected? It is not the purpose of this chapter to repeat all the facts and theories on the development of particularly severe pain following nerve damage, referred to as chronic neuropathic pain or causalgia: the literature discusses centrally located biochemical reactions and – with regard to the course of the sympathetic nerve system – newly occurring synaptic contacts between neighboring axons. Details can be derived from Wall's and Melzack's 1994 book showing that many unsolved questions remain for further research.

We will attempt to limit ourselves to experience derived from surgical treatment of peripheral nerve lesion-related pain. The possibility of ongoing severe pain after nerve injury was described very early by Mitchell in 1872, 1 year before the first efforts on nerve suture were tried by Hueter in 1873. Although theories, knowledge and rules on different types of nerve lesion and different types of tissue reaction following nerve injury were established (see Chap. 2), reliable explanations about the different intensities of pain resulting from such damage are totally lacking.

It is well known that nerve fibers after transsection regrow into the periphery or develop an amputation neuroma at a proximal nerve end, resulting in forces that run efferent. If we trigger these nerve ends or the neuroma by palpation or percussion transcutaneously, it causes electric-current-like pain that the patient localizes in the former distribution area of the injured nerve, known as neuroma pain, probably identical to the origin of the Tinel sign.

There is also evidence that injured peripheral nerves produce an abnormal biochemical and electrical activity in the afferent direction. These activities serve as a theoretical basis to explain why some patients, but not all, develop unusual and excruciating pain. Different individual dispositions, whose details are unknown, seem to be responsible for identical nerve lesions causing adverse reactions in some patients. Experiments done by Inbal and co-workers in 1980 on different types of rats revealed different measurable amounts of autotomy following identical procedures on nerves, and concluded that different genetic dispositions exist. If the normal nociceptive afferences change into hyperpathic nerve-related pain, this situation is referred to as neuropathic pain.

The term "hyperpathia" now means that a single stimulus may awaken no particular reaction, but if it is repeated or only slowly moved, it causes a sensation reaching intolerable levels for the patient. On the other hand, this type of pain sometimes needs more time than the stimulus itself takes to decrease or disappear.

"Allodynia" (complex regional pain syndrome, CRPS, according to the most recent taxonomy) means a slightly more severe situation: in these cases, a quite light stimulus applied to a small skin area provokes a highly painful sensation that spreads away from the actual stimulus location. The stimulus itself would be felt as innocuous when applied to unaffected skin. Allodynia is characteristically predisposed by nerve lesions located at high proximal levels (Sunderland 1991). It occurs in spite of measurable nerve regeneration in the normal motor and sensitive function. Frequently, there are sudden onsets, and it occurs earlier than neuroma pain does, which usually starts 6–8 weeks after injury.

In conclusion, we see three levels of pain following a nerve trauma or nerve transsection: (a) neuroma pain, a normally nonexistent pain, only occurring when triggered; (b) hyperpathic pain, a normally nonexistent pain, but of unbearable intensity if the skin in the distribution area of the injured nerve is repeatedly stimulated; and (c) allodynia, a pain which is permanently present as a burning sensation, for instance, and evocable by an innocuous stimulus. The last two levels of pain are referred to as neuropathic.

9.2 Treatment Modalities

9.2.1 Neurolysis and Nerve Repair

If the patient presents a situation that we evaluate as at level of neuroma pain, microsurgery, perhaps including the different steps of neurolysis, offers a chance of improving the patient's outcome. An additional nerve transposition such as in a case of non-transposed ulnar nerves can already improve the situation by embedding the hypersensitive nerve segment into a better sheltered area of the extremity. Microneurolysis requires that one is aware of the plexiform nerve structure because interchanging nerve fibers leave one fascicle group and join the surrounding group in numbers that differ from one patient to another (see Chap. 5). If nerve continuity was proved to be interrupted, restoration of continuity in order to improve motor function and sensitivity has priority. Following neurolysis, transposition, or nerve grafting, the neuroma pain is for the most part reduced by being extended over the entire nerve distance. The patient feels the trigger point and the occurrence of neuroma pain moving slowly downward into the periphery, where it finally disappears at the distal extremity end.

On relatively rare occasions, contrary to the above-described usual development, patients may suffer from a highly characteristic syndrome of ongoing pain and abnormal sensitivity in the area that the damaged nerve formally supplied. As has already been mentioned, this unusual pain level may show a sudden onset, starts earlier than neuroma pain, and, if evoked by perhaps normally innocuous stimuli, be more intense than expected. It is often difficult for the patient to describe the neuropathic pain. The literature is not very rich in experiments where microsurgical procedures were used with those special painful lesions. Noordenbos and Wall (1981) reported seven patients suffering from neuropathic pain who received surgical transsection and excision of the damaged nerve segment. Five of seven nerves were repaired by insertion of sural nerve grafts to bridge the nerve gap. The authors argued for nerve resection and restoration, with the well-known high rate of success in cases of nerve lesion where pain was not the dominant symptom. In two cases, the affected nerve was resected back into apparently normal and soft tissue so that the later expected neuroma would be better embedded. The authors came to the conclusion that, with one exception, all these special patients with hyperpathia or allodynia should not have been treated by secondary nerve resection. These interven-

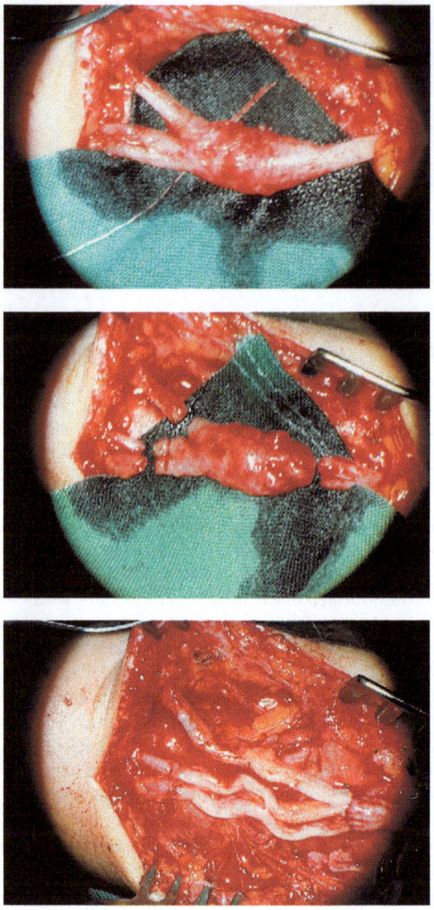

a

b

c

Figure 9.1 a–c

Painful neuroma of the superficial radial nerve branch at ramification level. a Neuroma in continuity; b transsection of all individual fascicles; c reconstruction with sural nerve pieces tions were deemed failures because the patients had pain recurrence or even duplication when examined 20–72 months after the nerve resection. It must be pointed out that the authors stressed that conclusions on expected therapy success can only be based on long-term follow-up, after a period of over 19 months on average for these seven cases. Our own experience does not differ.

In conclusion, it is of major importance to evaluate the type of pain first, and to distinguish between neuroma pain and neuropathic pain before surgery. Touching the nerve by means of neurolysis or nerve repair is only allowed in neuroma. Nevertheless, even in this case, a deteriorating development from neuroma pain toward "neuropathic" pain may be secondarily induced by the surgeon, a risk that should influence our preoperative explanations to the patient.

The location of the neuroma decides where to place the skin incision. The principles to be followed in its extension do not differ from those concerning other trauma cases and should be derived from Chaps. 5 and 6 (▶ Fig. 9.1).

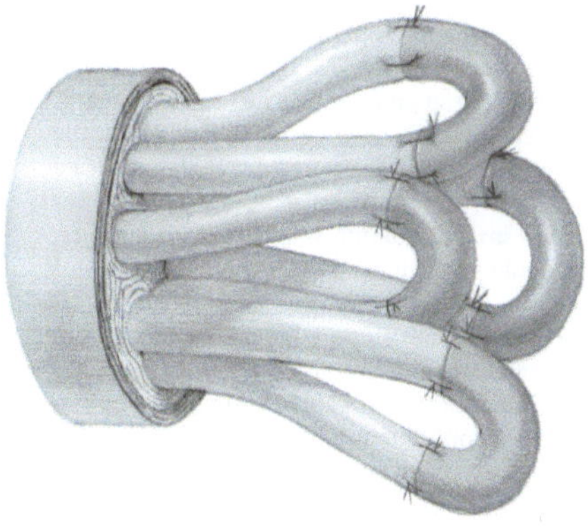

Figure 9.2

Principle of centro-central grafting to avoid terminal neuroma-associated pain

9.2.2 Centro-Central Grafting

Terminal neuromas result either from traumatic nerve sections or from limb amputations. In the latter case, nerve continuity cannot be restored; in the first case, nerve repair as treatment of neuroma pain should be the first priority, but it will probably not succeed when an injured skin nerve has less than a pencil lead diameter or when the nerve lesion involves its peripheral ramification.

It must be remembered that microsurgical procedures on terminal neuroma are reserved for neuroma pain cases exclusively. In contrast, neuropathic pain due to neuroma could be significantly worsened by microsurgery, whatever the type. The first and most important task therefore consists of excluding hyperpathia or even allodynia cases. The remaining normal terminal neuroma cases may be treated by nerve grafting if the anatomical situation allows it.

The alternative consists of a method that has been referred to as centro-central anastomosis or grafting. Earlier, Seddon tried to reduce terminal neuroma pain by end-to-end suturing two fascicles of the proximal nerve stump. Samii (1981) modified this procedure by interposing U-shaped grafts between two fascicles (▶ Fig. 9.2). Unfortunately, very little further research has been done on this interesting but again time-consuming method. A significantly reduced autotomy rate was found following centro-central grafting, then compared to simple nerve segment resection done in rat experiments, results that encourage extending this method in humans (Gonzalez-Darder et al. 1985). Histological investigations of centro-centrally interposed grafts were said to give evidence that the outgrowing sprouts entered the grafts from both sides and stopped at the second suture line (Barberá et al. 1988). Unknown factors obviously seemed to prevent the sprouts from entering fascicles from the distal to proximal direction. To avoid new neuroma, an exact fascicular alignment had to be achieved surgically to exclude fiber aberrations at both suture lines (▶ Fig. 9.3). The authors assumed a reduction in the above-mentioned efferent and afferent ongoing forces within the axons. It appears obvious that additional experiments could probably succeed in answering further questions: for instance, the experimental application of our earlier-mentioned method to visualize outgrowing sprouts directly (Becker and Penkert 2000) may also confirm the histologically proven observations that the axons seem to stop at the second suture line. In addition, quantitative studies of anterograde transport rates within nerve fibers, already done in primates by means of repeated recordings of its mechanosensitivity, a method described by Koschorke et al. (1991), may allow future monitoring of different afferent- and efferent-running reactions on axon disruption. Unfortunately, this method may require further technical improvements to enable similar studies on rat or rabbit nerves. A centro-central anastomosis at the nerve end should reduce the anterograde transports significantly and over the long term.

If centro-central grafting is to be used in humans, it is of great importance to decide beforehand if the fascicular pattern of the affected nerve allows such a microsurgical procedure at all. Cutaneous nerves such as the small abdominal wall nerves, for instance, are generally not suitable. The same holds true for digital nerves.

Patients with limb amputation are excluded from restoration of nerve continuity. They can experience several different types of pain affecting the amputation stump. Also, different combinations of pain types individually occur, including:

- Stump pain: a pain that remains localized at the stump. It includes several local sensory abnormalities of nonneural origin and the typical neuroma pain, which can be triggered by percussion and palpation of the peculiar neuroma.
- Phantom pain: a pain that is localized in areas of the amputated limb. Its occurrence used to be explained by centrally located alterations, but reliable explanations are lacking.
- Neuralgia: a pain that occurs like an attack in the peripheral nerve stump's distribution.
- Causalgia: a pain felt like a burning of the former distribution area of the affected nerve, more or less identical to what was described above as allodynia, but with the difference that the pain intensity is no longer susceptible to stimulating the affected skin area.

In terms of the neuroma pain component only, microsurgical centro-central grafting can succeed if an amputee requests treatment. Patients with the other pain types are candidates for intraspinal neuromodulation techniques. The usually difficult differentiation between the various types of pain associated with a stump may be supported by locally blocking injections, which stop the terminal neuroma pain only. It is the patient who then decides if this situation might be of help.

The fascicular pattern of the involved nerve stump following limb amputation (i.e., of the sciatic, femoral, peroneal, or tibial nerves) does not play as important a role as in cases of skin or terminal nerves. Nerve trunks have enough fascicle groups to interpose U-shaped grafts and to achieve sufficient interfascicular alignment (▶ Fig. 9.3b). There is no need for a sural nerve graft; instead, the grafts can be taken from the nerve stump itself. With interfascicular separation of several fascicle groups, about 4–5 cm of

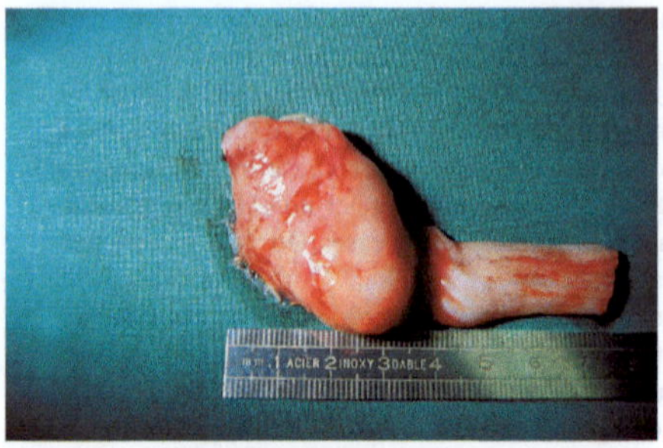

a

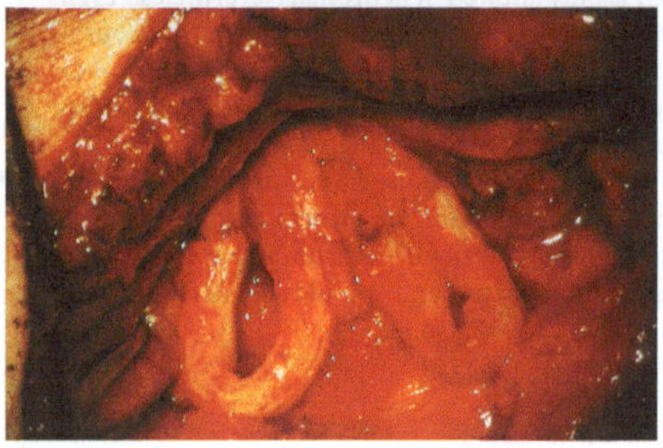

b

Figure 9.3 a, b

Amputation (terminal) neuroma, sciatic nerve. a Resected nerve with neuroma; b centro-centrally positioned grafts

the nerves can be resected so that they can be interposed in a U-shaped manner. Of course, this microsurgical procedure requires large-scale nerve exposure. The roughly 10- to 15-cm skin incision runs parallel to the well-known nerve trunk, with the patient either prone or supine. Simultaneous treatment on femoral and sciatic nerve stumps, for instance, is therefore impossible. The skin incision must not touch the limb stump end to avoid hypersensitive scars. After finishing the microsurgical procedure, the wound must be closed very carefully to avoid graft displacement, a delicate procedure during the final operating step. The primary surgeons use to preserve as much muscle tissue as possible around the stump end; this muscle mass often tends to displace grafts during wound closure. Finally, a period of 10 days of immobilization of the stump is mandatory so that the patient does not put weight on the stump at all.

9.2.3 Peripheral Neuromodulation

The last two chapters have dealt with microsurgical treatment modalities used on damaged nerves associated with pain within a tolerable range. In contrast, hyperpathia or allodynia pain is not treatable with reconstructive microsurgical methods. Clinical evidence reported by Noordenbos and Wall in 1981 has shown that microsurgery remained unsuccessful or even duplicated the pain level in a significant number of cases.

The idea of achieving pain relief by electrically stimulating the dorsal columns of the spinal cord (spinal cord stimulation, SCS) was derived from the gate control theory by Melzack and Wall in 1965. According to this concept, a stimulation of large afferent A-fibers of peripheral nerves should reduce the pain input to the brain via the small unmyelinated and thinly myelinated C-fibers. As the conduction velocity of A-fibers is faster than the that of C-fibers, A-fibers were said to have capacity to "gate out" pain stimuli from transmission to the cortex. Although since disproved, Melzack's idea also led to the concept of peripheral neuromodulation (peripheral nerve stimulation, PNS) which was first tested by Wall and Sweet in 1967. Fortunately, stimulation at high frequencies proved to stimulate A-fibers exclusively. Until further research provides further evidence, this is the only peripheral nerve surgery available in cases of different types of neuropathic pain of damaged nerves.

The operation technique is quite simple. In a first operation with general or even local anesthesia, the affected nerve is explored proximal or, in special situations, distal to the lesion. Using magnification, the nerve epineurium is pierced, and the quadripolar electrode is slightly pushed into the subepineurial space a few centimeters distal or proximal, depending on the affected nerve and its availability (▶ Fig. 9.4). After a test stimulation period of a few days, the external screener is changed into an internal one placed subcutaneously like a pacemaker. Technical details can be derived from Medtronic's guides on pacemaker lead implantation. In the US, flat leads with flat quadripolar electrodes are positioned inferior to the targeted nerve, and a flap of fascial tissue is placed between them to create a protective layer. In Europe, rod electrodes are placed in a subepineurial position.

The principle of both the first and second operations is very simple. Indeed, the main questions concerning this method involve the caliber and location of the target nerve and not in the principle of the procedure itself.

First, the affected nerve may be difficult to approach because situated within the retroperitoneal space (e.g., iliohypogastric, ilioinguinal, genitofemoral, and obturator nerves).

Second, cutaneous nerves may be small in diameter and localized rather far in the periphery and in the neighborhood of joints (e.g., the infrapatellar nerve) so that implanting a lead has a higher risk of later displacement.

It has sometimes proved of worth to expose the targeted nerve under local anesthesia, a situation making it possible to test the electrode and to prevent a displacement during the procedure. Additionally, some nerve divisions can distinguish between main motor and sensory branches. An approach under local anesthesia at the level of the radial nerve ramification, for instance, makes it possible to choose the superficial branch as the only target, a nerve which is quite often involved, and to exclude inadvertent side effects on motor fibers (▶ Fig. 9.4b–e).

It is also important to try to create situations where the electrical wire need bridge only one extremity joint.

In spite of some of the above-mentioned limitations, we should use neuromodulation techniques far more, as a method that, on the one hand, does not induce further damage to already neuropathically affected nerves, and on the other hand, has proved to be successful in pain relief or, at least, in pain reduction in more than 80% of cases, according to the published series of Hassenbusch et al. (1996) and Shetter et al. (1997).

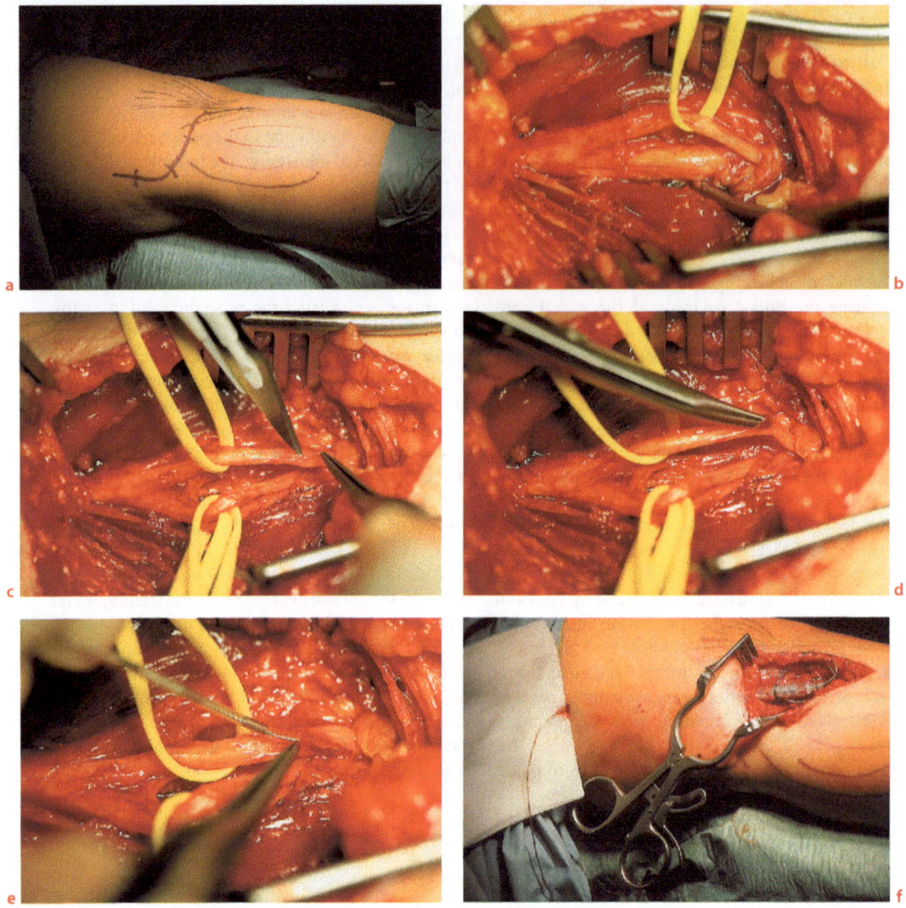

Figure 9.4 a–f

Peripheral nerve stimulation of the superficial radial nerve branch. **a** Skin incision, right arm, view from patient's head; **b** exploration of the superficial branch (*yellow loop*), deep branch, and motor branch to the short wrist extensor; **c, d** epineurotomy; **e** subepineurial positioning of the pad electrode; **f** placement of the connections

Part III

Muscle and Tendon Transfers in Peripheral Nerve Lesions

Muscle and Tendon Transfer

10.1 Introduction

This chapter aims to explain the standard operations in muscle and tendon transfer in reconstructive surgery. The operations are described in detail; however, the transfers should be performed by surgeons who are experienced with the presented techniques to offer the patient the best outcome.

The techniques of muscle and tendon transfer (MTT) were established mostly by orthopedic and general surgeons long before peripheral nerve surgery was introduced into clinical practice. MTT was established not only for reconstruction after nerve lesions, especially after gunshot wounds in the world wars, but to restore function after peripheral nerve diseases such as poliomyelitis and leprosy. While in poliomyelitis sensation remains normal, in leprosy and in most peripheral nerve lesions (depending on the level of lesion) sensation is absent. This underlines that sensation is not always a necessary prerequisite for motor reconstruction. However, with increasing vaccination programs, poliomyelitis has been eradicated in Europe and North America, and with popularization of microsurgical nerve reconstruction, the techniques of MTT were almost forgotten. After reconstructive surgeons and neurosurgeons realized that MTT should be an important part of the concept of how to treat patients with injured nerves, in the beginning of the 1980s MTT experienced a renaissance.

The principles of MTT are very simple, although special requirements must be considered before the operation. MTT is accompanied by a very special tool, called dynamic tenodesis: a tendon or tendon graft is fixed between the disturbed joint and a healthy joint. The motion of the healthy joint then activates the tenodesis, which acts on the disturbed joint and allows proper motion (for details see Fowler tenodesis in Chap. 11.4.5.2).

MTT aims to reconstruct dynamic muscle balance. Thus, operations with static results such as arthrodesis or static tenodesis are only considered as the last options in reconstructive surgery.

Today, indications for MTT include:

- Peripheral nerve lesions where either nerve reconstruction was not successful or nerve reconstruction is not indicated
- Trauma to muscles and tendons
- Functional loss due to vascular problems (such as ischemic contracture/compartment syndrome)
- Congenital malformations
- Tetraplegia
- Cerebral palsy
- Spasticity of muscles (in combination with other procedures)

This chapter presents the general principles of MTT and focuses on functional reconstruction after traumatic nerve lesions.

10.2 General Principles

10.2.1 Prerequisites

In addition to the technical considerations, MTT requires absolute compliance from the patient. It is mandatory for the surgeon to explain the complete procedure to the patient, benefits and pitfalls, duration of the postoperative course and possible problems. The surgeon and patient then have to decide whether they want to go the route of reconstruction together.

MTT is the final step in rehabilitation. Whether the original cause of imbalance has been traumatic, congenital, infectious, or vascular, the respective extremity must be evaluated in terms of function lost and function retained. This includes first a satisfactory range of passive joint motion. Immediately after loss of function, physical therapy and occupational therapy should start. The passive joint motion should be

Table 10.1. Evaluating muscles for transfer

Retained function	Muscle available for transfer	Needed function	Operation
Hip flexion (M4)	M. iliopsoas		
Hip extension (M4)	M. gluteus maximus		Single stage possible
Hip adduction (M3)	M. adductor		
Hip adduction (M4)	longus/magnus		
(No Trendelenburg)	M. gracialis		
Knee flexion (M4)	M. gluteus minimus		
Foot flexion (M4)	M. biceps femoris →	Knee extension	
Toe flexion (M4)	M. semitendinosus →	Knee extension	
Great toe extension (M5)	M. semimembranosus		
	M. triceps surae		
	M. tibialis posterior →	Foot dorsiflexion	
	M. flexor digiti longus		
	M. flexor hallucis longus		
	M. extensor hallucis longus		

retained and if necessary the extremity must be splinted to avoid contractures of functioning and stretching of denervated muscles (e.g., a splint for radial nerve injury). MTT that includes stiff joints makes no sense. An arthrolysis or tenolysis, if contractures are present, to improve the range of motion, may be required prior to any transfer (Beasly 1970).

Second, in some cases the extent of the initial trauma precludes MTT because of malalignment of bone or visible and subcutaneous scarring that would impair tendon function by adhering. Correction prior to a transfer might include osteotomy, bone grafts, and pedicled or free flaps. Thus, MTT should only be carried out in a scar-free area that allows the transferred muscles and tendons to move freely.

Third, it has always been noted that motor reconstruction should only be done after a loss of sensitivity has been restored. This allows moving the extremity without visual control. Of course, if possible, sensitivity should be restored prior to MTT. However, we found that even in an extremity with lost sensitivity, function can be restored satisfactorily. This requires that the patient is taught to use his extremity carefully and protect it from harm such as hot water, shoes that are too tight, etc. Programs are already in use, especially for diabetic patients, which can be easily adapted for patients with nerve lesions.

10.2.2 Evaluating Muscles for Transfer

Before selecting a muscle for transfer the lost function and the retained function have to be documented meticulously. It is important to know the function that is needed and all muscles that are available for transfer. It is therefore helpful to list all the available muscles and the functions that are to be restored. These lists can then be matched, which facilitates planning. For example, as illustrated in ▶ Table 10.1, the patient suffered from a right lumbosacral plexus lesion with loss of knee extension and foot dorsiflexion.

It is of importance to judge the expendability of a muscle for transfer. Restoring one major function at the expense of another major function is contraindicated. For example, using both intact wrist flexors (flexor carpi ulnaris muscle, FCU, and flexor carpi radialis muscle, FCR) for finger extension causes an imbalance, with an unstable, hyperextended wrist and the inability to extend the fingers completely (Zachary 1946).

The strength of the muscle that should be transferred must be evaluated very carefully. The muscle should not be reinnervated or fibrotic. Clinical examination usually allows isolated muscle testing and grading of strength according to the British Medical Research Council (BMRC) scale from 0 to 5.

0 No contraction
1 Only palpable contraction
2 Active movement without gravity (poor)
3 Active movement against gravity (fair)
4 Active movement against resistance (good)
5 Normal strength

A muscle that is transferred usually looses up to one grade of strength. Thus, the strength should be good or normal when used for transfer. If clinical testing is doubtful, electromyography (EMG), ultrasound or MRT might be helpful to evaluate whether the muscle is reinnervated or is fibrotic due to a trauma. However, in our experience clinical testing and if necessary intraoperative assessment (color of muscle, intraoperative direct stimulation) are more predictable.

Although it was stated that it is not important whether the transferred muscle acts as a synergist or an antagonist, we found that re-education and rehabilitation is less difficult when the transfer is synergistic, for example, transfer of a wrist flexor to restore finger extension (▶ Fig. 10.1). These functions, wrist flexion and finger extension, and on the other hand wrist extension and finger flexion are considered synergistic, these combinations of movements are what make a functional hand! A flexed wrist never comes with flexed fingers! Thus synergistic movements are not just extension or flexion, but combinations of both functions that are memorized as movements.

Therefore, transferring a muscle within its synergistic group offers better results. If not available, an antagonist muscle can be used. We strongly recommend training the muscles that are to be transferred prior to the operation to improve strength and, more important, the consciousness for this special movement. This facilitates postoperative therapy considerably. Children can easily learn how to use the new function after MTT. However, the older the patient with a transfer is, the more difficult the postoperative learning process is.

The power of the muscles for transfer is determined as working capacity (WC). WC is defined as absolute muscle power (physiological cross-section) by amplitude of the respective muscle (in meters per kilogram, mkg; × 9,807=Joule). For transfers at the hand there are tables, established by Curtis (1974) and Brand (1974, 1988) that allow a preoperative assessment of the lost and retained function, and show whether the planned transfer will restore or hinder muscle balance.

Besides absolute muscle power, the amplitude of excursion should be sufficient for satisfactory function (Brand et al. 1981). The brachioradialis (BR) muscle, for example, is not sufficient to restore finger flexion due to its limited motion. However, excursion, especially of the BR, can be increased by dissecting its tendon proximally and freeing all of its fascial attachments. It then can be used to restore the long thumb flexor. In some cases, muscle excursion can be made sufficient by adding a dynamic tenodesis to the transfer (Buck-Gramcko and Nigst 1991).

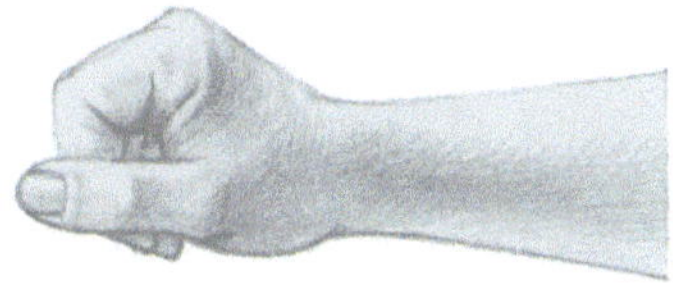

a

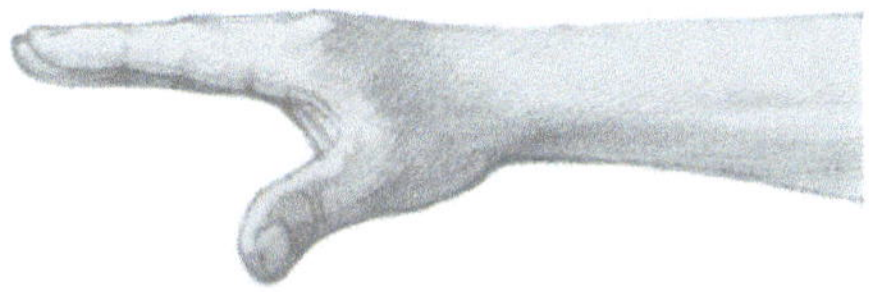

b

Figure 10.1

a Wrist extension and finger flexion are synergistic. b Wrist flexion and finger extension are also synergistic movements. A flexed wrist never comes with flexed fingers! Thus synergistic movements are not just extension or flexion, but combinations of both functions that are memorized as movements

10.2.3 Technical Considerations

Wherever possible, we prefer a bloodless situation. If intraoperative evaluation of the transferred muscle and its nerve is necessary, we avoid a tourniquet (leading to a nerve conduction block) and relaxation of the patient until diagnosis is made. As in all incisions, the relaxed tension lines should be respected. And straight incisions crossing joints are of course avoided. For identifying, dissecting and mobilizing, a short transverse incision is helpful; for suturing of the tendon or muscle, a greater incision might be necessary such as a lazy-S or L-shaped incision. The tendons can be easily identified underneath the fascia using a tendon hook, which makes it possible to atraumatically pull the respective tendon and to control the function by vision.

The transferred tendons should be routed subcutaneously. The tendons can be tunneled with special blunt forceps or a tendon weaver. When freeing the

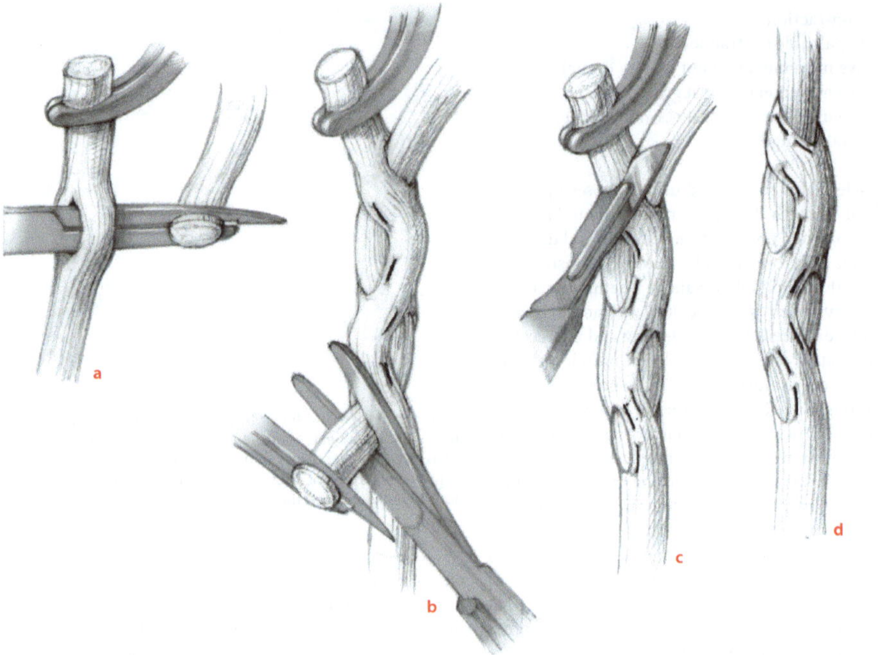

Figure 10.2 a–d

The transferred tendon is woven into the original tendon using the tendon weaver according to Buck-Gramcko. The suture knots are placed inside so as not to impair the gliding of the tendon. The ends of the tendons are resected and sutured. This type of tendon suture is according to Pulvertaft

muscle, keep in mind where the neurovascular bundle crosses the dissection. Prevent stretching, rotation, or other damage to nerve and vessels. Usually, the neurovascular bundle enters the muscle in the proximal third. Raw bone and fascia might impair gliding; thus care must be taken to avoid such obstacles.

The muscle and its tendon should not make an acute angle between origin and new attachment. This would impair the WC of the muscle, creates a bowstring effect, produces adherence, or it might injure the transferred tissue. However, when an acute angle is necessary, a pulley must be created.

Should it be necessary to split the transferred tendon and to anchor it to separate points, the muscle will, of course, act primarily on the tendon under greatest tension. This must be avoided by equalizing the tension on the split tendons (Smith 1980).

The new attachment is usually (especially in the hand) made by suturing the transferred tendon to the tendons of the paralyzed muscles. If a reversible transposition is made, the end-to-side suture is preferred. However, if no regeneration is anticipated the suturing is done in an end-to-end manner. Suturing is best done by weaving the transferred tendon into the original one (▶ Fig. 10.2). Other forms of suture are periosteal fixation, pull-out sutures, transosseous suture or transosseous tunneling. In transfers for the shoulder and lower extremity, if possible we transpose the muscle or tendon with its bony attachment, big enough to fix it with a screw. This preserves the natural tendon-bone attachment, which can only in parts be reconstructed by the surgeon. The place of the new attachment is then carefully roughened and the bone is fixed with a screw. Newly developed anchor systems such as cork-screw anchors are most helpful in fixating the rest of the tendon or the muscle. However, in our experience the sole use of anchors is not sufficient to create a long-lasting attachment when high forces are acting. Sutures should be nonabsorbable. In the hand, monofil material is sufficient; in transfers at the shoulder or knee, stronger polyfil material is required. The strength should follow the thickness and force of the transferred tendon. In the hand, for example, we use 3–0, 4–0 and 5–0 nylon sutures. For transfers at the shoulder, the sutures must be stronger, such as 0 or 2.

In some transfers, the correct tension of the transferred tendons and muscles is not important, as they are elongated as much as possible. However, especially in transfers for the injured hand, and when the muscle is completely detached from its origin and insertion, care should be taken to insert the muscle in correct tension. It is necessary to bring the distal part in to the function that is to be restored (e.g., to flex the elbow, when elbow flexion is restored), and then to suture the tendon or muscle under mild tension. An intraoperative dynamic control (moving the distal extremity carefully) is always mandatory. In transfers where the muscle is completely detached (then the muscle shrinks!), the correct tension of the muscle has to be marked prior to detachment, for example, by a running suture with a knot every 5 cm. After transfer, the correct tension is measured by these knots. Another method is (after inserting the muscle) simulation of function by carefully applying an electrical stimulus to the nerve (start with a low mode and increase step by step). If tension is too little, function is not sufficiently achieved.

The easier the transfer, the better the function. Thus, keep it as simple as possible.

10.2.4 Postoperative Course

Immobilization is the key to success in this kind of surgery. Splints are always applied to relax the transferred muscles and tendons as well as the sutures. Immobilization should last as long as it takes the tendon sutures or the transferred bony fragments to heal, from 3 to 6 weeks. One should avoid immediately removing the splint after the immobilization period. This would stretch the immobilized muscle and might impair the outcome. Thus, a light splint in reduced relaxation for the respective muscles is applied after rigid splinting. A night splint for protection is necessary in some transfers. In restoration of shoulder abduction for example, we lower the arm every week by 10–15°.

Usually, movement is not consciously done. As in most transfers, the new function has to be learned consciously: preoperative training of the muscle that is used for transfer is very important. This facilitates postoperative learning greatly (Wintsch 1972). Physical therapy and occupational therapy, especially in transfers at the hand, are mandatory after the splint has been removed. We found it very useful to establish a personal communication with the physical therapist. In some centers the therapists are informed about the transfer in the operating room. However, as these kinds of operations are done in special centers and therapists are usually near the patient's residence, we prefer personal contact (e.g., by phone). It is important to meticulously explain the lost function and the function of the transferred muscles prior to transfer. Thus a standard movement can be created by telling the patient to move the transferred muscle (old movement), relaxing the antagonists of the new movement and changing the position of the joint to increase the movement of the transferred muscle. For example, after using the superficial flexor (FDS) of the ring finger to restore the opposition of the thumb, physical therapy should begin with the hand hanging relaxed in the carpal joint. The patient is told to flex the ring finger (old movement) and to oppose the thumb (new movement) and to extend the carpal joint, which enforces the new movement.

In conclusion, we think that intensive postoperative training is as important as the operation itself. If the patient is not willing to spend this time (up to 6 months) after the operation for training, one should not operate on this patient.

10.2.5 Timing of Operation

Basically, MTT should be performed as early as possible in order to restore functional activity and prevent the development of poor patterns of motion. However, if a nerve is reconstructed one should estimate the recovery time. If 3 months after the time of expected recovery no signs of reinnervation are detectable, MTT should be done (Omer 1988). If initial exploration reveals an irreparable nerve or muscle loss, early transfer should be considered. In some cases it might be helpful to restore function with MTT parallel to the nerve reconstruction. This is especially favored in isolated proximal distal nerve lesions (e.g., radial, ulnar, or peroneal nerves). The transfers then act as an internal splint, preventing joint deformities and allowing other muscles to act properly. In very special cases (long recovery time, old patient, or patient with malignant tumor) we do not explore the nerve, but immediately perform a MTT to allow early function.

There are some transfers that can be done in a single-stage operation. In the hand, however, multiple stages are necessary when more than one function is to be restored. This is due to the needed operation time and the mandatory splinting. It is advised to start with the flexors and to restore the extensors in a second stage. Usually, we start with the most desired function and/or the function that can be restored easily. This very much increases patient's motivation for training and surgery.

Transfers for Functional Reconstruction

In this chapter we will describe the standard procedures of MTT in functional reconstruction. There will always be a patient that does not fit into this standard pattern. In these, the decisions on transfer must be made after careful examination, listing of all retained function and listing of the functions that are to be reconstructed (see Chap. 10). Thus, combinations and modifications of all possible transfers are to be considered.

We will present the transfers that aim to reconstruct special functions, not nerves. Therefore, the individual chapters will not always match the respective nerve lesions described in Chap. 2.

11.1 Scapula Muscles

Paralysis of the muscles of the scapula such as the trapezius, serratus anterior, levator scapulae and the rhomboid muscles make the scapula unstable and impair shoulder function. Additionally, their missing function may be responsible for a secondary scoliosis of the cervical and thoracic spine.

11.1.1 Shoulder Abduction (Accessory Nerve)

Depending on the level of nerve lesion, loss of function differs, especially because innervation is not as clear as always described. A proximal lesion involves paralysis of the sternocleidomastoid muscle. This weakens the ability to move the head away from the affected site. To our knowledge there is currently no indication to reconstruct this function by a transfer.

Involvement of the trapezius muscle, however, may lead to a general weakness in the affected shoulder girdle and arm, the inability to abduct the shoulder above 90°. The scapula rotates distally and laterally and flares slightly. Its inferior angle is closer to the midline than its superior angle. In abduction, this position is accentuated, while by moving the shoulder anteriorly the flaring disappears.

Rarely, if the functional loss has resulted in severe disability and nerve reconstruction has failed, reconstruction can be achieved by grafting fascial strips (for example taken from the fascia lata of the thigh) from the spine of the scapula to the distal cervical and proximal thoracic spinous processes. These static operations can be combined with a transfer of the levator scapulae muscle to the acromial part of the spina scapulae. However, if possible, the following dynamic operation is preferred, because its results are usually better.

Preferred Transfer. Dynamic reconstruction can be achieved by transferring the levator scapulae muscle laterally on the spine of the scapula to a point adjacent to the acromion. Other authors describe a lateral transposition of the rhomboid muscles under the infraspinatus muscle. The patient is positioned prone. Two incisions are made, one parallel to the lateral spina scapulae and one parallel to the medial scapular border. The trapezius muscle is dissected from the medial scapula, and the levator scapulae and the rhomboid muscles are identified. The muscles are detached from their origin with a small piece of bone, and dissected proximally, leaving the dorsal scapular nerve intact. Care must be taken not to injure the attachment of the serratus anterior and the subscapular muscle. The infraspinatus muscle is medially detached. The rhomboid muscles are then fixed with nonabsorbable sutures through drill holes (or anchors, e.g., corkscrew anchor systems) in the scapula as far lateral as possible. At this moment, the shoulder girdle is held dorsally, and the arm is abducted 90°. After reattachment of the infraspinatus muscle to its origin by nonabsorbable sutures, the lateral spina scapulae (as close to the acromion as possible) is freed from the trapezius muscle and the supraspinatus and deltoid muscles are carefully detached. Holes are drilled again or anchors are placed in the lateral spina scapulae (close to the acromion) and the levator scapulae muscle is tunneled through the paralyzed trapezius muscle and fixed to the drill holes or anchors with nonabsorbable sutures (Rudigier 1991).

Postoperatively, arm and shoulder are immobilized in a 90° abduction position with slight retroversion for 6 weeks. Mobilization starts with isometric contraction and then abduction.

11.1.2 Dorsal Scapular and Thoracodorsal Nerves

A dorsal scapular nerve lesion results in paralysis of rhomboid and levator scapulae muscles. Usually, an isolated paralysis (of levator scapulae muscle) is well compensated by the trapezius muscle. If the paralysis of the rhomboid muscles leads to functional problems, fascial grafts can be anchored between the medial border of the scapula and the distal cervical and proximal thoracic spinatus processes. Others describe a dynamic fixation of the inferior scapula angle with a strip from the cranial portion of the latissimus dorsi muscle (see Sect. 11.1.3).

The thoracodorsal nerve innervates the latissimus dorsi muscle, whose function is the internal rotation of the arm. The latissimus dorsi is dispensable and often used for reconstruction of other functions, as its function is compensated by pectoral, subscapular and teres major muscles.

11.1.3 Scapular Winging (Long Thoracic Nerve)

Winging the scapula is usually the result of a paralyzed long thoracic nerve. Abduction and anteversion of the arm accentuate the winging. Loss of the serratus anterior muscle results in an unstable scapula with an impaired abduction as the inferior angle cannot move ventrally. Many operative procedures have been described to restore scapula stability. None of these procedures were performed in large populations. Thus, the results are mainly based on case reports. The transfer of the sternal part of the greater pectoral muscle with or without a fascial strip, and the transfer of the minor pectoral muscle try to simulate the original serratus anterior muscle.

If intact, the transfer of the teres major muscle is preferred (Hass 1931). The teres major muscle (n. subscapularis) originates from the inferior angle of the scapula and attaches with the latissimus dorsi muscle at the crista tuberculi minoris. The internal rotation is well compensated by other muscles. The patient is placed on the healthy side, the arm is abducted 90°, but remains free for intraoperative movement. From an incision parallel to the ventral axillary fold, the serratus anterior muscle is exposed around the 5th and 6th rib. The teres major muscle is then dissected more dorsally, underneath the latissimus dorsi muscle and freed from its attachment at the humerus (leave tendon at the muscle). Care must be taken to avoid a lesion of the axillary nerve that runs through the lateral axilla space. The teres major can then be dissected very carefully (not to injure the supplying vessels) and is then pulled ventrally/caudally, where it can be periosteally sutured to the ribs and the remaining serratus anterior (▶ Fig. 11.1). Immobilization is required for 6 weeks in 90° abduction.

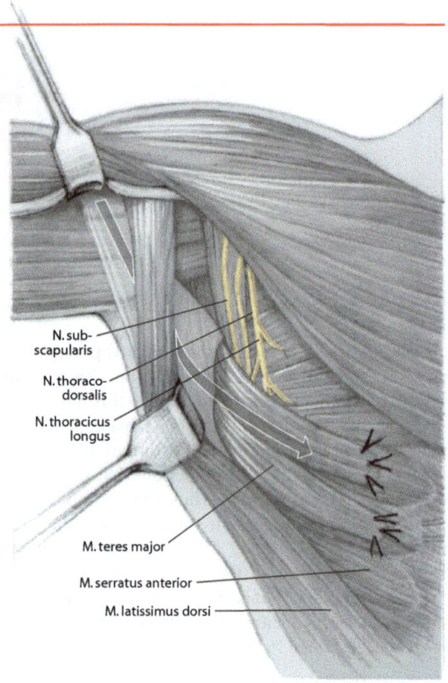

Figure 11.1

The teres major muscle is dissected under the latissimus dorsi muscle and freed from its attachment at the humerus and is then pulled ventrally/caudally, where it can be periosteally sutured to the ribs and the remaining serratus anterior muscle

Another popular method is the transfer of the contralateral latissimus dorsi muscle. However, there are still no long-term results available (Terzis and Papakonstantinou 2002). A static reconstruction is the connection of the injured scapula to the normally functioning scapula (at the level of the spina) by fascia lata strips. Both scapulae are fixed with the medial border parallel to the spine.

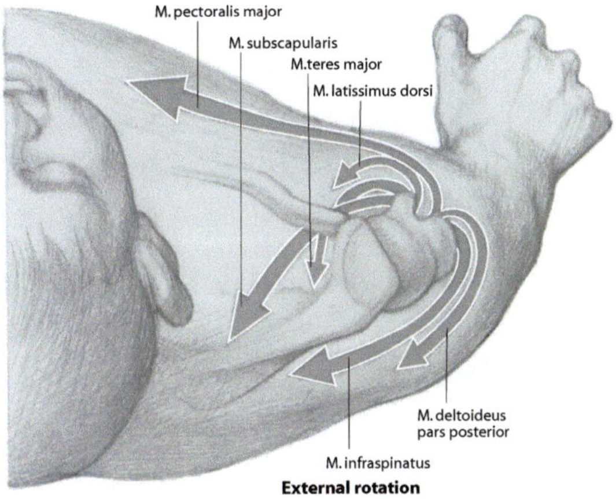

Figure 11.2

The main movers for internal and external rotation of the shoulder. External rotation is supported to some extent by the teres minor and supraspinatus muscles

11.2 Shoulder

The disability caused by paralysis of the muscles about the shoulder can be decreased to some extent by tendon and muscle transfers. The pattern and severity of the paralysis determine which method is most appropriate. The described methods, of course, aim for a near normal result. However, in some cases it is simply not possible to restore normal function. The goal here is to make the arm as useful as possible.

The deltoid and the clavicular part of the pectoral major muscles are the prime movers. They participate in lifting and exert forces in the three directions at the junction of the proximal and middle thirds of the humeral shaft axis. The subscapular, supraspinatus, infraspinatus muscles are the steering group. These muscles exert forces at the junction of the axes of the humeral head and neck and humeral shaft (▶ Fig. 11.2). As the arm is elevated, the humeral head, by rolling and gliding movements, constantly changes its point of contact with the glenoid cavity. Although these muscles exert a little force in lifting the arm, their chief function is stabilizing the humeral head as it moves in the glenoid. The pectoral major (sternal part), latissimus dorsi, teres major and minor muscles belong to the depressor group. They are intermediately located and exert their forces on the proximal fourth of the humeral shaft axis. During elevation they rotate the shaft, and in the last few degrees they depress the humeral head. They exert only minimal steering action on the head. Their absence does not cause apparent disability except that performance of the limb in lifting weights above the head is decreased.

11.2.1 Shoulder Abduction (Axillary and Suprascapular Nerves)

The deltoid (axillary nerve) and the supraspinatus (suprascapular nerve) muscles abduct the arm. The functions of these muscles are absolutely necessary for shoulder movement. An isolated paralysis of the supraspinatus can be compensated if all other muscles are intact. However, the loss of the deltoid muscle requires reconstruction.

The preferred method is the transfer of the trapezius muscle (Saha 1967). As this operation is very easy, results are very good and predictable. Of course, the trapezius has to be intact for this procedure. We found that the utilization of distal branches of the accessory nerve to neurotize other nerves (suprascapular or musculocutaneous nerves) does not impair the innervation for the transferred part (pars horizontalis) of the trapezius muscle. The patient is placed on the healthy side, the arm is left free for intraoperative movement. We prefer a lazy-S or Y-shaped incision over the acromion, spina and humerus (▶ Fig. 11.3). Others recommend a saber-cut incision beginning in

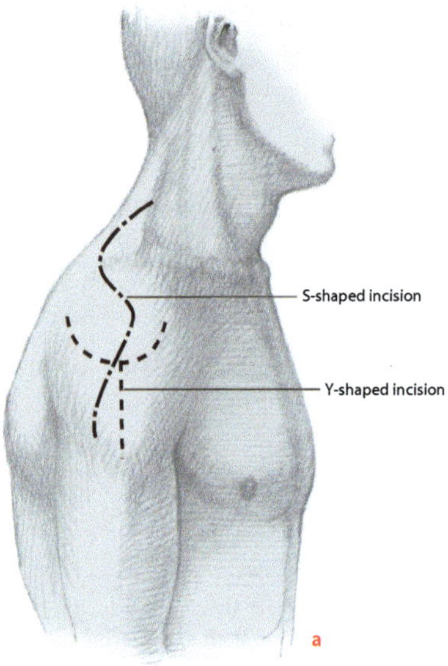

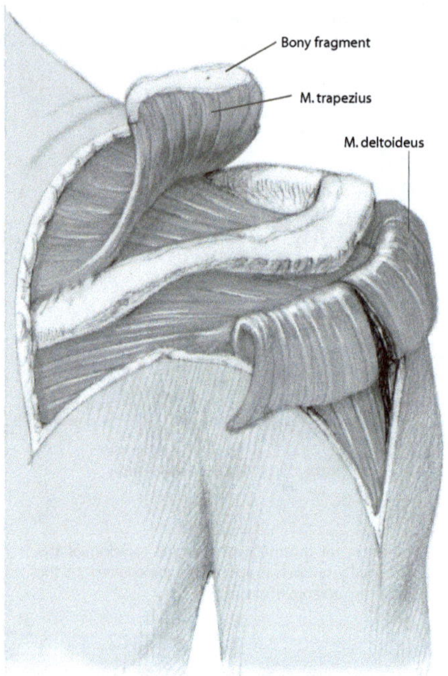

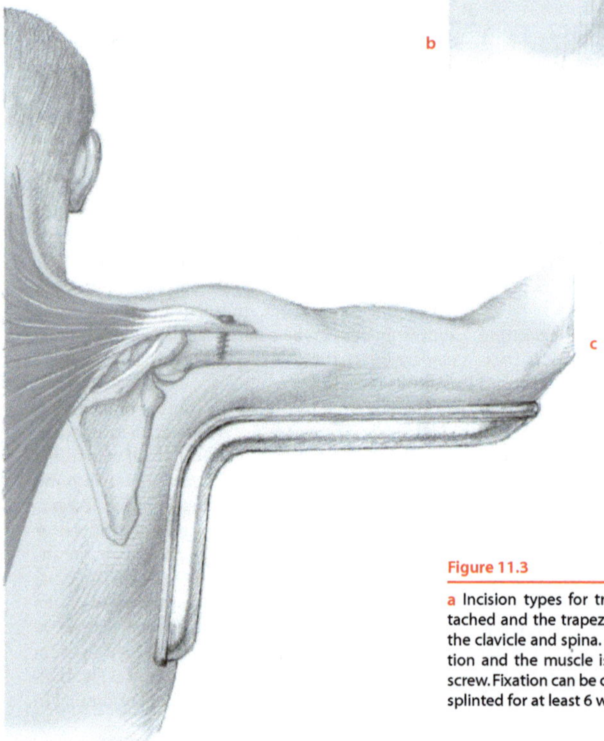

Figure 11.3

a Incision types for trapezius transfer. b The deltoid is detached and the trapezius is harvested with the bony part of the clavicle and spina. c The arm is placed in maximal abduction and the muscle is inserted as distal as possible with a screw. Fixation can be completed using anchors. The patient is splinted for at least 6 weeks in abduction the axillary fold and extending to scapular spine (2 cm lateral to the vertebral border; Harmon 1950). The complete horizontal part of the trapezius is exposed, leaving the muscle fascia intact. The deltoid origin is then detached and reflected laterally. The humeral head is exposed. Then the acromial attachment of the trapezius is osteotomized and elevated with bony parts of the clavicle and spina in an obliquely distal and lateral plane. The coracoclavicular ligament should be left intact. The complete trapezius is detached from clavicle and spina, and these parts are sutured to the main part to maintain correct tension. The muscle is then freed from the deep cervical fascia to allow adequate transposition. (When indicated, transfers to reconstruct the function of the subscapular, supra- or infraspinatus muscles are performed at this time of the operation; see below and Sect. 11.2.2.) Before the trapezius is inserted, the arm is placed in the 90° position and the correct position estimated. In the area where the bony fragment is fixed, a distally based periosteal flap is elevated; the bone should then be roughened. If an external rotation is desired, the fragment is placed more anteriorly, if an internal rotation is needed more dorsally. Then the hole is drilled into the humerus, and two corkscrew anchors are placed anteriorly and posteriorly. The trapezius muscle insertion is fixed with an appropriate spongiosa screw and the remaining parts are sutured to the anchors. Then suture the periosteal flap on top of the trapezius insertion. We immobilize the arm in 90° abduction for 6 weeks. Then the arm is lowered 10–15° every week. Physical therapy then starts with trapezius training.

Some authors recommend reconstructing supraspinatus function by transposition of the levator scapulae muscle. However, from our experience this muscle cannot always be transposed adequately. Alternatively, the transposition of the sternocleidomastoid muscle was described. In this operation the muscle is detached from its insertion via a separate incision, freed and tunneled underneath the cervical fascia and fixed at the major tubercle (Rudigier 1991). The operation is then completed with the trapezius transfer. The functional result is considered good; however, this transfer usually results in severe esthetic problems.

Other transfers for deltoid reconstruction are the complete transposition of the pectoral major muscle (reconstructing the anterior and middle part of the deltoid) and the teres major muscle (for the posterior part). The muscles are detached from the origin and insertion, transposed solely on their neurovascular pedicle, and then sutured with the correct tension in 90° abduction. The complete transposition of the latissimus dorsi muscle is more difficult. Although it keeps the acromioclavicular joint intact, the results are not as good as the trapezius transfer. This might be due to the partial antagonistic function of the latissimus dorsi muscle. Additionally, it has to be considered that the latissimus is a versatile muscle for other reconstructive options.

If the deltoid muscle is only partially denervated, the intact parts of the muscle can be transferred to restore the lost function. Especially if the posterior portion can be transposed more ventrally, function is considered good, preventing anterior dislocation of the shoulder. Postoperative treatment is similar to that after trapezius transfer.

11.2.2 External Rotation (Suprascapular and Axillary Nerves)

The infraspinatus muscle is the most powerful external rotator of the arm. The dorsal part of the deltoid muscle, the teres minor (both axillary nerves) and to some extent the supraspinatus muscle, can compensate infraspinatus paralysis. However, if more than one of these muscles is paralyzed or the patient is young and/or athletically active we recommend a reconstruction of external rotation.

If possible, the latissimus dorsi muscle should preferably be transferred. This is very easy and reliable. However, as the latissimus dorsi is a powerful internal rotator, we strongly recommend preoperative physical therapy to learn an isolated contraction of the muscle. Again the patient is placed on the healthy side, the arm in 90° abduction, but free for intraoperative movement. Via a mid-axillary incision extended to the posterior axillary fold and the dorsal arm (a straight incision crossing the joint should be avoided) the latissimus dorsi is identified, the thoracodorsal vessels and nerves are isolated (▶ Fig. 11.4). If no other transfer is planned, the ramifications to teres major and serratus anterior muscles can be ligated to facilitate the harvesting of the muscle. The insertion of the muscle is identified, and detached as close to the bone as possible. As in some cases the insertion of latissimus and teres major are conjoint, they can be harvested as one tendon (Phipps and Hoffer 1995). Identify the tubercle at the inferior end of the greater tuberosity via a blunt dissection in the interval between the deltoid and long head of the triceps muscle. Care should be taken not to injure the axillary nerve (running through the lateral axillary space) when passing the muscle beneath the deltoid. At least two

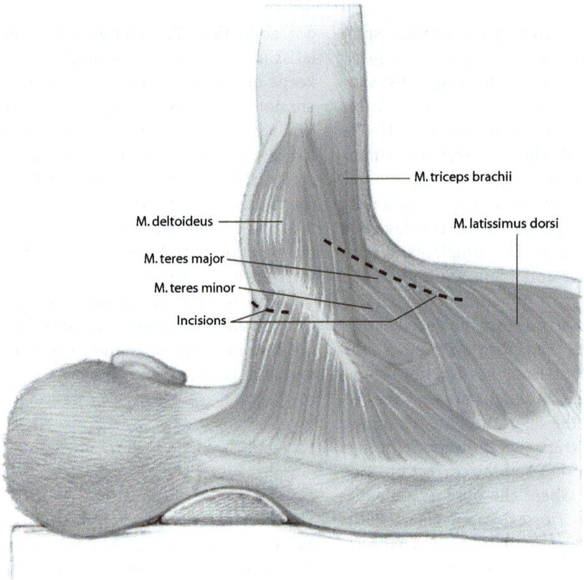
M. triceps brachii
M. deltoideus
M. latissimus dorsi
M. teres major
M. teres minor
Incisions

a

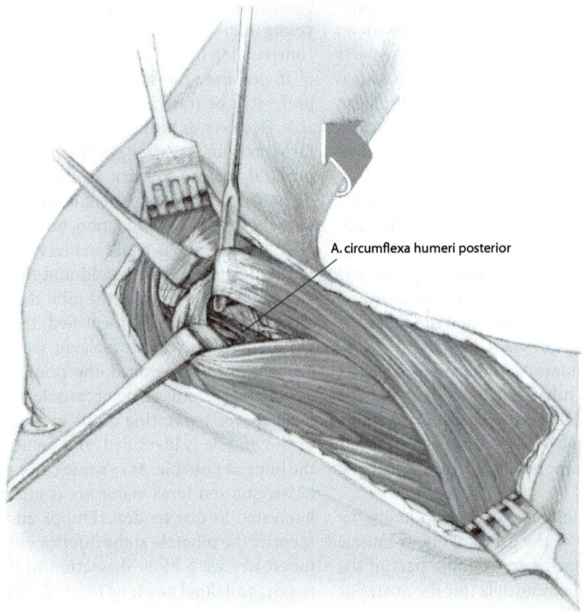
A. circumflexa humeri posterior

b

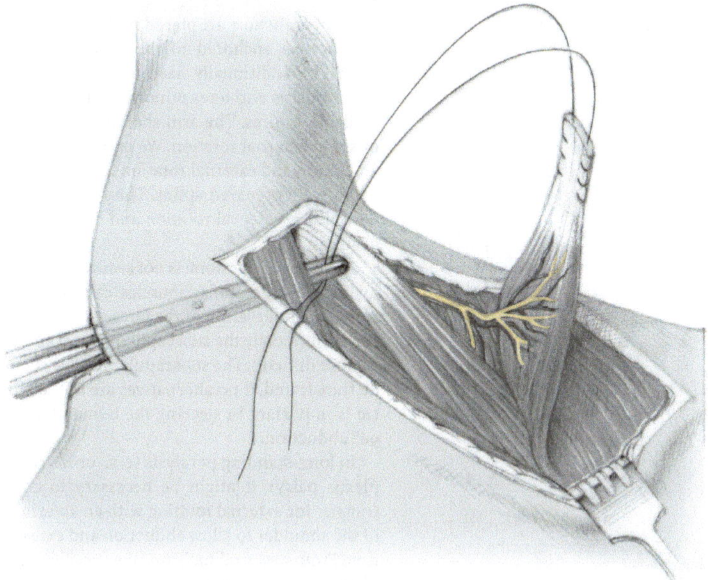

c

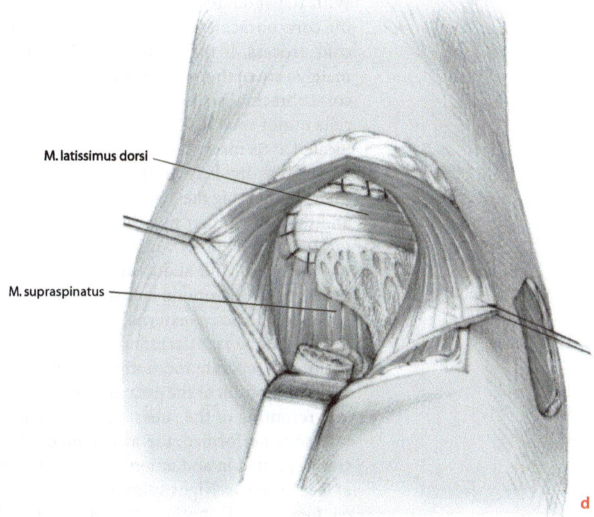

d

Figure 11.4

a Incisions for latissimus transfer to restore external rotation. b The insertion is identified and released. c The muscle is then rerouted under the deltoid muscle and (d) sutured to the tubercle (with anchors) and to the rotator cuff muscles

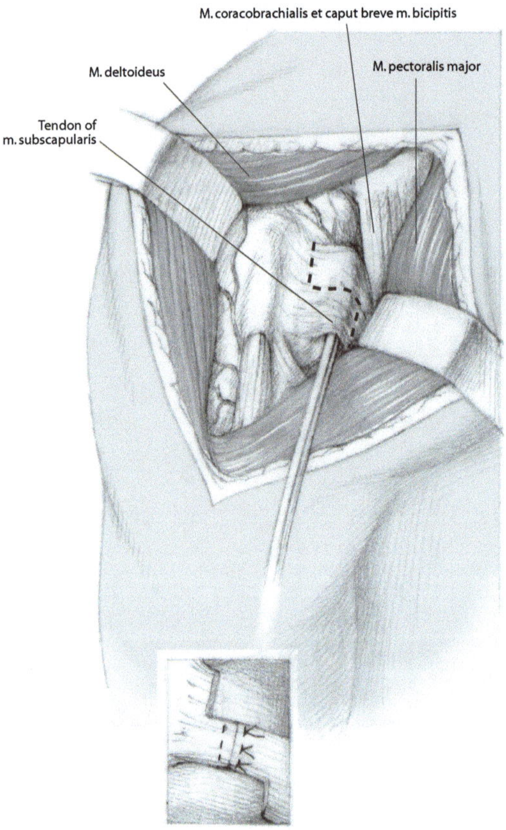

Figure 11.5

Anterior release with elongation of the subscapular tendon

corkscrew anchors are placed, and then the latissimus insertion is anchored to the tubercle; the muscle should be additionally fixed periosteally and to the infraspinatus and teres minor insertion with nonabsorbable sutures. The arm should be held in neutral or slight external rotation. We immobilize the arm in adduction and external rotation for 6 weeks in a preoperatively prepared splint. The transferred muscle now allows external rotation and holds the humeral head caudally.

If the latissimus dorsi is not available, the teres major or the subscapular muscles can be transferred. However, innervation of the teres major is not always constant (mostly the subscapular nerve) and training is more difficult. The subscapular muscle should only be transferred, if no alternatives are left, as this muscle is important in steering the humeral head above 90° abduction.

In long-standing paralysis (e.g., obstetric brachial plexus palsy), it might be necessary to combine a transfer for external rotation with an anterior release of the shoulder to allow abduction and external rotation. From a ventral incision (the coracoid process to distal part of pectoralis major insertion) in the deltopectoral groove, the pectoralis tendon is divided. With the shoulder rotated externally and abducted, the coracobrachialis is traced superiorly to the coracoid process. If the coracoid is elongated, approximately 1 cm of the tip is resected with the insertion of coracobrachialis, short head of biceps and the pectoralis minor muscles. Then the subscapular tendon is located at its insertion on the lesser tuberosity and is completely divided without incising the capsule. We prefer elongating the insertions of the major pectoral and the subscapular muscle, rather than only dividing them (▶ Fig. 11.5). In some cases, the acromion may interfere with abduction and reduction of subluxation. The acromion is then divided and elevated. If there is no active external rotator, the subscapular muscle can be transferred for external rotation. This requires a separate incision in the posterior axillary fold, exploration of the greater tuberosity (see above) and rerouting of the subscapular insertion. If only a release is performed, the arm should be postoperatively splinted in abduction and external rotation for at least 2 weeks. Night splinting is then recommended for at least another 4 weeks. Physical therapy should start as soon as possible.

In severe fixed rotation contracture, some authors recommend an external rotational osteotomy of the humerus. After osteotomy 5 cm distal to the joint, the distal fragment is externally rotated for approximately 60–90°. This can be combined with a transposition of other muscles to restore external rotation. Some authors describe the utilization of the major pectoral muscle. The clavicular part is used for external rotation, the sternal part for adduction.

11.2.3 Internal Rotation (Medial and Lateral Thoracal, Thoracodorsal, and Subscapular Nerves)

Loss of internal rotation is usually not complete. If one muscle is paralyzed, function is well compensated by others. The problem is rather the internal rotation contracture then the loss of internal rotation. However, the loss of the subscapular muscle should be compensated if the supraspinatus and infraspinatus muscles are also paralyzed, as these muscles are necessary to fix and steer the humeral head, especially in abduction over 90° (see above).

The subscapular muscle function is preferably reconstructed by a transfer of the proximal parts of the serratus anterior muscle. This is usually combined with a trapezius/levator scapulae muscle transfer for restoration of abduction (see Sect. 11.2.2). Extend the Y-incision or saber-cut ventrally, identify two cranial segments of the serratus anterior and dissect bluntly underneath the serratus. The preparation is difficult as the serratus is attached to the origin of the subscapularis and has to be dissected very carefully beginning from the medial border of the scapula. The arm is then held in about 100° abduction and the scapula is held away from the thorax. Avoid injury to the thoracodorsal nerve and vessels, and retract the axillary vessels and distal brachial plexus parts. The rerouted serratus anterior parts can then be attached to the lesser tubercle with corkscrew anchors and nonabsorbable sutures to the insertion of the subscapularis muscle. Postoperative treatment is similar to the trapezius transfer (Sect. 11.2.2).

Alternatively to the serratus anterior transfer, the transposition of either the pectoralis minor or the latissimus dorsi was described.

11.3 Elbow

Most operations are designed to restore active flexion and in some cases active extension of the elbow. If the functions of the hand are good or restored by tendon transfers, an active motion of the elbow should be desired. However, even if function of the hand remains poor, some patients demand control of elbow flexion to use the hand for simple procedures (Chuang et al. 2002).

The most important muscles for flexion are the biceps and the brachial muscles (both musculocutaneous nerve). The brachioradial (BR, radial nerve) is not as powerful, but allows flexion against gravity. The forearm and hand muscles that origin at the humerus (extensor carpi radialis longus/brevis, pronator teres, flexor carpi ulnaris/radialis, flexor digitorum superficialis muscles) can help with elbow flexion. Extension is provided by the triceps and the anconeus muscles.

11.3.1 Elbow Flexion (Musculocutaneous and Radial Nerve)

If the brachioradialis (radial nerve) is working and the patient does not require a powerful flexion, no operation should be done. If none of the flexors are working, a transfer should be considered. The best and preferred method is the complete transposition of the latissimus dorsi muscle (Schottstaedt et al. 1958; Zancolli 1973). The patient is placed on the side, the arm abducted 90° (▶ Fig. 11.6). The latissimus dorsi is exposed via a mid-axillary incision, the thoracodorsal vessels and nerve are identified and isolated (to subscapular artery). The muscle is then elevated with a skin island in direction of the muscle fibers (about 15 cm long and 6 cm wide), avoiding a lesion of the fascia. Before the origin (with thoracolumbar fascia) and insertion are divided, the tension of the muscle is marked with a running suture, with a knot every 5 cm (about four times). The muscle, now completely detached (except the neurovascular bundle) is kept ventrally and the donor site is primarily closed, only a small hole for the vessels and nerve is kept open. The patient is then placed on the back, the arm placed on an arm table. The recipient bed is prepared by incising the area over the biceps. Sometimes it is necessary to remove the biceps muscle to allow the transposed muscle to fit in the bed. Distally, the insertion of the biceps is prepared and proximally the coracoid process is roughened. The muscle is then transposed ventrally (if necessary, divide the intercostobrachial nerves) and inserted into the bed; care must be taken not to twist the neurovascular bundle, sutured to form a roll, and then sutured to the distal biceps tendon and the lacertus fibrosus with nonabsorbable sutures. The skin in the elbow is then closed, and the elbow is flexed and from this point continuously held in 90° flexion. Then the muscle is placed in the desired tension (see principles in Chap. 10: knot

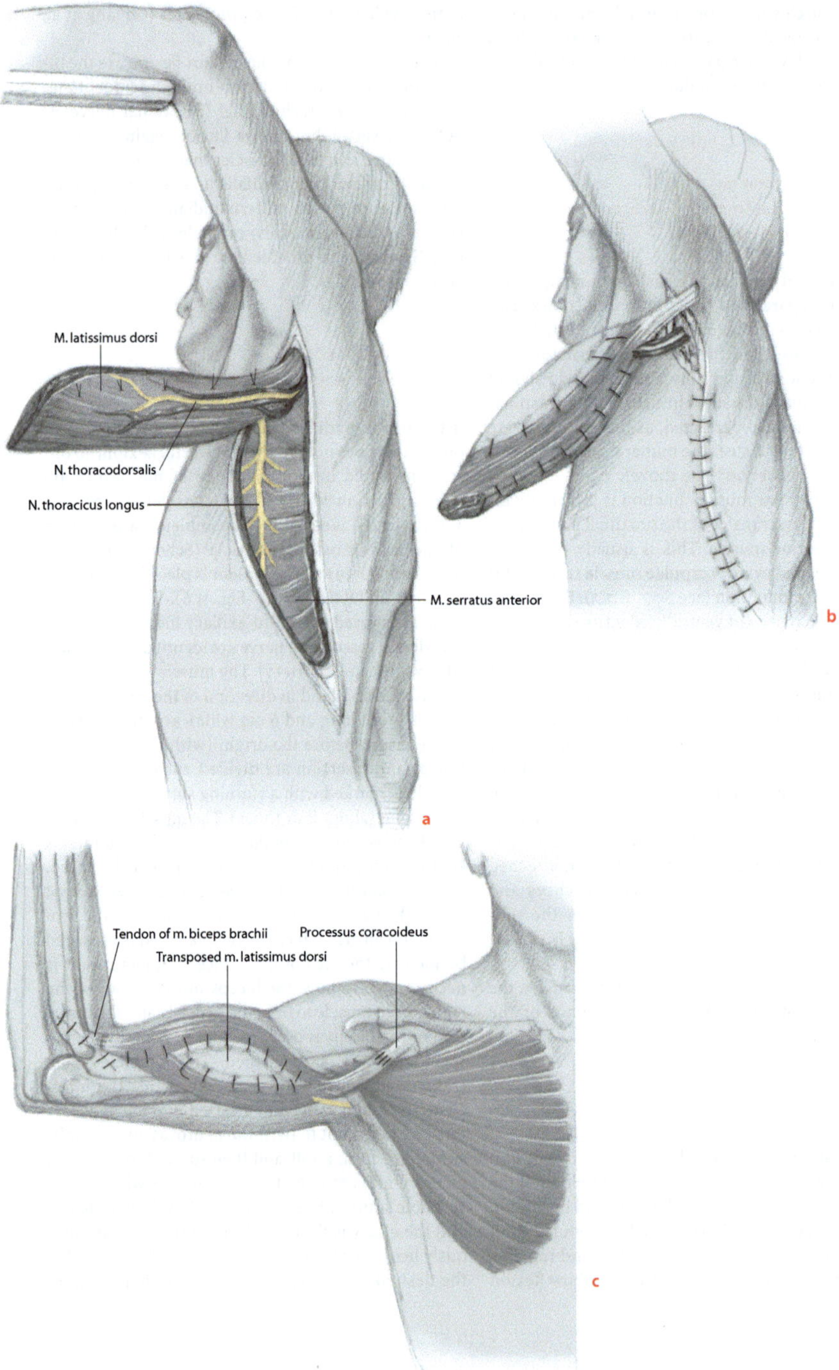
M. latissimus dorsi
N. thoracodorsalis
N. thoracicus longus
M. serratus anterior
a
b
Tendon of m. biceps brachii
Processus coracoideus
Transposed m. latissimus dorsi
c

◀ Figure 11.6a–c

Transfer of the latissimus for elbow flexion. a Harvesting the muscle with a skin island. To estimate correct tension a knot is placed every 5 cm prior to detaching the muscle. b The muscle is sutured to itself and transposed ventrally. c The muscle is sutured with the proper tension distally to the biceps tendon and proximally to the coracoid process. The elbow is kept in flexion

sutures every 5 cm) and fixed with the former insertion to the coracoid process. Use corkscrew anchors and nonabsorbable sutures to fix it to the short head of the biceps muscle. If the patient is not relaxed the correct tension of the muscle can be estimated by allowing the elbow to extend and then stimulating the thoracodorsal nerve. Postoperatively, shoulder and elbow (in 90°, mild pronation of forearm) are immobilized by bandaging the arm to the thorax for 6 weeks. After releasing the bandage immediate extension of the elbow must be avoided so as not to injure the transferred muscle. Physical therapy for the wrist and hand starts early. Physical therapy for the transferred muscle should start first with re-education (relaxing the triceps and allowing former movement of latissimus, internal rotation/adduction, in about 60° of flexion). After an additional 2 weeks the muscle can be fully trained.

If the latissimus is not available for reconstruction, the triceps tendon can be transferred ventrally (Caroll 1952). This very easy method offers very good and powerful results. The triceps tendon is detached at the olecranon and rerouted around the radial epicondyle and sutured to the biceps tendon (▶ Fig. 11.7). Postoperative treatment is as described above. In this operation, the elbow extension is considered of little importance, since gravity will extend the elbow. However, there are special indications where elbow extension is necessary. A good triceps function is essential in crutch walking or shifting the body weight to the hands during such activities as moving from bed to wheelchair because elbow extension is then locked. Additionally, in thrusting and pushing motions with the forearm a functioning triceps is necessary (see Sect. 11.3.2).

There are several other methods to restore elbow flexion. However, none gives as good results as the latissimus transfer. Clark (1946) and others described a transfer of the pectoralis major muscle. The tendon, however, has to be extended either by the sheath of the rectus abdominis muscle or the long head of the biceps muscle. In addition, the flexorplasty according to Steindler (1930) can restore flexion, although not powerful flexion. In this operation the pronator teres

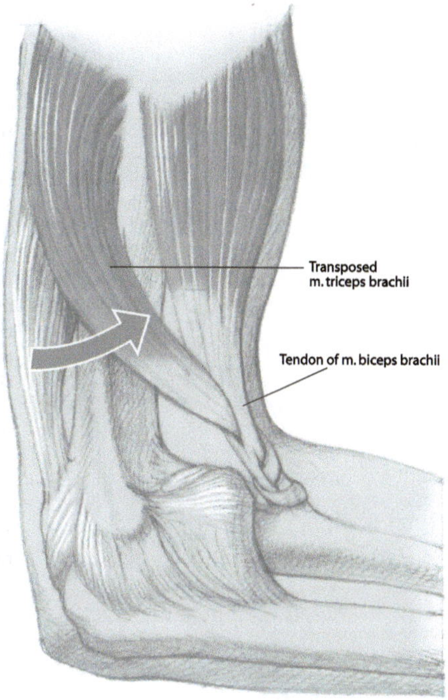

Figure 11.7

Transfer of triceps tendon to restore elbow flexion, according to Caroll

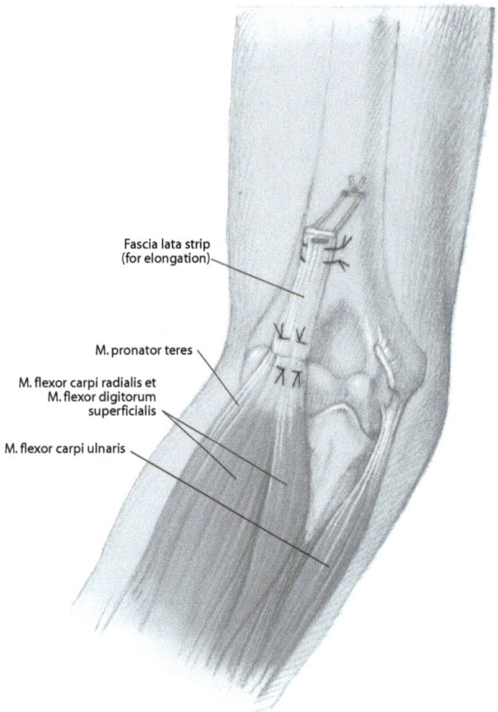

Figure 11.8

Steindler flexorplasty. The pronator teres (PT), the flexor carpi radialis (FCR), the flexor digitorum superficialis (FDS), and the flexor carpi ulnaris muscle (FCU) muscles are detached from their origin and transposed proximally. If the muscles are too short, a transosseously fixed fascia lata strip can be used for elongation

(PT), the flexor carpi radialis (FCR), the flexor digitorum superficialis (FDS), and the flexor carpi ulnaris (FCU) muscles are detached from the medial epicondyle, freed distally for about 5 cm and then transposed proximally (either with or without fascia lata strip) to the lateral humerus (▶ Fig. 11.8). If a pronation contracture persists, the FCU tendon can be transferred around the ulna to the distal radius. In addition, for restoration of elbow flexion, transfers of the sternocleidomastoid muscle or a reversed transposition of the FCU have been described in special cases.

11.3.2 Elbow Extension (Radial Nerve)

As described in the preceding section, there are special indications (e.g., tetraplegia) where elbow extension is necessary such as in crutch walking or shifting the body weight to the hands. It therefore might be necessary to reconstruct elbow extension. For this operation, a flexion contracture of the elbow has to be corrected before, as it would significantly impair the result.

Again the transposition of the latissimus dorsi muscle is preferred. The method is similar to flexion reconstruction. However, in this technique the insertion of the latissimus can be kept in situ and the muscle is placed "over the top." If not possible, extension can be achieved by transposing the BR. The ventral parts are detached, and then dorsally transposed over the top and sutured to the triceps tendon.

Additionally, Moberg (1987) described the transposition of the spinal part of the deltoid muscle (C5). This must be elongated by a free tendon graft (in tetraplegia, e.g., the tibialis anterior tendon) and sutured into the triceps aponeurosis.

11.4 Wrist and Hand

Motion of the hand is necessary for the highly adaptive functions of pinching, grasping and hooking. It is made possible by the many joints among the 29 bones in the hand, wrist and forearm and by the 50 muscles that act as motors and stabilizers. Five control supination and pronation, seven move the hand at the wrist, 18 flex or extend the fingers, and 20 small muscles of the hand contribute to precise movements of the thumb and fingers. Tendon transfers undertaken to correct imbalance in such a coordinated and precise system must have limited objectives: to replace a nonfunctioning basic motion, to eliminate the deforming force of a strong muscle pulling against a paralyzed antagonist, and to improve stability of the extremity through better balance.

Especially in the hand, the principles of MTT must be respected, as one wrong transfer impairs hand function severely. Muscles are controlled at the unconscious level and by conscious effort. Synergistic muscles such as wrist extensors, finger flexors and digital abductors act in coordination; likewise wrist flexors, finger extensors and digital adductors are synergistic. To ease postoperative action, these movement patterns should be respected if possible (Tubiana 1969).

11.4.1 Extension of Wrist, Fingers, and Thumb (Radial Nerve)

Tendon transfers for radial palsy are among the most frequently performed transfers. In high radial palsy, the wrist extensors are involved, whereas in low palsy (interosseous posterior nerve), the wrist extensors (extensor carpi radialis longus and brevis muscles, ERCL/B) are intact. Functional testing thus will present whether a wrist extension also needs to be restored. As wrist extension is one of the most important functions, this must be done very carefully. In radial nerve palsy, finger extension is for the most part not active in the metacarpophalangeal joints (MP joints). Extension in the proximal and distal phalangeal joints (PIP and DIP) depends on the ulnar nerve.

The preferred method for reconstruction of wrist extension is transfer of the pronator teres muscle (PT). The PT acts as a synergist of wrist extension. This transfer is combined with the reconstruction of finger extension with the flexor carpi ulnaris muscle (FCU) and the transfer of the palmaris longus (PL) for thumb extension (extensor pollicis longus, EPL). This transfer is known as Merle d'Aubigné transfer (1946, popular in Europe; ► Fig. 11.9). Brand (1988) advocated the use of the flexor carpi radialis muscle (FCR) to avoid a radial deviation caused by the unopposed pull of the radial wrist extensors, and thus to maintain the FCU as the strong wrist flexor that keeps the hand in a more ulnar plane, necessary for most manual work. Basically, we use the transfer according to Merle d'Aubigné, and the results are very good. In combined lesions, sometimes the FCR is used for finger extension (passed through the interosseous membrane). Whatever transfer is done, it is absolutely mandatory to keep one of the wrist flexors intact. If the PL is unavailable the flexor digitorum superficialis of the ring finger (FDS) is used. If in a combined lesion no other donors than the PT and FCU or FCR are available, the EPL can be sutured to the finger extensors.

The operation is performed in a bloodless field. To better understand the procedure, we describe the operation transfer by transfer; however, it is easier to identify all structures for all transfers first, and then suture the tendons. An incision is made on the radial side (middle third) of the forearm (► Fig. 11.10). The ECRL/B, the BR and the superficial radial nerve are identified. The PT is located under the BR (palmar) and the ERCL (dorsal). The insertion is freed with a periosteal slip to extend the length of the tendon and is dissected proximally. The PT slip is then passed

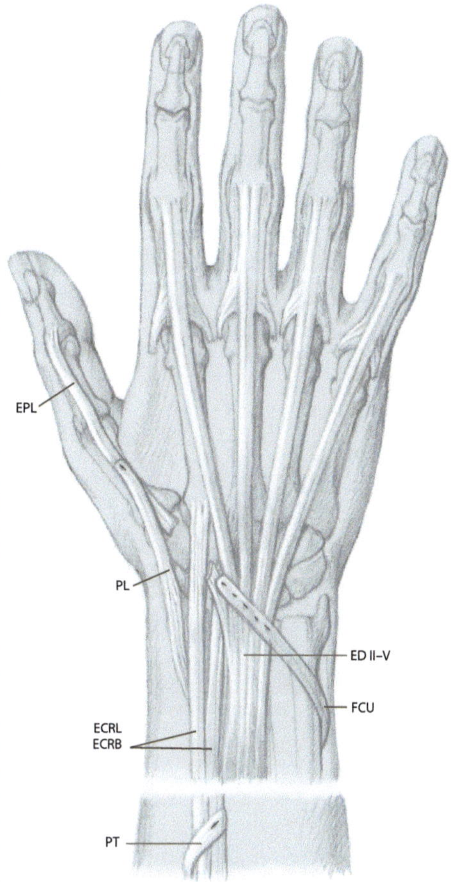

Figure 11.9

Principle of Merle d'Aubigné transfer. PT is transferred to the extensor carpi radialis longus and brevis (ECRL/B), FCU for ED2–5 and the palmaris longus (PL) for extensor pollicis longus (EPL)

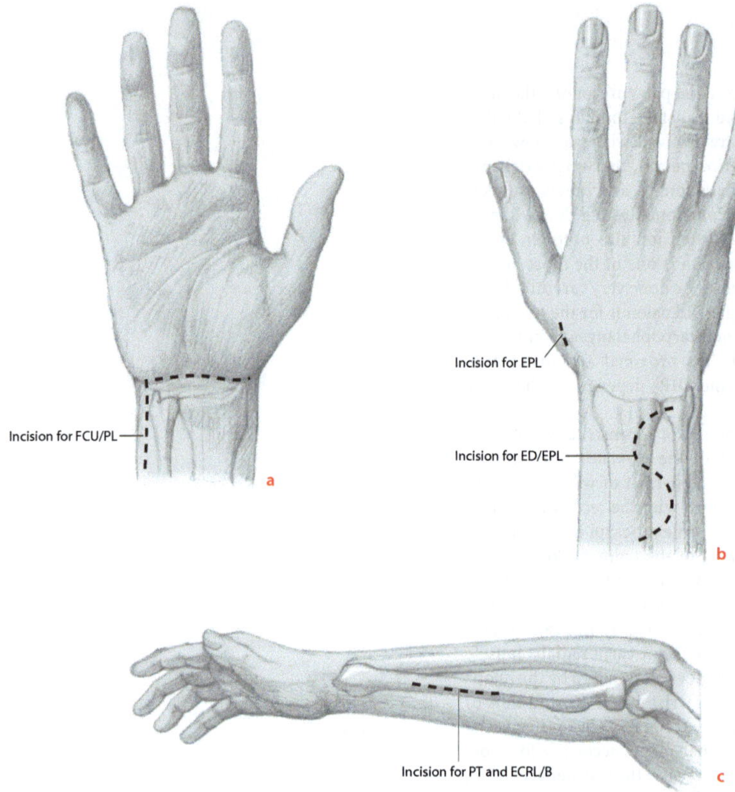

Figure 11.10

a Incision an the palmar aspect to identify FCU and PL. b Incision on the dorsal side to dissect the extensor digitorum (ED) and EPL. c Incision to free the PT and ERCL/B

through the ERCL/B under full extension of the wrist. The wrist must from now on be held in this position. The PT tendon is sutured with nonabsorbable sutures. The distal part of the slip is then sutured to itself (▶ Fig. 11.11a,b). From a distal ulnar palmar incision, the FCU tendon is dissected far proximally; if necessary a proximal ulnar incision is added. Then the extensor digitorum (ED) is exposed from a separate incision proximal to the extensor retinaculum. The FCU is subcutaneously tunneled dorsally, and the fingers are held in maximal extension. The FCU tendon is passed through the ED tendons from ulnar to radial, taking care to increase extension toward the radial tendons. The FCU is then sutured with nonabsorbable sutures and the distal slip is again sutured to itself (▶ Fig. 11.11c,d). Then the PL is identified from a distal palmar incision freed proximally to the muscle belly. The EPL is identified from a dorsal incision at the level of the metacarpal bone, and divided as proximal as possible (proximal of the retinaculum), subcutaneously rerouted to the palmar side. Avoid a lesion of the radial artery and superficial radial nerve (if intact). An incision for the suture might be necessary. Again the tendons are passed through themselves and sutured with nonabsorbable material (▶ Fig. 11.11e,f). The thumb is held in full extension.

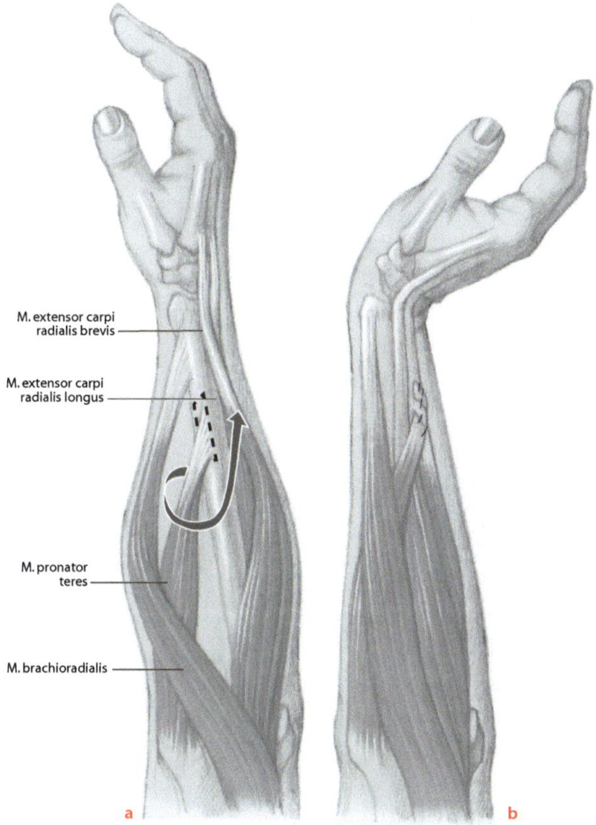

Figure 11.11 a, b

a The PT is harvested with a periosteal strip and then (b) sutured to the ECRL/B.
c–f see next page

If the PL is absent, the FDS of the ring finger is identified through a palmar incision at the PIP joint level and also identified at the palmar aspect of the wrist. The tendon is then distally divided (watch the chiasm of FDS/P) and rerouted to be sutured with the EPL. We found the route via the interosseous membrane to be the best. The tourniquet is open, with hemostasis achieved, and then the skin is closed. The hand is immobilized in a splint that includes the upper arm (elbow 90°), forearm, thumb and the fingers; the PIP and DIP joints are left free. Wrist and fingers are maintained in full extension. The splint is left for 4 weeks, a light splint is used for 2 weeks and physical therapy started with care. It has proved to be successful to talk to the therapist personally, explain the transfer and advise proper movements. For example, for the wrist, start in the hand in supination (dorsum downward) and tell the patient to pronate (old movement) and extend the wrist.

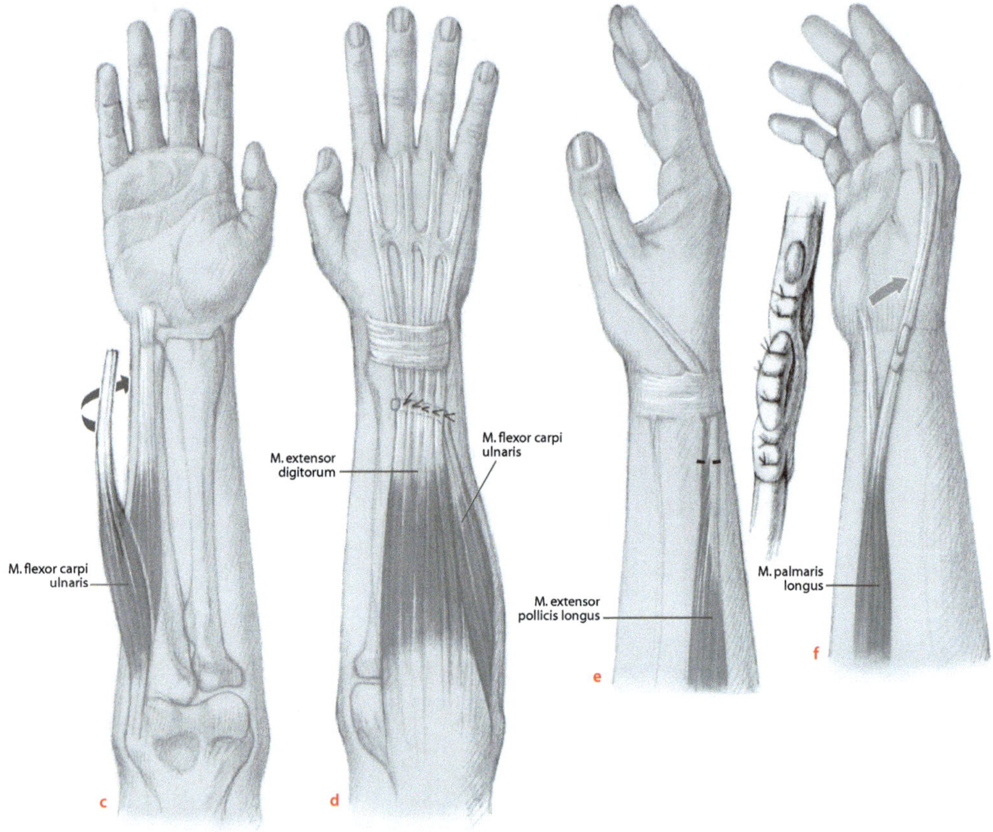

Figure 11.11 c–f

c The FCU is harvested and subcutaneously tunneled to the dorsal side and (d) sutured into the ED (e) The PL is harvested and sutured to the proximally cut EPL (f)

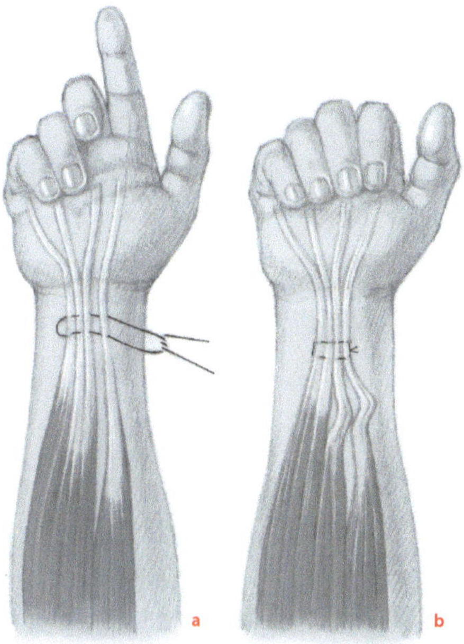

Figure 11.12a,b

In a high median nerve palsy, the flexor digitorum profundus (FDP) of the index and middle fingers is sutured to the FDP tendons of the ring and little fingers

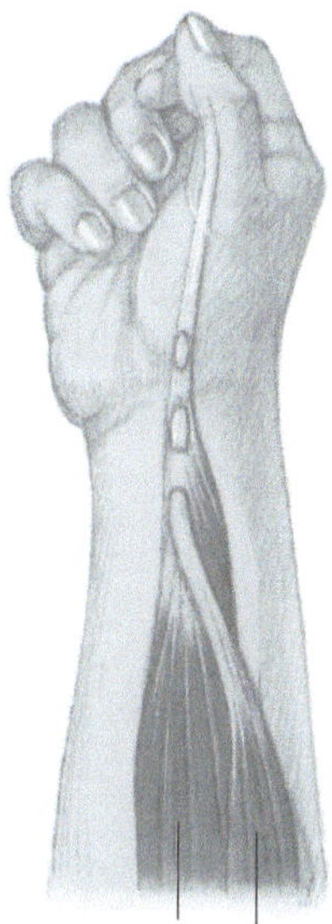

Figure 11.13

The FPL is restored using the brachioradialis (BR) as motor

11.4.2 High Median Nerve Palsy

A high, isolated median nerve paralysis is rare. If no innervation anomalies are present, the patient has loss of pronation at the forearm, weakened wrist flexion, loss of flexion of the thumb, index and middle finger. Opposition of the thumb is also lost. Sensitivity in the median nerve sensory distribution is also lost. The function can only be restored partially. Usually, the flexor digitorum profundus (FDP) tendons of the index and middle fingers are sutured to the FDP tendons of the ring and little fingers (▶ Fig. 11.12). The flexor pollicis longus muscle (FPL) is reconstructed by a transfer of the BR. This requires a meticulous dissection of the BR to free it from all adhesions and thus achieve an adequate excursion (▶ Fig. 11.13). Alternatively, if muscles for transfer are not available, the arthrodesis of the IP joint of the thumb does not cause major impairment. The loss of opposition is discussed in Sect. 11.4.3 (low median paralysis). Very often, function is not as impaired as anatomically described. This is related to innervation anomalies, where the ulnar nerve innervates the flexor pollicis brevis (FPB) and abductor pollicis brevis (APB) muscles.

11.4.3 Opposition of Thumb (Median Nerve)

Opposition of the thumb is necessary for a pinching grip. The complex motion consists of abduction of the thumb from the palmar surface of the index finger, flexion of the metacarpophalangeal joint of the thumb, internal rotation or pronation of the thumb, radial deviation of the proximal phalanx of the thumb on the metacarpal, and motion of the thumb toward the fingers. This motion requires intact APB, opponens and FPB muscles. There are several tech-

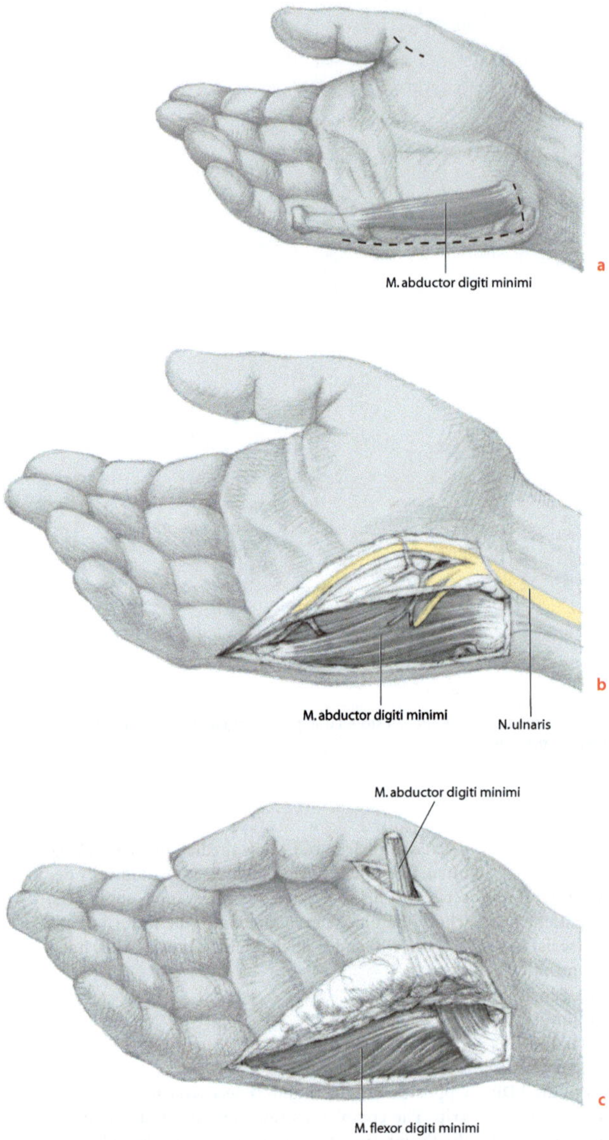

Figure 11.14a–c

The abductor minimi muscle (ADM) is used to restore opposition of the thumb. a The ADM is exposed from the ulnar, the muscle is harvested from distal to proximal, leaving vessels and innervation intact (b). The muscle is then subcutaneously tunneled and fixed to the insertion of the APB and dorsal EPL slip (c) niques to restore opposition. All the following techniques achieve good results. The selection should be made based on accompanied injuries and the resulting innervation loss. An adduction contracture of the thumb must be prevented by proper splinting. If present, it is necessary to release any adduction contracture prior to the transfer operation.

Transfer of the abductor minimi muscle (ADM) is preferred. However, this transfer requires an intact ulnar nerve. The advantage over the other methods is that no pulley is required to direct the transferred tendon in the proper angle (approaching the thumb from the ulnar side of the palm or wrist). In a bloodless field, an incision is made over the direction of the ADM, ulnar aspect of wrist (▶ Fig. 11.14). The ADM is identified distally and divided with a long tendinous slip. Sometimes it is difficult to respect the correct border to the flexor digiti minimi and the opponens digiti minimi, both radial and underneath the ADM. The ADM is freed proximally to the pisohamate ligament and the pisiform bone. Care must be taken not to injure the neurovascular bundle that enters the muscle in that region. Then the palm is tunneled subcutaneously to the insertion of the abductor pollicis brevis (APB). The distal tendon of the ADM is divided, and the ADM slip fixed with nonabsorbable sutures to the insertion of the APB and to the dorsal slip of the EPL to achieve a mild extension in opposition. After operation, a cast is provided with mild flexion of the wrist and opposition of the thumb for 4 weeks. A light cast is then used for the night. Then physical therapy starts: the standard movement is to hold the hand in a relaxed position with the wrist flexed, then tell the patient to abduct the little finger and oppose the thumb and extend the wrist.

In case the ulnar nerve is also injured, opponens reconstruction can be performed by transferring the FDS of the ring or middle finger. For this method, the FDS has to be intact from innervation and no additional tendinous lesion should be present. The tendon is harvested as described in Sect. 11.4.1 and then rerouted dorsal/ulnar around the FCU and then through the palm to the insertion of the APB at the metacarpophalangeal level (▶ Fig. 11.15). Alternatively, pulleys are used to create a slip from the FCU, a hole in the retinaculum flexorum or the pisiform bone. As the transferred tendon is longer than the ADM tendon, different insertion techniques have been developed. The Brand method is safe and thus described here. Both FDS strips are divided further proximally. One strip is then passed through the APB insertion, then passed around the EPL tendon and sutured to itself. The other strip is passed dorsal proximal around the MP joint and sutured to the insertion of the adductor pollicis (AP) and periosteally to the phalanx of the thumb. Both strips are to be fixed in similar tension to prevent inefficiency. Postoperative treatment is identical to the ADM transfer, but in physical therapy the patient must be told to flex the ring finger.

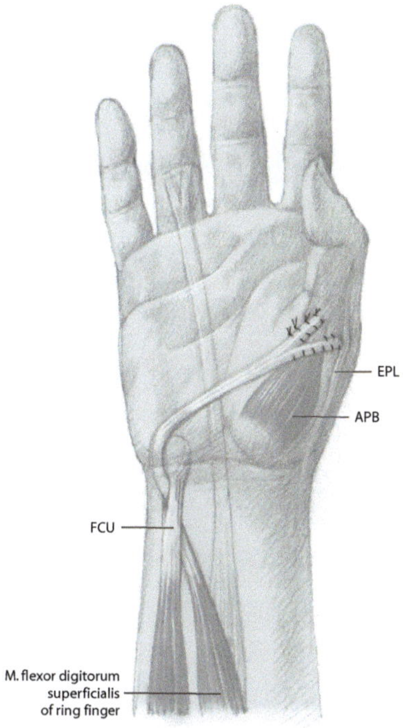

Figure 11.15

Alternatively to the ADM, the FDS of the ring finger can be used to restore opposition. The FCU is then used as a pulley

If neither the ADM nor the FDS are available because of lesions of the median, ulnar nerves or tendons themselves, the transfer of the radial nerve innervated extensor indicis (EI) is suggested. As this tendon has a separate motor, it is well suited for transfers (▶ Fig. 11.16). The EI is identified through a dorsal incision at the MP joint of the index finger. The EI lies ulnar to the ED. It is then divided, and the extensor hood reconstructed with a nonabsorbable suture. Through a second incision proximal, the EI is freed from the fascia and subcutaneously transposed su-

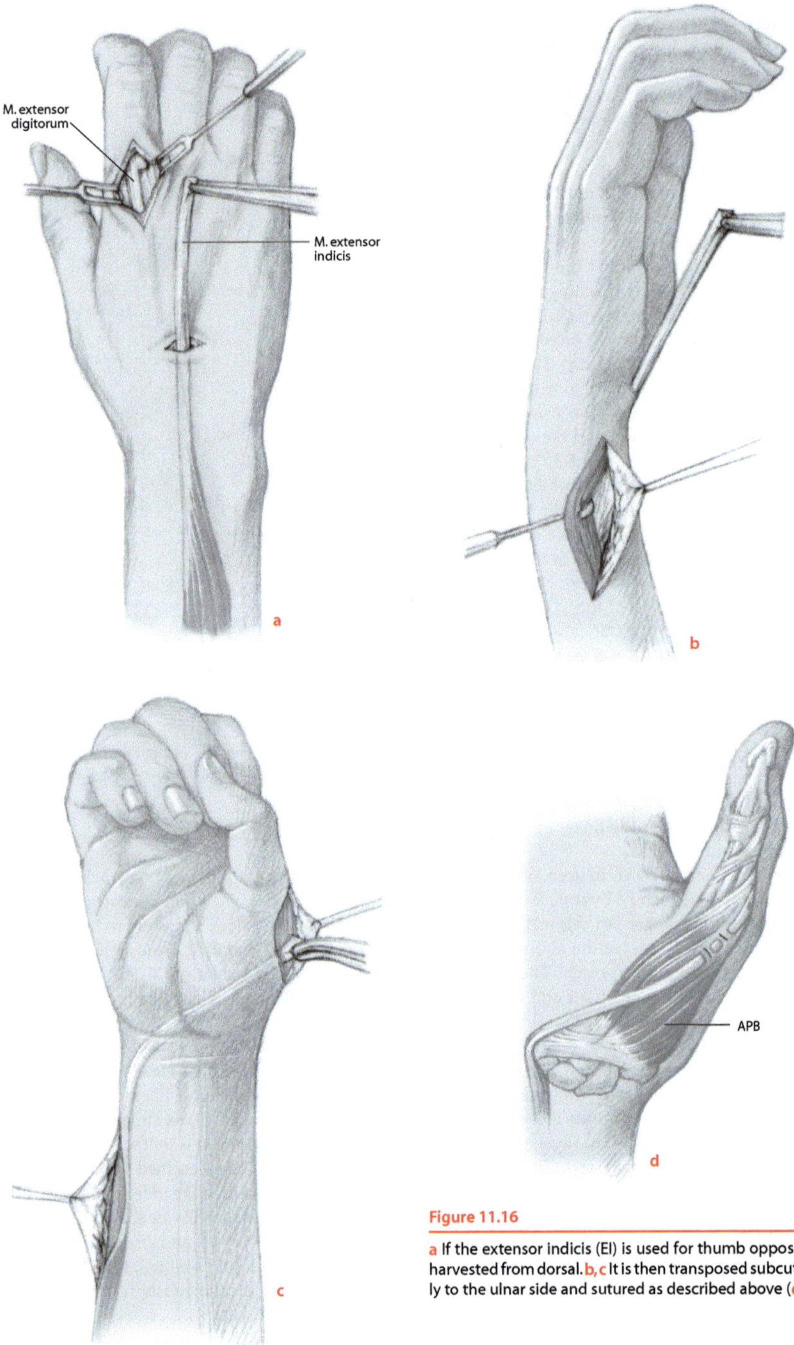

Figure 11.16

a If the extensor indicis (EI) is used for thumb opposition it is harvested from dorsal. b, c It is then transposed subcutaneously to the ulnar side and sutured as described above (d) perficial to the extensor carpi ulnaris muscle (ECU) to the pisiform bone (third incision) and then placed like the ADM tendon (see above). Postoperative treatment is similar; physiotherapy, however, appears more difficult as the EI is an antagonist to the thumb opposing muscles.

11.4.4 High Ulnar Nerve Palsy

In addition to the loss of finger abduction and adduction, adduction of the thumb and a claw hand (distal palsy), an isolated high ulnar nerve palsy results in a loss of function of the FDP of the ring and little fingers, and the FCU. Innervation anomalies might alter the presentation. The corrections of the functional deficits of distal palsy are extensively discussed in the following chapters as they are more important. In accordance with high median nerve palsy, the loss of FDP of the ring and little fingers are corrected by suturing the respective tendons to the FDP tendons of the middle finger. If more power is required an extensor muscle (such as ECRL) may be transferred to the ulnar FDP tendons. The loss of the FCU is well tolerated if another wrist flexor is present.

11.4.5 Distal Ulnar Nerve Palsy

The functional deficits caused by distal ulnar nerve palsy are weakness of pinch resulting from paralysis of the adductor pollicis and first dorsal interosseous muscles, weakness of grip produced by paralysis of most of the finger intrinsics, and sometimes clawing of the ring and little fingers associated with paralysis of all their intrinsics. Innervation anomalies of the intrinsic can present either a more severe paralysis or a more moderate loss of function.

11.4.5.1 Adduction of Thumb and Abduction of Index Finger

The paralysis of the adductor pollicis results in a major loss of function that should be corrected when possible by the appropriate tendon transfer. However, this transfer should be accompanied by restoration of abduction of the index finger. Several transfers have been advised to achieve functional results. Again we describe our preferred methods; however, other techniques must be remembered to provide the best possible results in combined nerve palsies.

For thumb adduction we prefer the transfer of the superficial flexor of the ring finger (▶ Fig. 11.17). To avoid a deformity of the PIP joint, the tendon is sectioned at the base of the proximal phalanx of the ring finger, brought out at the mid-palm, ulnar to the thenar crease. It is then passed through the natural opening of the fascia between the ring and middle fingers at the distal third of the palm. The tendon is now passed subcutaneously and fixed at the radial side of the thumb at the level of the MP joint. The tendon is placed in 30° wrist flexion, the thumb in mild flexion and adduction. Some authors prefer a transosseous pull out suture. This, however, is not necessary from our experience. After operation, immobilization is carried out for 4 weeks in adduction of the thumb and mild flexion of the wrist. Other transfers are the transposition and elongation of the BR or the ERCL/B with a tendon graft. The BR, however, is preferred and elongated with the PL tendon rerouted through the third interosseous space (▶ Fig. 11.18). This transfer is advised in a proximal palsy. The same result can be achieved using the EI, passed through the interosseous membrane or, like the BR, through the third interosseous space (▶ Fig. 11.19). The extensor digiti minimi has also been described as a transfer tendon (Burkhalter 1974).

Thumb adduction should be restored in one operation combined with the reconstruction of the index finger radial abduction (Bruner 1946): for this, we prefer the transfer of the extensor pollicis brevis (EPB; ▶ Fig. 11.20). This provides a stable pinch. From a curved incision over the MP joint of the thumb the EPB is divided, the extensor hood reconstructed, the EPB tendon is then rerouted from an incision over the tabatière, subcutaneously tunneled, and passed through the insertion of the first dorsal interosseous tendon (separate incision). Immobilization is as described above. Physical therapy should aim to enforce the new movements and relax the antagonists, depending on the transferred tendons.

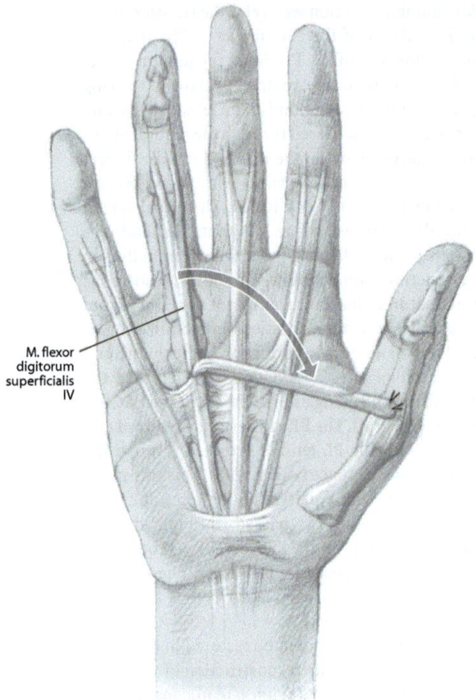

Figure 11.17

The FDS of the ring finger can be used for thumb adduction. The palmar fascia acts as a pulley

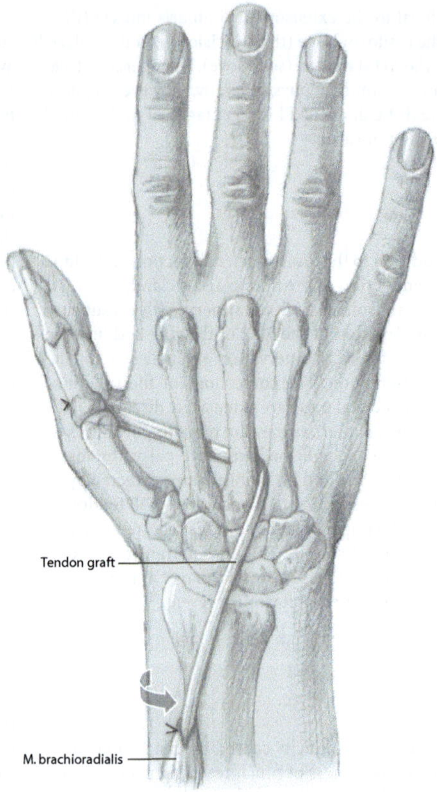

Figure 11.18

The brachioradialis (BR) can be elongated with a tendon graft and acts as a thumb adductor when passed through the third interosseous space

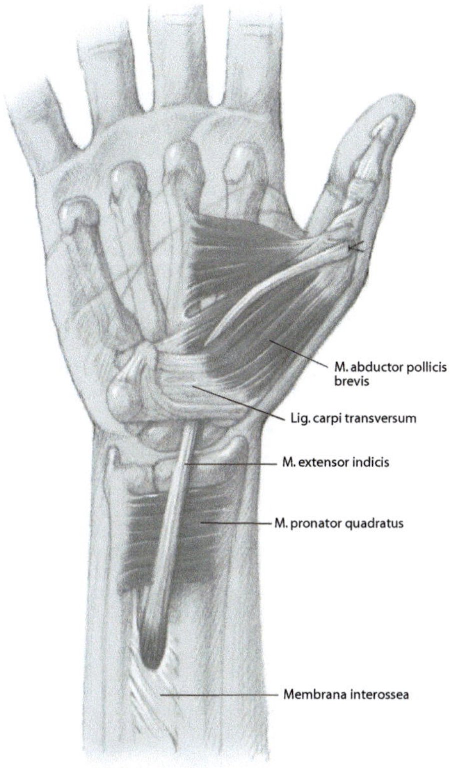

Figure 11.19

The extensor indicis (EI) can also be used for thumb adduction. The tendon can either be passed through the interosseous membrane or through the third interosseous space (see Fig. 11.18)

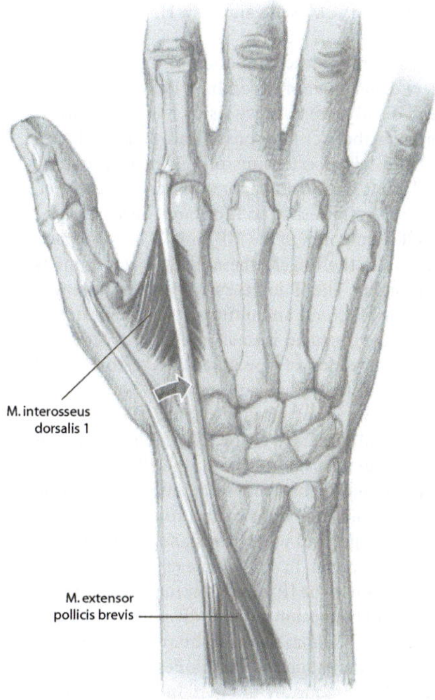

Figure 11.20

The index finger abduction should be restored in the same operation as thumb adduction. The transfer of the extensor pollicis brevis (EPB) is preferred

11.4.5.2 Intrinsic Muscles and Claw Hand

Loss of intrinsic muscle function of the fingers as a result of distal ulnar or in combination with distal ulnar and distal median nerve lesion has intact extrinsic muscles that act unopposed and thus produce a claw hand. Hyperextension of the metacarpophalangeal joints is the primary or most disabling aspect. The grasp is diminished 50 % or more because of the lack of flexion power in the MP joints. The movement in flexion of the fingers themselves is additionally asynchronous. The IP joints must flex first, followed next by the MP joints and ultimately by full flexion of fingers. Thus the hand is unable to grasp a large object. The correction of claw hand and restoration of intrinsic muscles is a staged procedure. Many simple procedures are based on the fact that if hyperextension in the MP joints is corrected, extrinsic muscles are able to extend the fingers in the IP joints sufficiently. Therefore, the proper operation depends on muscles available for transfer, the amount of passive motion in finger and wrist joints and on the experience of the surgeon. In a moderate claw hand that allows extension in the IP joints after manually correcting the hyperextension of the MP joints (metacarpophalangeal stabilization test; Bouvier maneuver), simple procedures such as capsulodesis, tenodesis or the "lasso" technique are advised. In severe clawing, transfers of active tendons may be required (▶ Figs. 11.21, 11.22).

- Capsulodesis (modified Zancolli 1979). From a transverse incision in the palm (at the level of the distal flexor crease), expose tendon sheaths, do not damage neurovascular bundles. Incise over each MP joint longitudinally, retract the flexor tendons, create a distally based U-shaped flap, achieve a 20°–30° flexion of the MP joints and fix the flaps transosseously through a drill hole. Alternatively, a spindle-shaped excision can be performed, to achieve flexion of the MP joints (▶ Fig. 11.23). Immobilize in 30° flexion of the MP joints in dorsal splint for 3 weeks, but allow motion of IP joints. Physical therapy starts after 3 weeks.
- Dynamic tenodesis (Fowler). In this easy procedure a tendon graft twice as long as the distance from the dorsum of the wrist to the PIP joints (e.g., PL or plantaris tendon) is used (▶ Fig. 11.24). Expose the dorsal retinaculum of the wrist from a transverse incision, pass the graft distal to the proximal edge through the retinaculum, and split each end into two equal slips (correction of all fingers). Then transfer each slip to the fingers by rout-

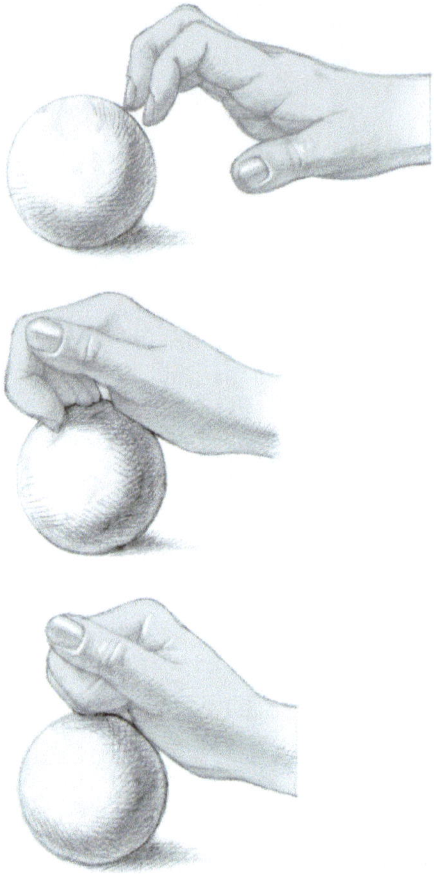

Figure 11.21

In a claw hand resulting from an ulnar nerve lesion, hyperextension of the metacarpophalangeal joints is most disabling. The grasp is diminished because of the lack of flexion power in the metacarpophalangeal (MP) joints. The movement in flexion of the fingers themselves is additionally asynchronous. The phalangeal (IP) joints must flex first, followed next by the MP joints and ultimately by full flexion of fingers. Thus the hand is unable to grasp a large object

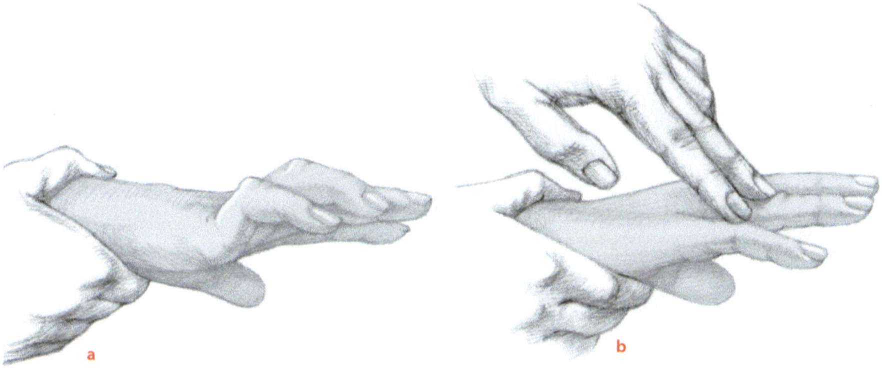

Figure 11.22a,b

Bouvier maneuver. In a moderate claw hand that allows extension in the IP joints after manually correcting the hyperextension of the MP joints (metacarpophalangeal stabilization test; Bouvier maneuver), simple procedures such as capsulodesis, tenodesis or the lasso technique are advised

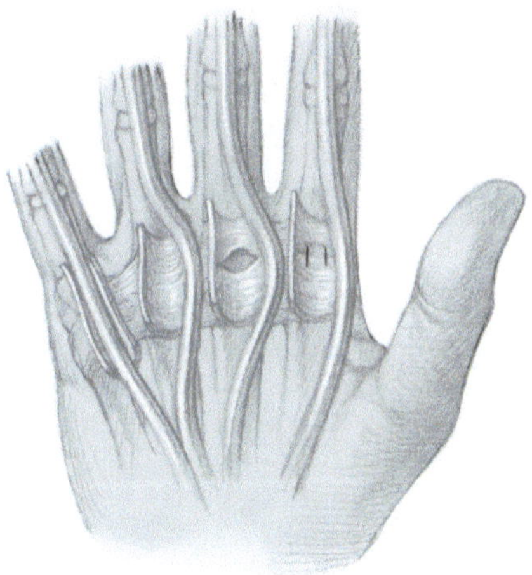

Figure 11.23

In a moderate claw hand, it might be sufficient to only excise a spindle-shaped part of the capsule of the MP joint and to suture it in a flexed position

ing them palmar to deep transverse metacarpal ligament and attach on the ulnar side of extensor aponeurosis (index finger) and the radial side of extensor aponeurosis of the other fingers (alternatively to the A2 pulley). Suture the grafts so that when the wrist is flexed, force will be exerted on the extensor mechanism so as to extend the IP joints without hyperflexing the MP joints (Buck-Gramcko and Nigst 1991).

- Lasso technique (Zancolli). This very easy method is preferred as it focuses on flexion of the MP joints. However, for this technique an active motor is required. If available, the FDS of the ring finger is used (direct operation); if not, ECRL or BR are extended with grafts and rerouted (indirect operation). Either method is fixed similarly. The FDS tendon is harvested and extracted to the mid of the palm, divided into the needed number of slips (ideally two slips) and then routed from proximally underneath the A1 pulley, transferred distally again and sutured to itself (▶ Fig. 11.25). The wrist should be in a neutral position, the fingers extended (neutral position). Immobilization is carried out in a splint with 30° flexion in the MP joints for 3 weeks. Immediate active movement of the IP joints is advised. If only the ring and little fingers are affected, Zancolli (1979) advised the use of the EI tendon, rerouted through the interosseous membrane and the carpal tunnel.

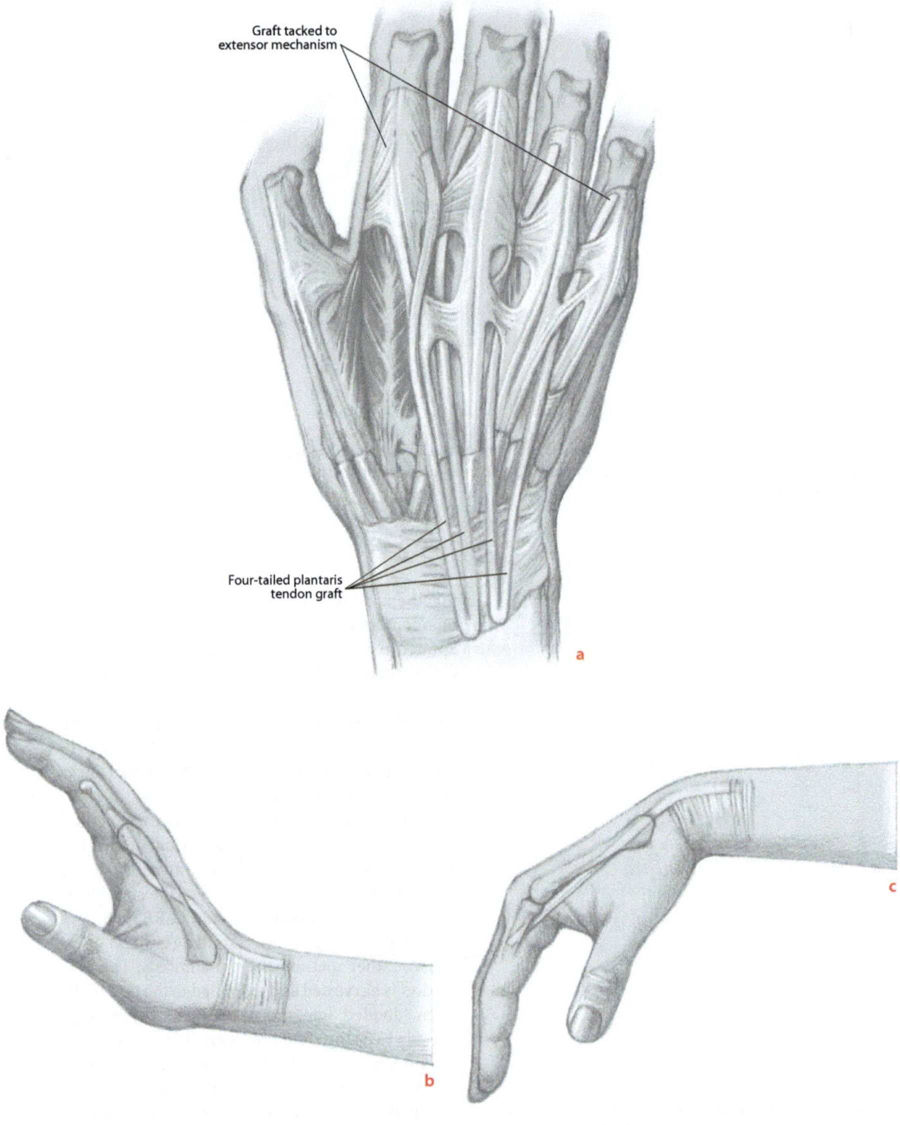

Figure 11.24a–c

Fowler tenodesis. A tendon graft twice as long as the distance from the dorsum of the wrist to the PIP joints is placed to correct hyperextension. The transfer is routed palmar to the deep transverse metacarpal ligament and attached to the ulnar side of extensor aponeurosis (index finger) and the radial side of extensor aponeurosis of the other fingers (alternatively to the A2 pulley). The grafts are sutured so that when the wrist is flexed, force will be exerted on the extensor mechanism so as to extend the IP joints without hyperflexing the MP joints

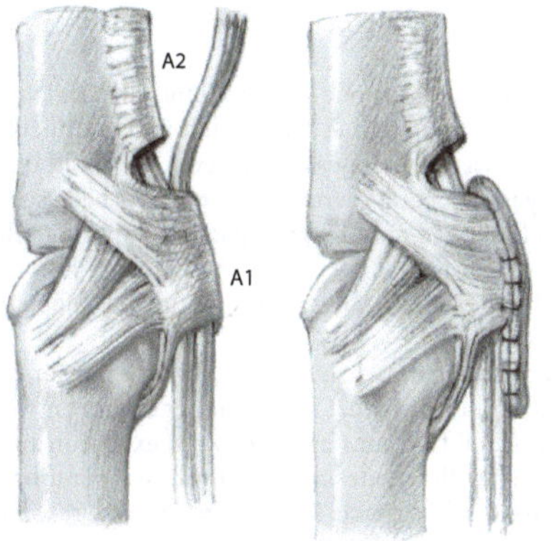

Figure 11.25

Lasso technique. The FDS tendon is harvested and extracted to the middle of the palm, divided into the needed amount of slips (ideally two slips) and then routed from proximally under the A1 pulley, transferred distally again and sutured to itself

- Transfer of ERCL/B (Brand). This technique is more difficult but is more powerful. The ERCB or ERCL is detached and elongated with grafts (as many as necessary, up to four for all fingers, many-tailed grafts). The tendon is routed under the BR palmarly and runs through the carpal tunnel (Brand II route). The grafts are then inserted to the extensor aponeurosis as described above under the proper tension. Problems encountered can involve a possible median nerve compression in the carpal tunnel and adhesions of the grafts. In some cases, a swan neck deformity has been described due to too much tension.

11.4.5.3 Abducted Little Finger (Wartenberg Sign)

Permanent abduction of the little finger is not a major functional problem, but frequently disturbs patients. The position is best corrected by transferring the extensor digiti minimi muscle (EDM) either palmarly (if a MP joint hyperextension is to be corrected) or dorsally to the radial extensor aponeurosis. Alternatively, a split tendon from the extensor tendon of the ring finger can be used. This does not cause an extension deficit for the little finger.

11.4.6 Combined Nerve Palsies

Combined nerve lesions increase the functional loss, and decrease the number of tendons available for transfer. In the following we will describe possible transfers in combined palsies of the major nerves of the hand, assuming the worst case scenario. These are suggestions and must be modified for the individual patients and their personal needs. However, if nerve reconstruction was carried out, it is likely that some function of these regenerated muscles (if they achieve at least an M4) can be used to correct imbalance and to focus on the important functions of the hand.

11.4.6.1 Combined Distal Median and Ulnar Nerve Palsy

This severe functional loss requires enormous efforts, not only operatively, but also in conservative treatment such as physical therapy, correct splinting and skin treatment:

- For thumb adduction use the FDS of the ring finger. (If the flexor tendons were injured in a trauma, use elongated BR transfer).
- For thumb opposition use EI transfer.
- For index abduction use the EPB.
- For intrinsic restoration use the lasso technique with a superficial flexor (e.g., FDS of the middle finger). If superficial flexors are injured, use capsulodesis (when the Bouvier sign is positive) or Brand transfer of ECRL with graft elongation.
  Still available for transfer are the ECU and EDM.

11.4.6.2 Combined Proximal Median and Ulnar Nerve Palsy

- For restoration of all deep flexors (FDP) use the ECRL.
- For FPL use the BR; alternatively the IP joint arthrodesis.
- For thumb adduction then use the BR.
- For thumb opposition use EI transfer.
- For index abduction use the EPB or EDM.
- For intrinsic restoration use capsulodesis or ECU with grafts.

It might be necessary to fuse the MP joint of the thumb or to correct the position by transposition of the radial sesamoid, if a hyperextension of this joint is present (accentuated, if the EPB is used).

11.4.6.3 Combined Proximal Median and Radial Nerve Palsy

This lesion in not likely to occur as a distal lesion; a proximal palsy is very difficult to treat, as only the ulnar nerve innervated muscles are available for transfer. If no innervation anomalies or reinnervated muscles are present, an arthrodesis of the wrist and IP joint of the thumb are advised.

- For finger and thumb extension (MP joints) the FCU is used.
- The FDP of the index finger is fixed to the FDP of the middle (or ring) finger.
- For opposition of the thumb use the ADM.

11.4.6.4 Combined Proximal Ulnar and Radial Nerve Palsy

The classic transfers can be applied in these lesions and offer a good prognosis.

- For wrist extension use the PT.
- For extension of the fingers use the FDS of the middle finger (do not use the FCR, as one strong wrist flexor should be maintained).
- For thumb extension use PL.
- For flexion of the ring and little fingers (FDP) the tendons are fixed to the FDP of the middle finger.
- For the claw hand use capsulodesis or tenodesis.

To stabilize the thumb an arthrodesis of the MP joint might be necessary.

11.4.6.5 Special Pattern of Paralysis

In special cases only one or two motors are available for restoring function at the hand. It is very difficult to give advice in these cases; however, we would like to suggest an operation method, which has been successfully applied to tetraplegic patients, knowing full well that peripheral nerve and central nerve lesions have different approaches in reconstruction (Moberg 1987; Nigst 1991).

If one potent muscle is left, e.g., a wrist extensor, or the BR, or any other that allows proper excursion, the muscle should be transferred for wrist extension and combined with tenodesis and arthrodesis operations to achieve a key pinch. This operation was recommended by Moberg and later modified by Brand (▶ Fig. 11.26). First the muscle is transferred to allow extension. If the BR is used the tendon can easily passed through the ERCB at the middle third of the forearm. To achieve a key pinch, the FPL tendon is routed around the palm (leaving the A1 pulley intact), beneath the flexor tendons and trough Guyon's canal before applying tenodesis to the distal radius (pass the tendon through drill holes and suture to itself). The tension is adjusted so that during extension of the wrist the thumb firmly contacts the side of the index finger. To obtain a stable thumb, the IP joint must be fused (using Kirscher wire), and tenodesis of the EPL tendon to the first metacarpal bone (through drill holes) is necessary in approximately 20° flexion of the MP joint. Other operations such as the Bruner "winch" technique allow key pinch with supination (the FPL is fixed to the ulna).

If wrist extension is preserved and two tendons are available, they should be used for finger extension (ED and EPL), and the FDP tendons. The FPL receives tenodesis as described above or fixed to the wrist extensor (▶ Fig. 11.27a–c).

These are the only possible methods available, which must be tailored for each patient and may be combined with other arthrodesis or tenodesis operations, according to the patients needs.

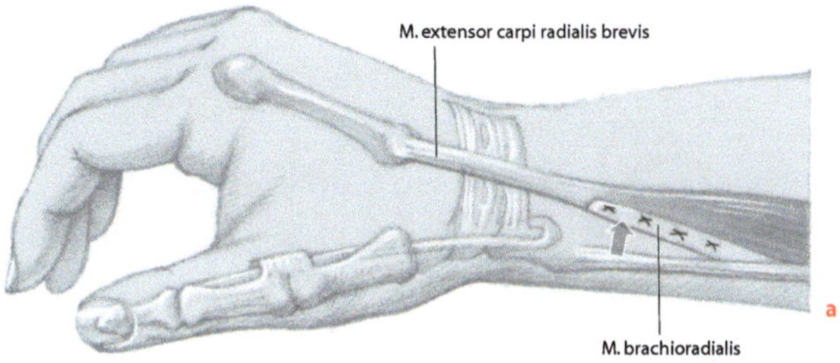

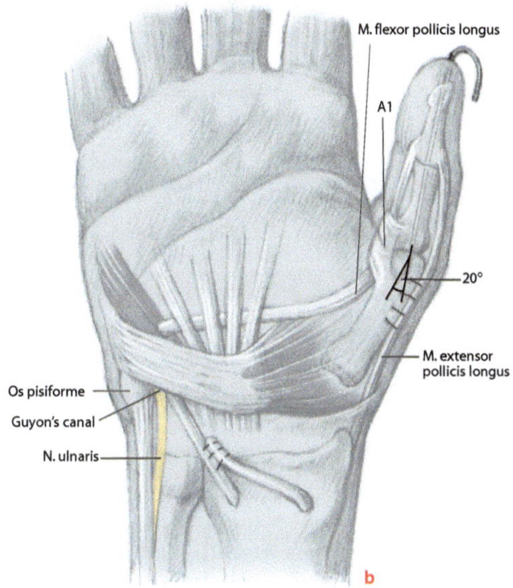

Figure 11.26a, b

Key pinch operation according to Moberg/Brand. a The BR is transferred to allow extension. b For key pinch the flexor pollicis longus muscle (FPL) tendon is routed around the palm (leaving the A1 pulley intact), beneath the flexor tendons and trough Guyon's canal before tenodesis to the distal radius (pass the tendon through drill holes and suture to itself). The tension is adjusted so that during extension of the wrist, the thumb firmly contacts the side of the index finger. For a stable thumb, the IP joint is fused, and the EPL tendon undergoes tenodesis to the first metacarpal bone in approximately 20° flexion of the MP joint

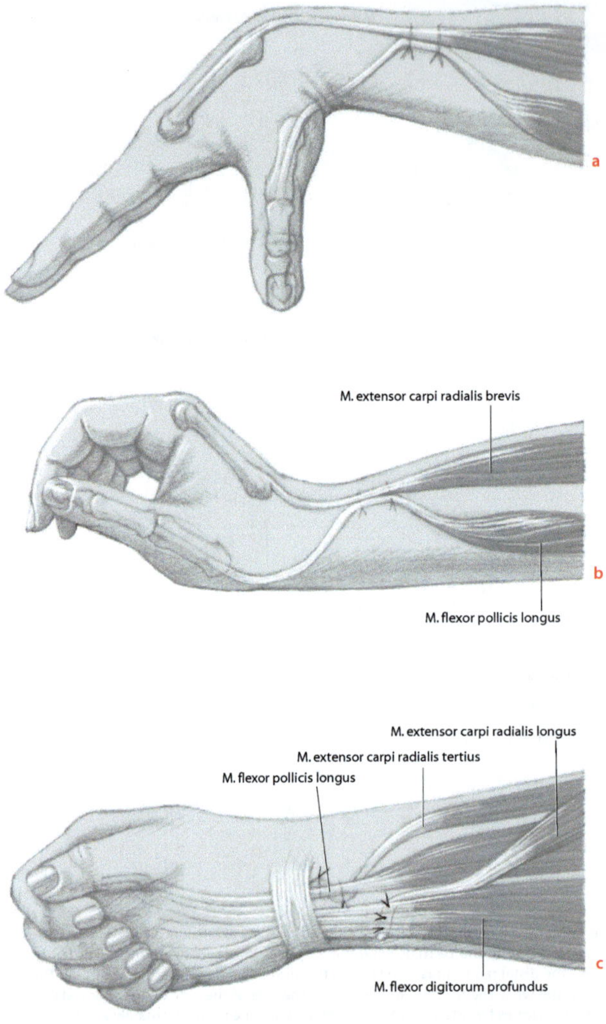

Figure 11.27 a–c

If wrist extension is preserved the FPL can also be fixed to the wrist extensor (a, b), thus producing a key pinch when extending the wrist. If two tendons are available (c), they should be used for finger extension (ED and EPL), and the FDP tendons. In some cases, an extensor carpi radialis tertius is present; it can be used for restoration of FPL function

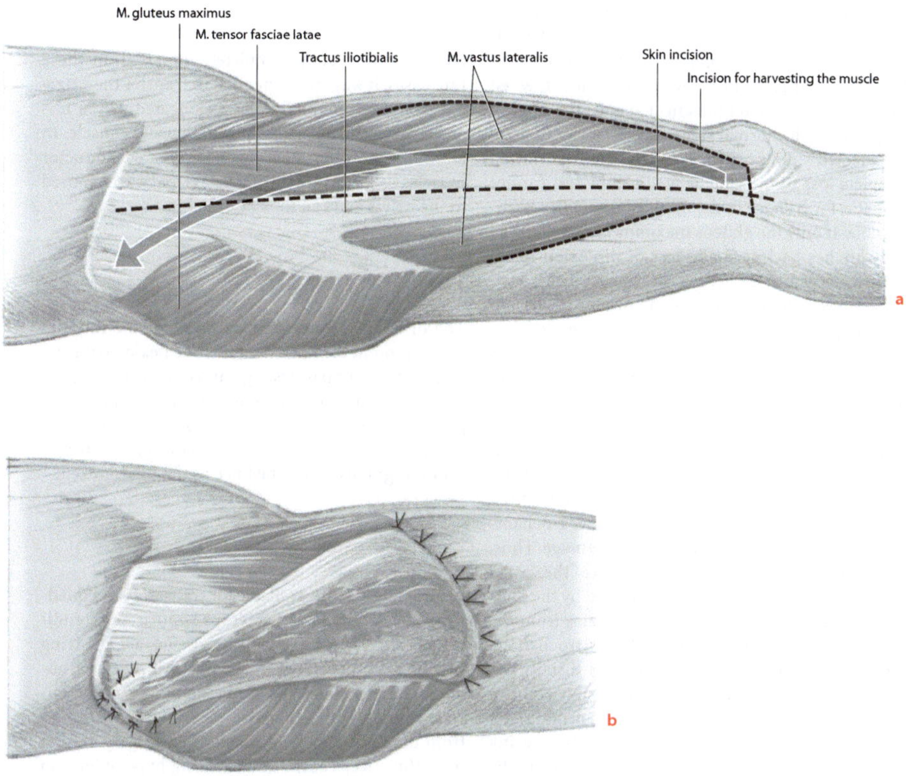

11.5 Hip

Several muscles act on the hip to achieve flexion, extension, abduction and adduction. Paralysis usually causes severe impairment, including flexion and abduction contractures of the hip, hip instability and limping are caused by paralysis of the gluteus maximus and medius muscles.

11.5.1 Abduction, Extension of the Hip (Superior and Inferior Gluteal Nerves)

A palsy of the superior gluteal nerve causes a weakness of abduction due to the paralysis of the gluteus medius and minimus and the tensor fascia latae muscles. The result is an unstable hip and an unsightly and fatiguing limb. Due to weakness of the gluteus

Figure 11.28a, b

To restore hip abduction, the vastus lateralis muscle is transposed. a Over a straight incision, the muscle is harvested from distal to proximal. The nerve and vessels entering from medial in the proximal third are left intact. The muscle can be transposed proximally to the origin of the gluteus medius (b). If the vastus is too short (because of irregularities of the neurovascular bundle) it can be elongated with fascial strips from the TFL. The muscle is fixed with nonabsorbable sutures (through drill holes) in the pelvis. Alternatively, corkscrew anchors are used. The tension should allow an overcorrection with abduction of the hip. In long-standing paralysis, it might be necessary to combine this procedure with a myotomy of the adductor muscles medius during weight bearing on the affected side, the trunk sways toward the affected side and the pelvis elevates on the opposite side (compensated Trendelenburg gait). In a severe impairment, when the weight is borne on the affected side, the level of the pelvis on the normal side will drop lower than on the affected side (positive Trendelenburg gait). In a complete loss of the gluteus medius, the test cannot be made, for balance in the disabled extremity is impossible. If only the gluteus maximus is impaired the body lurches backward and loss of hip extension is present, necessary for getting up from a sitting position or for ascending steps. To stabilize the pelvis and improve gait, a muscle transfer is recommended.

If the gluteus medius is paralyzed and gluteus maximus is intact, the transposition of the latter more ventrally (toward the trochanter major) might improve the instability. There have been several suggestions to stabilize the hip by other transfers. However, all previously published transfers such as the transfer of the external oblique muscle or the transfer of the iliopsoas (with iliacus) muscle to the grater trochanter are either too weak or cause severe damage. Thus, we prefer the over-the-top transposition of the vastus lateralis muscle (▶ Fig. 11.28). Innervated by the femoral nerve, this powerful muscle originates from the insertion of the gluteus medius (lesser trochanter) and is easy to transpose. The muscle is distally detached with its tendon and proximally removed from the quadriceps group, if possible up to its origin at the greater trochanter. The nerve and vessels entering from medial in the proximal third are left intact. The muscle can be transposed proximally to the origin of the gluteus medius. If the vastus is too short (because of irregularities of the neurovascular bundle) it can be elongated with fascial strips from the tensor fasciae latae (TFL). The muscle is fixed with nonabsorbable sutures through drill holes in the pelvis; alternatively corkscrew anchors are used. The tension should allow an overcorrection with abduction of the hip. In long-standing paralysis, it might be necessary to combine this procedure with a myotomy of the adductor muscles and a varus femoral osteotomy. The patient is immobilized for 6 weeks in a cast in hip abduction. Physical therapy should focus on the difficult education (hip flexor and knee extensor for hip abduction) by relaxing hip adduction and flexion.

11.5.2 Hip Flexion (Femoral Nerve)

Hip flexion is rarely completely impaired. In these rare cases, it was recommended to transfer the external oblique abdominal muscle elongated with a fascial strip to the insertion of the iliopsoas muscle. In addition, the obturator nerve-innervated adductor muscles (e.g., the gracilis muscle) can be transposed to the pelvis and can thus flex the hip.

11.6 Knee

The disabilities caused by paralysis of the muscles acting around the knee joint include flexion contracture, quadriceps paralysis, genu recurvatum, and flail knee. Only the impaired knee extension can be improved by tendon transfers. Transfers for the hamstring muscles are usually not necessary, because in walking, gravity flexes the knee as the hip is flexed.

11.6.1 Knee Extension (Femoral Nerve)

Several muscles are available for transfer to the quadriceps tendon and patella: biceps femoris, semitendinosus, and tensor fascia latae. Using a hamstring muscle for transfer, the power of the hip flexors, abductors and the triceps surae should be fair (Schwartzmann 1948). Otherwise, clearing the extremity from the floor may be difficult after surgery. Both a powerful triceps surae and avoiding hyperextension immobilization after surgery can prevent a possible genu recurvatum.

The preferred transfer is the combination of the biceps femoris muscle and semitendinosus muscle; the latter serves more as a rein on the patella to prevent its dislocating laterally (▶ Fig. 11.29). In a bloodless field, the distal insertion of the biceps femoris tendon is identified from a lateral incision. The biceps tendon is freed with an osteotome from the fibula along with a piece of bone, preserving the peroneal nerve and the fibular collateral ligament. The biceps is freed proximally as far as possible (till the vessels enter the muscle) to create a pull that is as oblique as possible. Also, the origin of the short head of biceps must be freed. A subcutaneous tunnel is created ventrally, and an incision is made over the distal quadriceps tendon and patella. The iliotibial band and the fascia of the vastus lateralis and the intermuscular septae are divided. From a third incision over the posteromedial aspect, the semitendinosus insertion is identified posterior to the sartorius and distal to the

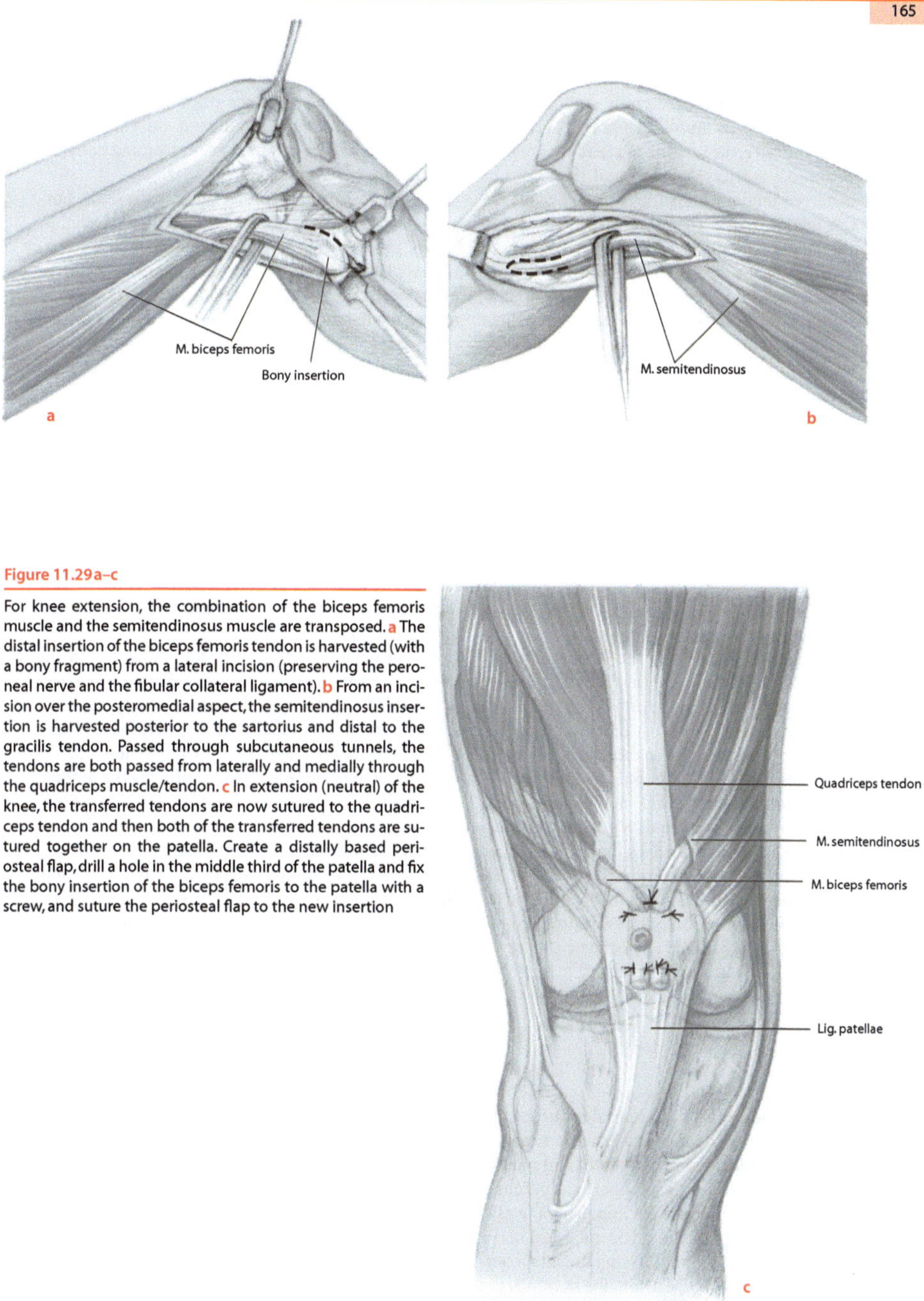

Figure 11.29a–c

For knee extension, the combination of the biceps femoris muscle and the semitendinosus muscle are transposed. **a** The distal insertion of the biceps femoris tendon is harvested (with a bony fragment) from a lateral incision (preserving the peroneal nerve and the fibular collateral ligament). **b** From an incision over the posteromedial aspect, the semitendinosus insertion is harvested posterior to the sartorius and distal to the gracilis tendon. Passed through subcutaneous tunnels, the tendons are both passed from laterally and medially through the quadriceps muscle/tendon. **c** In extension (neutral) of the knee, the transferred tendons are now sutured to the quadriceps tendon and then both of the transferred tendons are sutured together on the patella. Create a distally based periosteal flap, drill a hole in the middle third of the patella and fix the bony insertion of the biceps femoris to the patella with a screw, and suture the periosteal flap to the new insertion gracilis tendon. The muscle is detached and freed to the middle third of the thigh. Reroute subcutaneously and pass both muscles laterally and medially through the quadriceps muscle/tendon. In extension (neutral) of the knee, the transferred tendons are now sutured to the quadriceps tendon and then both of the transferred tendons are sutured together on the patella. A distally based periosteal flap is created, a hole drilled in the middle third of the patella and the bony insertion of the biceps femoris fixed to the patella with a screw, and the periosteal flap sutured to the new insertion. Alternatively, a transverse hole through the patella can be created. The postoperative treatment is immobilization for 6 weeks in knee extension (neutral position) in a cast. The hip is left without movement (biceps extends in hip) for 3 weeks. Weight bearing starts after 8 weeks. Apply a knee brace in extension for a total of 3 months. Physical therapy should start after the eighth week with relaxing the knee flexors and moving the preoperatively trained biceps femoris.

11.7 Foot and Ankle

Long-standing paralysis usually causes severe deformities of the foot and ankle, they are the most dependent parts of the body and are subjected to greater strain than other parts. The most common deformities include claw toes, cavovarus foot, dorsal bunion, talipes equinus, talipes equinovarus, talipes cavovarus, talipes equinovalgus, and talipes calcaneus. These deformities are corrected by tendon transfers to restore muscle balance and by bony procedures such as osteotomy and arthrodesis. However, we would like to focus on the transfers that restore movement. That is the restoration of dorsiflexion and pronation of the foot, in order to correct peroneal nerve palsy. Only rarely is a transfer necessary to correct a loss of plantar flexion.

11.7.1 Dorsiflexion of the Foot (Peroneal Nerve)

A complete peroneal palsy causes paralysis of the tibialis anterior, extensor hallucis longus and extensor digitorum longus (deep peroneal nerve) and paralysis of the peroneal muscle group (superficial peroneal nerve). This results in a drop foot, impairing the gait. A palsy of one of the branches of the peroneal nerve can easily be corrected by transferring the intact tendons into a more dynamic position, for example, the peroneal muscles (peroneus longus) more medially (base of second metatarsal), or the tibialis anterior tendon more laterally (second or third metatarsal). If the extensor hallucis longus presents hyperactivity the tendon should be lengthened (in children) or transferred to the metatarsal neck, avoiding bony deformities of the first metatarsal.

In complete palsy we prefer the transfer of the posterior tibial muscle. This transfer is easy and reliable. Again, preoperative training is mandatory. The patient is placed on his back, and in a bloodless field, the insertion of the tibialis posterior tendon is exposed from a medial incision; the tendon is then harvested with a bony fragment, and dissected proximally along the medial border of the tibia until the distal parts of the muscle are mobilized (▶ Fig. 11.30). An anterior incision over the distal third of the leg is made, lateral to the tibialis anterior tendon. Deeply dissect between the tibialis anterior and the extensor hallucis longus. Injuries to the tibialis anterior vessels should be avoided, and a generous window cut in the interosseous membrane. The tibialis posterior tendon is rerouted through this window, and care taken not to kink the tendon. Make an incision over the middle cuneiform and the third metatarsal, reroute the tendon underneath the retinaculum extensorum (take a thick silicon drain for routing the tendon with the bony fragment). Create a periosteal flap over the base of the third metatarsal and insert the bony fragment with the screw. The distal tendon is sutured periosteally as is the periosteal flap back over the tendon. The foot should be held in 90° when suturing the tendon. Alternatively, some authors describe splitting the tendon and suturing under equal tension medially and laterally. As we see more complications than advantages with this technique, we abandoned this method. Immobilization should last for 6 weeks, with weight bearing after the 3rd week in a cast. Physical therapy, relaxing plantar flexion and training the tibialis posterior muscle follow. A peroneal splint (L-shaped) should be left for 3 months.

In cases with a flexion contracture of the ankle, it might be necessary to perform an arthrolysis prior to this transfer. As an arthrolysis requires immediate movement, we do not recommend a single-stage operation.

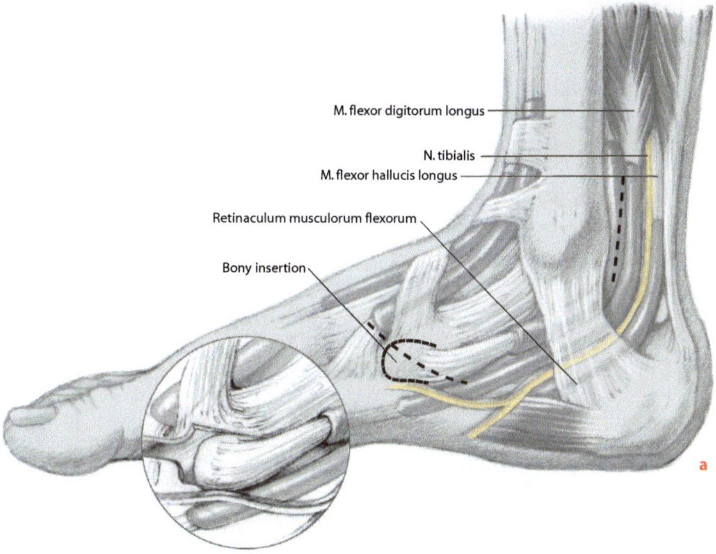

Figure 11.30a–d

Transfer of the posterior tibial muscle. a The insertion of the tibialis posterior tendon is exposed from a medial incision, the tendon is then harvested with a bony fragment, and dissected proximally along the medial border of the tibia.

Figures b–d: see next pages

11.7.2 Plantar Flexion (Tibial Nerve)

The loss of plantar flexion is usually well compensated because gravity acts on flexion if the foot is elevated. However, in rare cases, it might be necessary to restore plantar flexion, mainly by reconstruction of triceps surae function. The anterior tibial tendon should be preserved and may be transferred on the dorsum. Then only the peroneal nerve innervated peroneal and extensor muscle groups remain for transfer. However, as this operation may require several secondary procedures, the indication should be discussed carefully and an arthrodesis may be more appropriate.

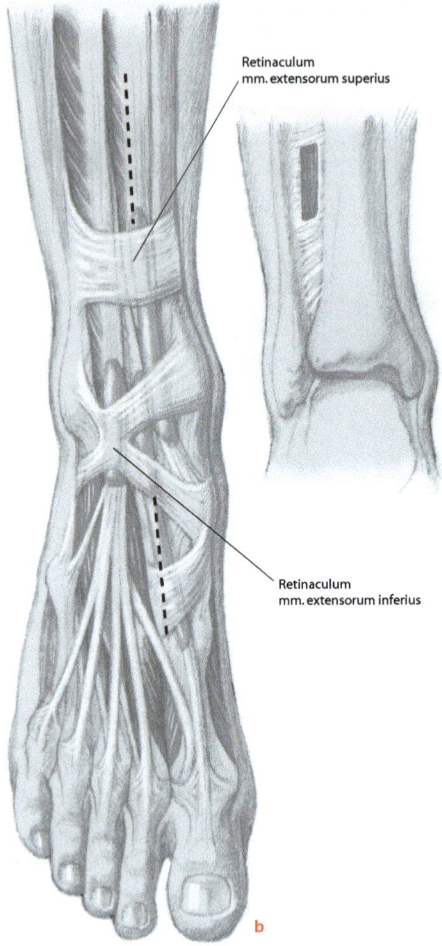

Figure 11.30a–d

Transfer of the posterior tibial muscle. **b** The tendon is then rerouted anteriorly through the distal third of the leg via a generous window in the interosseous membrane (avoiding injuries to the tibialis anterior vessels). **c, d** Reroute the tendon under the retinaculum extensorum (take a thick silicon drain for routing the tendon with the bony fragment) and fix the bony fragment with a screw at the middle cuneiform or base of the third metatarsal. The foot should be held in 90° when suturing the tendon

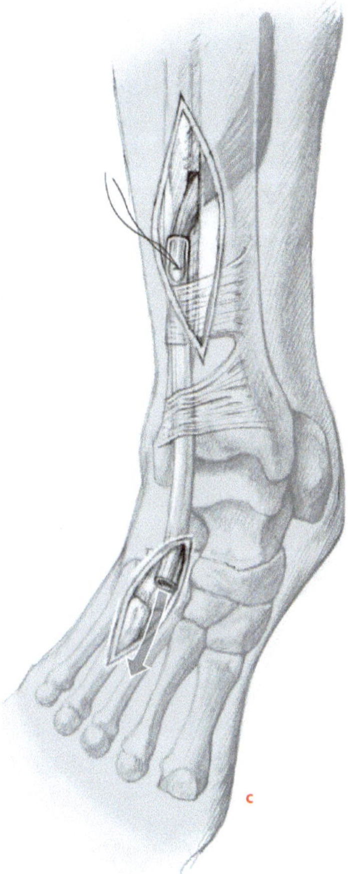

c

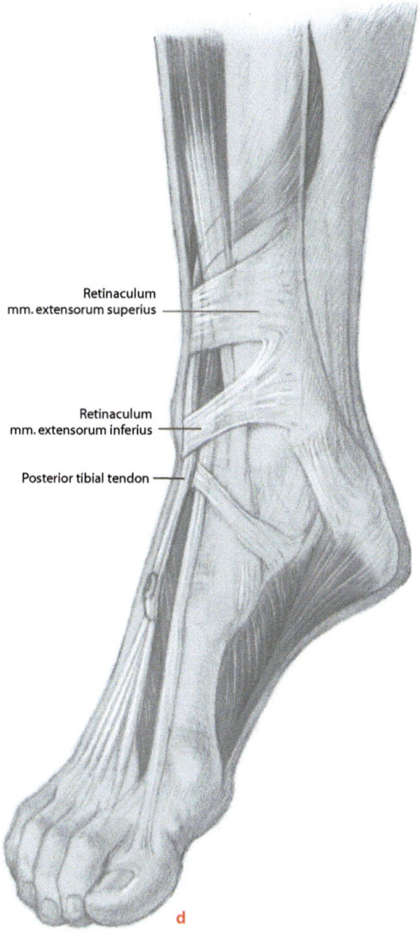
Retinaculum
mm. extensorum superius
Retinaculum
mm. extensorum inferius
Posterior tibial tendon

d

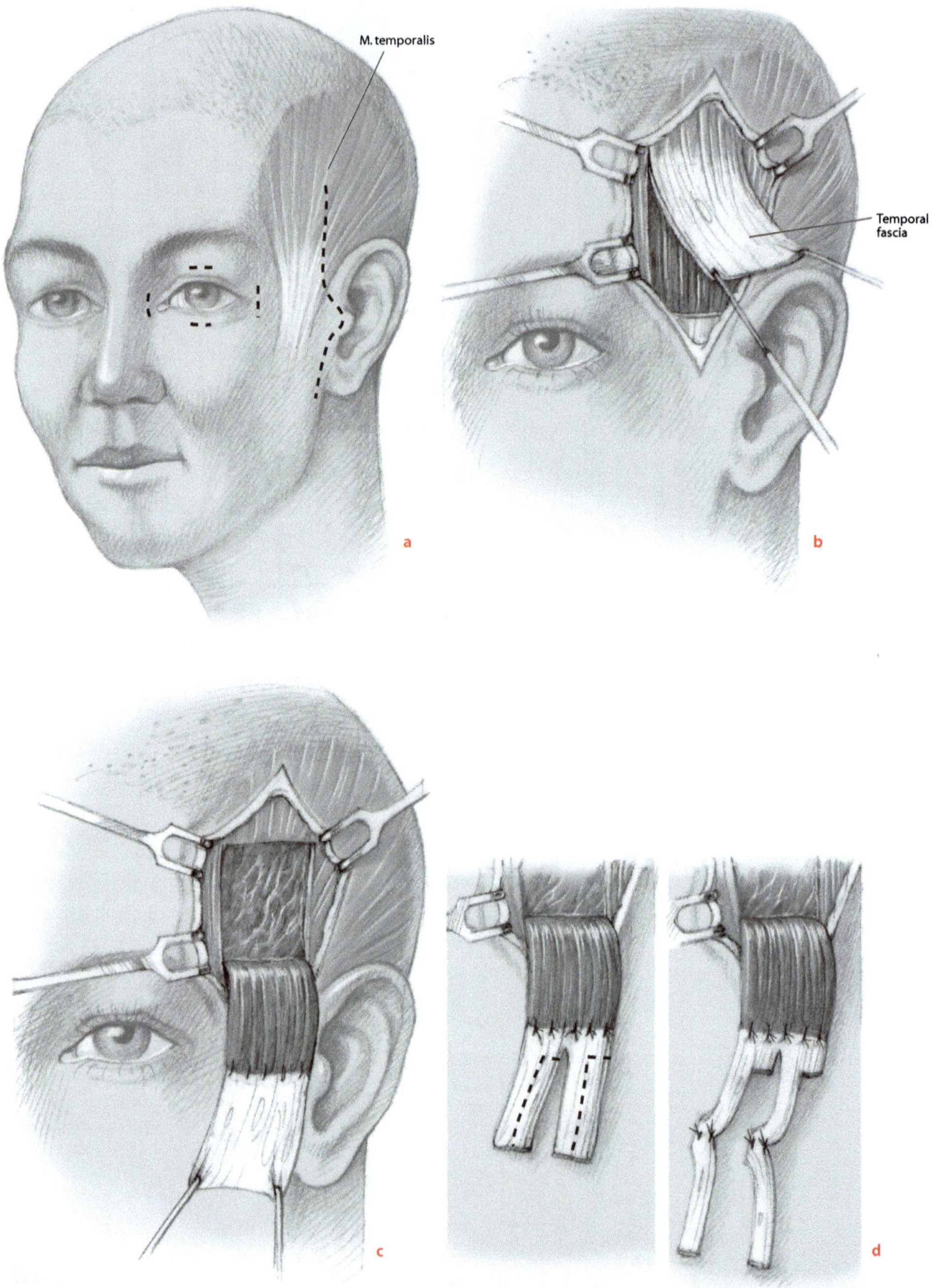
M. temporalis
Temporal fascia
a
b
c
d

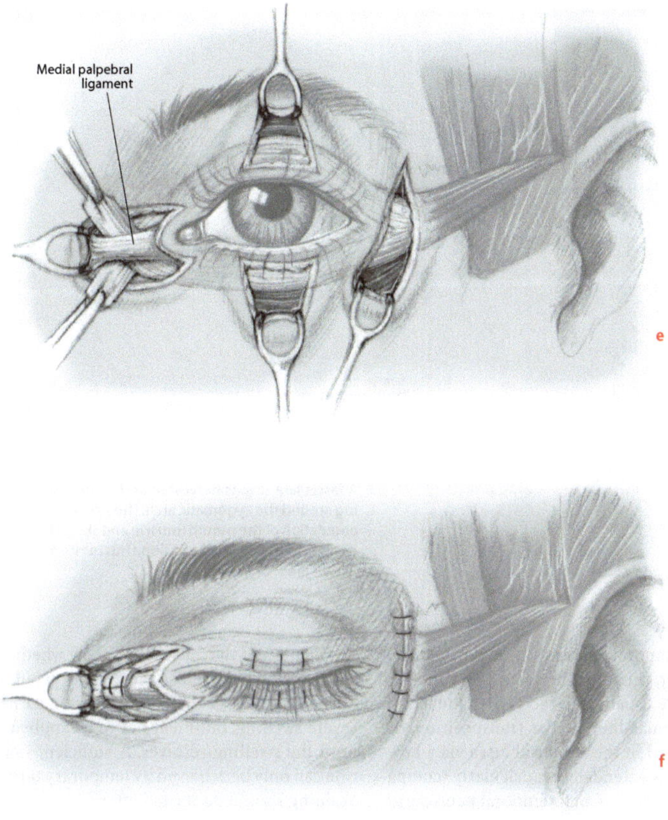

Figure 11.31 a–f

Transfer of the temporal muscle for closure of the eyes. a Incisions. b Harvest the superficial temporalis fascia from caudal to cranial, leaving the attachment to the muscle intact. c Then harvest the muscle from cranial to caudal. The area where the fascia is attached to the muscle is reinforced with nonabsorbable sutures. d The partial muscle is then divided into two narrow slips. If the strips are to short, an elongation with fascial strips (best from temporal fascia itself, or fascia lata) may become necessary. e A subcutaneous tunnel is dissected in the upper and lower eye lid, the fascial strips are then passed through and (f) fixed with nonabsorbable sutures at the medial aspect of the eye (medial palpebral ligament). Stimulation of the muscle will show whether the tension is correct to close the eyes

11.8 Facial Nerve

In failed facial nerve reconstruction, or nerve palsies that cannot be repaired by facial nerve surgery (Bell's palsies, tumors, etc.), several options for surgery are available. Besides the previously described hypoglossal facial anastomosis (see Chap. 7), the facial nerve of the healthy side can be used as a donor (see Chap. 12). However, this requires intact muscles on the affected side or muscle transplantation. As this is only indicated for particular patients, we describe the transposition of muscle to restore closure of the eyes, and if necessary elevation of the lips and the lateral commissure.

The transfer of the temporal muscle was first described by Gillies in 1934 and then modified by Anderson in 1961. As the temporal muscle is innervat-

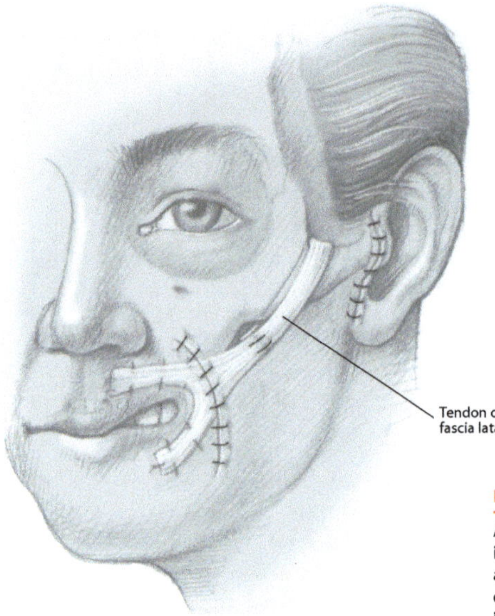

Figure 11.32

A fascia lata strip is harvested and sutured to itself after routing around the zygomatic arch. The strip is then sutured to the angulation of the mouth (muscle and skin). The incision can be done as a lunar shaped excision, thus removing the excess skin in that area

ed by the deep temporal nerves (V/3), it is usually not affected. However, this must be tested very meticulously. The muscle usually contracts when the mouth is closed and retracts the jaw. For transposition, the muscle is identified in the temporal fossa via a bow-like incision that is extended preauricularly (comparable to that for a classic frontotemporal neurosurgical approach). If the muscle is only used for closure of the eyes, the frontal part is elevated from cranial to caudal, leaving the superficial temporal vessels (both branches) and the deep branches of the temporal nerve intact that arise from beneath (▶ Fig. 11.31). The partial muscle is then divided into two narrow slips. If the strips are too short, an elongation with fascial strips (best from temporal fascia itself, or fascia lata) may become necessary. A very elegant method is to harvest the superficial temporalis fascia from caudal to cranial, leaving the attachment to the muscle intact. The area where the fascia is attached to the muscle is then reinforced with nonabsorbable sutures, and then the muscle is harvested from cranial to caudal. A subcutaneous tunnel is dissected in the upper and lower eye lid, the muscle strips are then passed through and fixed with nonabsorbable sutures at the medial aspect of the eye (medial palpebral ligament). Stimulation of the muscle will show whether the tension is sufficient to close the eyes. To avoid postoperative adhesions of the conjunctiva or cornea due to severe swelling, ointment has to be applied every 2 h until the swelling resolves. A sufficient immobilization can only be achieved by temporary tarsorrhaphy. Training should be started after 2 weeks. The patient is told to chew, the muscle then contracts and closes the eye. The patient has then to learn to transfer the movement for eye closure to an unconscious level.

Several modifications of this transfer have been presented, including a S-shaped elongation of the fascia to reach the medial eye and, when additionally used for the mouth, the lateral commissure where the strips are fixed transcutaneously. The commissure then must be immobilized with a hook or taped cranially to relax the transferred muscle. However, we found the transfer of the temporal muscle more reliable when only used for the eye. Several methods have been developed to correct the asymmetrical angulation of the mouth, mostly static techniques that include fascia lata (▶ Fig. 11.32) or cartilaginous grafts. These methods can be combined with a hemi-face lifting to achieve a certain extent of symmetry.

Principles of Free Neurovascular Muscle Transplantation

If no intact muscle is available for transfer, but a nerve is, the functional transplantation of a muscle must be discussed. This procedure has to be considered especially after ischemic or fibrotic changes of muscles, for example, in Volkmann's contracture. If no muscle is available to reconstruct flexion of wrist and hand, a muscle such as a gracilis muscle, can be harvested with its neurovascular bundle (▶ Fig. 12.1). The vessels are anastomosed to radial vessels at the level of the proximal forearm. The branch of the obturator nerve, which usually supplies the gracilis muscle, is then sutured to the interosseous anterior nerve (which contains only motor fibers), and the muscle is then inserted with the correct tension into the defect. Tension during recovery is avoided, and after approximately 3 months (depending on the length of nerve distal to suture) reinnervation can be detected, and physiotherapy can start. A secondary tightening of the muscle might become necessary. It was shown that the physiological structure of the muscle follows the nerve according to the fiber type. Although after reinnervation the number of motor units is decreased and their size are increased (both up to 50%), strength, however, is sufficient for regular movements, and can be trained postoperatively.

12.1 Facial Nerve

A special case of neurovascular muscle transplantation is the facial cross-nerve graft. As described in Chap. 7, primary suture of the facial nerve in case of a peripheral lesion provides the best results. To achieve symmetry in smile, however, a cross-facial nerve graft in addition with neurovascular muscle transplantation may become an option of therapy. The indication must be discussed very carefully, and as long grafts are required and several complications might occur, younger patients are more suitable for this kind of reconstruction. In the first stage, one or two nerve grafts are sutured to a branch of the healthy facial nerve (▶ Fig. 12.2). Usually, the right branch (r. zygo-

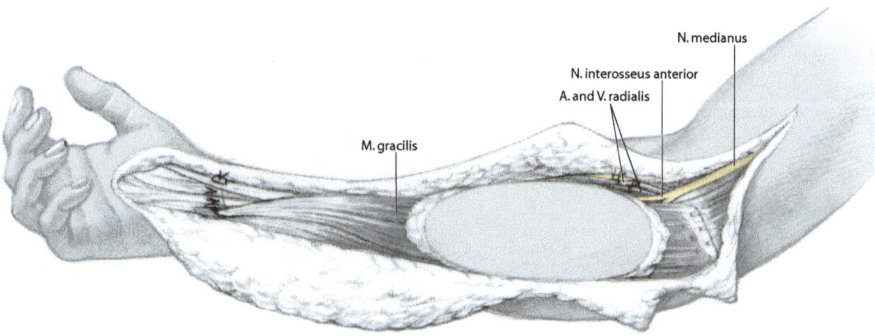

Figure 12.1

Example of a functional neurovascular muscle transplantation to restore finger flexion. The harvested muscle (gracilis muscle with skin island) is sutured into its new position. The vessels are anastomosed and the nerve is coapted to a donor nerve (N. interosseous anterior)

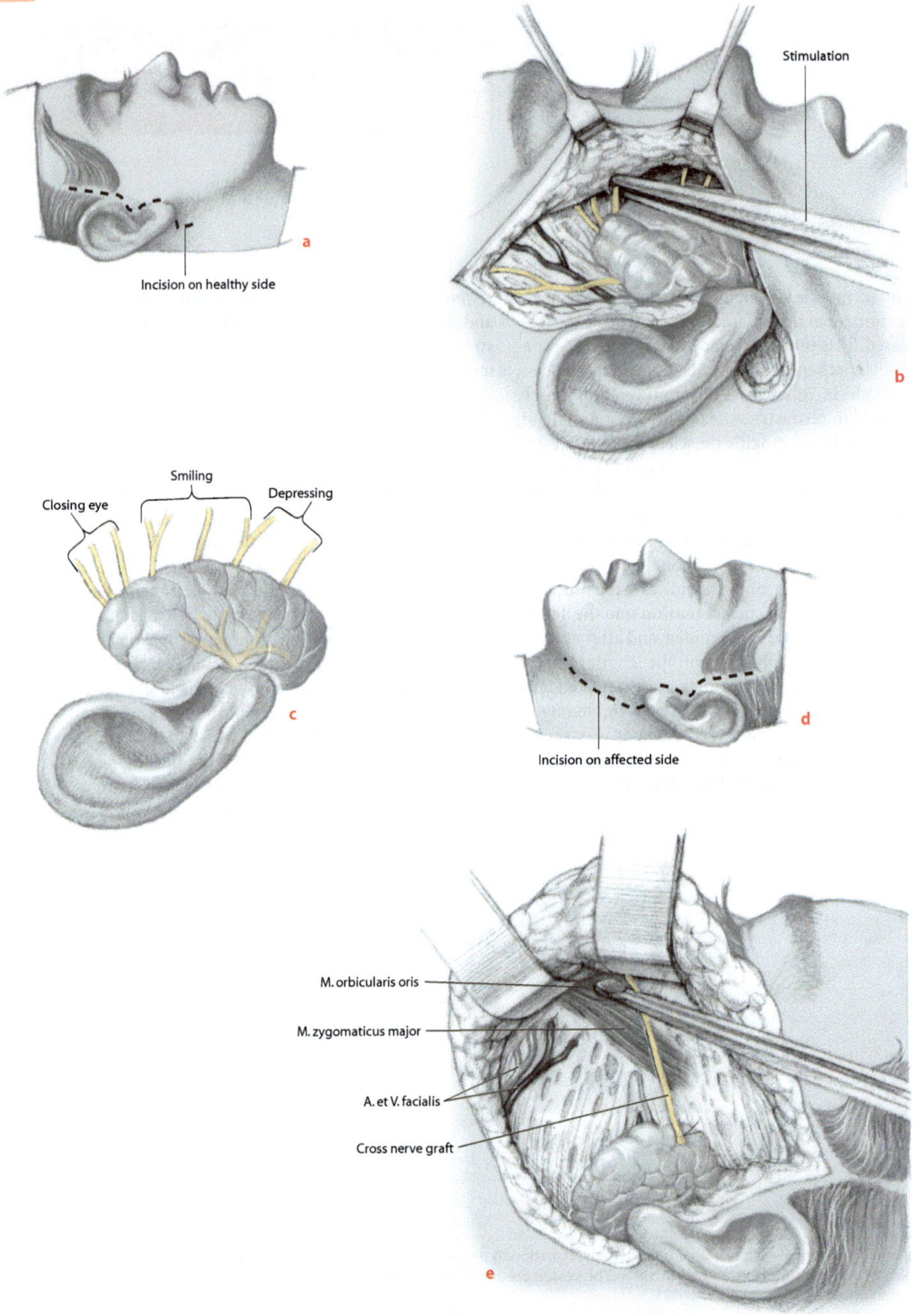
Incision on healthy side
a
Stimulation
b
Smiling
Closing eye
Depressing
c
Incision on affected side
d
M. orbicularis oris
M. zygomaticus major
A. et V. facialis
Cross nerve graft
e

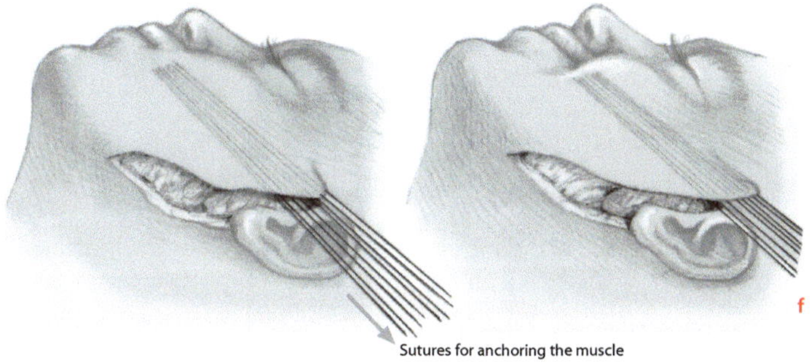

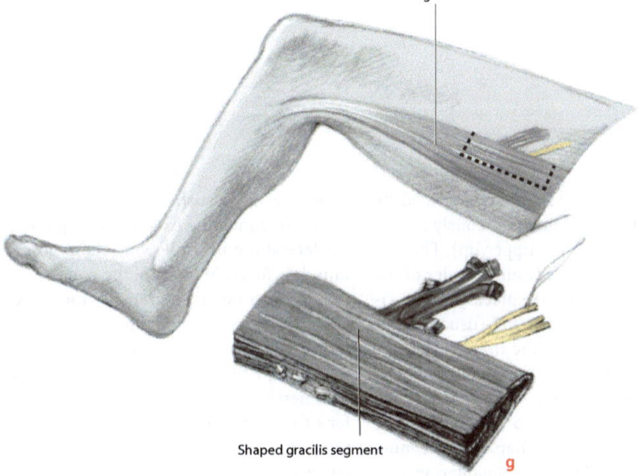

Figure 12.2 a–h

Cross-facial nerve graft in addition to neurovascular muscle transplantation. First stage. a Incision on the healthy side. b The right branch (r. zygomaticus n. facialis) is intraoperatively identified by stimulation. c Distribution of branches. A sural nerve graft is coapted to this branch and then subcutaneously routed to the contralateral side (via the upper lip). The end of the graft is placed near the frontal border of the ear and marked. Regeneration is allowed to take place until the Tinel sign reaches an appropriate level (usually after 6–9 months). In the second stage, the affected side is explored (incision, d), and nerve and donor vessels for muscle transplantation are identified (e). f The sutures for attaching the muscle are carefully placed to allow smiling (intraoperative testing is mandatory). g A segmental, shaped gracilis muscle is harvested and the vessels are anastomosed to the facial artery and vein. The cross-nerve graft is used to neurotize the obturator branch entering the gracilis muscle. h The muscle must be fixed at the zygomatic bone and the lateral mouth (following the zygomatic major muscle)

Figure 12 h: see next page

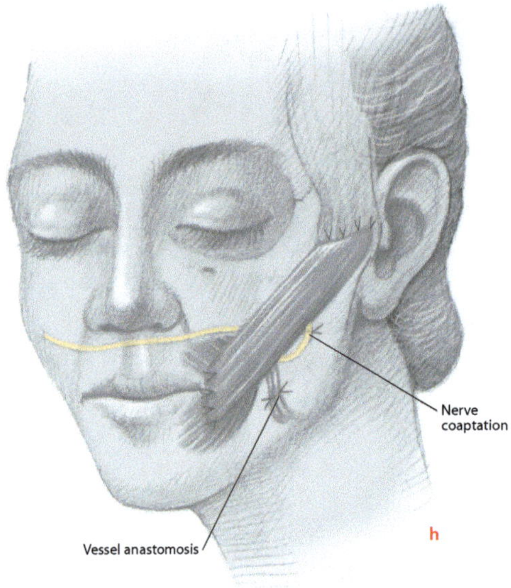

maticus n. facialis) is intraoperatively identified by stimulation. The graft is then subcutaneously routed to the contralateral side (via the upper lip). The end of the graft is placed near to the frontal border of the ear. Regeneration is allowed to take place until the Tinel sign reaches an appropriate level (usually after 6–9 months). If the muscles on the injured side are still intact [intraoperative inspection and pathological spontaneous activity in the electromyography (EMG)], the grafts can be used to intramuscularly neurotize the facial muscles (see Chap. 4). If the muscles show no sign of activity a transplantation of a healthy muscle is mandatory. The segmental gracilis muscle has shown to be sufficient for this purpose. The vessels are anastomosed to the superficial temporal or preferably to the facial artery and vein. The cross-nerve graft is used to neurotize the obturator branch entering the gracilis muscle. The muscle has to be inserted in such a manner that it allows smiling: the muscle must be fixed at the zygomatic bone and the lateral mouth (following the zygomaticus major muscle). To avoid tension, the commissure of lateral mouth must be taped cranially for 3 weeks. Physical therapy starts with beginning of reinnervation. It might become necessary to fix the muscle again after it is completely reinnervated. The restoration of a symmetrical smile should be combined with a transfer of the temporal muscle (innervated by the deep temporal nerves, V/3) to restore closure of the affected eye.

In Moebius syndrome where bilateral facial nerve aplasia is evident, Zuker and co-workers (2000) described the use of the masseteric nerve as a donor for a transplanted gracilis muscle, achieving a symmetrical contraction that is transferable to unconscious level.

Intramuscular Neurotization

As in some lesions where the branches of the nerve that enter the muscle are destroyed or are too small for coaptation, and in special cases where restoration of the original nerve is not advised, the technique of intermuscular neurotization according to Becker and co-workers (2002) is a valuable tool in reconstruction.

For this method a long nerve graft (e.g., sural nerve) is orthogradely sutured to the proximal nerve stump. The nerve graft is then longitudinally dissected proximally, leaving behind the cut small junctions between the little fascicles. These tiny branches (at least four or five) from the nerve graft are now inserted into the longitudinally split muscle like a fan. The grafts must contact the muscle over a long distance. Thus, at the nerve endings (where the junctions between the fascicles have been, and the real nerve end), a contact to the muscle is created, re-establishing neuromuscular junctions. Compared with the old technique, more nerve–muscle junctions are created, resulting in better reinnervation of the muscles.

References

Albert E (1885)Einige Operationen am Nerven. Wien Med Presse 26:1285

Allieu Y, Privat JM, Bonnel F (1982) Les neurotisations par le nerf spinal dans les avulsions radiculaires du plexus brachial. Neurochir 28:115–120

Anderl H (1973) Reconstruction of the face through cross-face-nerve transplantation in facial paralysis. Chir Plastica (Berl) 2:17–46

Anderson JG (1961) Surgical treatment of lagophthalmos in leprosy by the Gillies temporalis transfer. Br J Plast Surg 14: 339

Ballance CHA (1909) A Case of facial palsy treated by facio-hypoglossal anastomosis. Lancet 1:1675–1677

Ballance CHA (1924) Results obtained in some experiments in which the facial and recurrent laryngeal nerves were anastomosed with other nerves. BMJ 2:349–354

Barbera J, Gonzales J, Gil JL et al (1988) The quality and extension of nerve fiber regeneration in the centrocentral anastomosis of the peripheral nerve. Acta Neurochir (Wien) [Suppl 43]:205–209

Beasly RW (1970) Principles of tendon transfer. Orthop Clin North Am 1970 1:433–438

Becker MJH Lassner F, Fansa H, Mawrin C, Pallua N (2002) Refinements in intramuscular neurotization. Muscle Nerve 26:362–366

Becker S, Penkert G (2000) In vivo visualization of the neuromuscular junction before and after autologous nerve transfer in the rat. J Reconstr Microsurg 16:111–120

Birch R (2001) Medial rotation contracture and posterior dislocation of the shoulder. In: Gilbert A (ed) Brachial plexus injuries. Martin Dunitz, London

Birch R, Bonney G, Parry CBW (1998) Surgical disorders of the peripheral nerves. Churchill Livingstone, Edinburgh

Brand PW, Beach RB, Thompson DE (1981) Relative tension and potential excursion of muscles in the forearm and hand. J Hand Surg 6A:209–219

Brand PW (1974) Biomechanics of tendon transfer. Orthop Clin N Am 5:205–230

Brand PW (1988) Biomechanics of tendon transfers. Hand Clin 4:137–154

Brooks D (1955) The place of nerve-grafting in orthopaedic surgery. J Bone Joint Surg 37A:299–305

Bruner JM (1948) Tendon transfer to restore abduction of the index finger using the extensor pollicis brevis. Plast Reconstr Surg 3:197–201

Buck-Gramcko D, Nigst H (eds) (1991) Motorische Ersatzoperationen der oberen Extremität, vol. 2. Hand und Unterarm. Hippokrates, Stuttgart

Burkhalter WE (1974) Early transfer in upper extremity peripheral nerve injury. Clin Orthop 1974 104:68–79

Caroll RE (1952) Restoration of flexor power to the flail elbow by transplantation of the triceps tendon. Surg Gyn Obstet 95:685–688

Carvalho GA, Nikkhah G, Matthies C, Penkert G, Samii M (1997) Diagnosis of root avulsion in traumatic brachial plexus injuries: value of computerized tomography myelography and magnetic resonance imaging. J Neurosurg 86:69–76

Chuang DCC, Hattori Y, Ma HS, Chen HC (2002) The reconstructive strategy for improving elbow function in late obstetric brachial plexus palsy. Plast Reconstr Surg 109:116–126

Clark JMP (1946) Reconstruction of biceps brachii by pectoral muscle transplantation. Br J Surg 34:180–181

Curtis RM (1974) Fundamental principles of tendon transfer. Orthop Clin N Am 5:231–242

Curtis RM, Eversmann WW (1973) Internal neurolysis as an adjunct to the treatment of the carpal tunnel syndrome. J Bone Joint Surg 55A:733–740

Cushing H (1903) The surgical treatment of facial paralysis by nerve anastomosis. Ann Surg 37:641–659

de Abreu LB (1989) Early restoration of pinch grip after ulnar nerve repair and tendon transfer. J Hand Surg 14B:309–314

Donner TR, Voorhies RM, Kline DG (1994) Neural sheath tumors of major nerves. J Neurosurg 81:362–373

Edshage S (1964) Peripheral nerve suture. Acta Chir Scand [Suppl] 331:1–104

Falconer M, Weddell G (1943) Costoclavicular compression of the subclavian artery and vein: relation to the scalenus anticus syndrome. Lancet 2:539–543

Fansa H, Keilhoff G, Horn T, Altmann S, Wolf G, Schneider W (2000) Stimulation of Schwann cell proliferation and axonal regeneration by FK 506. Restor Neurol Neurosci 16:77–86

Fansa H, Keilhoff G, Wolf G, Schneider W (2001) Tissue engineering of peripheral nerves: a comparison of veins and acellular muscle grafts with cultured Schwann cells. Plast Reconstr Surg 107:485–494

Fansa H, Schneider W, Wolf G, Keilhoff G (2002) Influence of insulin-like growth factor-I (IGF-I) on nerve autografts and tissue engineered nerve grafts. Muscle Nerve 26:87–96

Fansa H, Plogmeier K, Feistner H, Schneider W (1997) Plasticity and function – the fate of a free neurovascular latissimus dorsi muscle graft ten years post-reconstruction. J Reconstr Microsurg 13:551–554

Ferner RE, Gutmann DH (2002) International consensus statement on malignant peripheral nerve sheath tumors in neurofibromatosis 1. Cancer Res 62:1573–1577

Foerster O, Vortrag TAG (1916) der Dtsch. Orthop. Ges. Berlin Münch med Wschr 63:283

Frerichs O, Fansa H, Ziems P, Schneider W, Keilhoff G (2001) Regeneration of peripheral nerves after clenbuterol treatment in a rat model. Muscle Nerve 24:1687–1691

Gaitzsch G, Chamay A (1986) Paralytic brachial neuritis or Parsonage-Turner syndrome with anterior interosseous nerve involvement. Report of three cases. Ann Chir Main 5: 288–294

Gilbert A (2001) Brachial plexus injuries. Martin Dunitz, London

Gillies HD (1934) Facial paralysis. Proc R Soc Med 27:1372

Girsch W et al (2001) Endoscopic versus open carpal tunnel release: setup of a prospective randomised study. In: Frey M (ed) Endoscopy and microsurgery. Springer, Berlin Heidelberg New York, pp 47–58

Gonzalez-Darder J, Barbera J, Abellan J, Mora A (1985) Centro-central anastomosis in the prevention and treatment of painful terminal neuroma. An experimental study in the rat. J Neurosurg 63:754–758

Gu YD, Zhang GM, Chen DS et al (1992) Seventh cervical nerve root transfer from the contralateral healthy side for treatment of brachial plexus root avulsion. J Hand Surg 17B:518–521

Hardy RC, Perret G, Meyers R (1957) Phrenicofacial nerve anastomosis for facial paralysis. J Neurosurg 14:400–404

Harmon PH (1950) Surgical reconstruction of the paralytic shoulder by multiple muscle transplantation. J Bone Joint Surg 32A:583–595

Hass J (1931) Muskelplastik bei Serratuslähmung. Z Orthop Chir 55:617–622

Hassenbusch SJ, Stanton-Hicks M, Schoppa D, Walsh JG, Covington EC (1996) Long-term results of peripheral nerve stimulation for reflex sympathetic dystrophy. J Neurosurg 84:415–423

Hiller F (1951) Nerve regeneration in grafts. J Neuropath Clin Neurol 1:5–14

Huber GC (1919) Transplantation of peripheral nerves. Arch Neurol Psychiat 2:466–480

Hueter K (1873) Die allgemeine Chirurgie. Vogel, Leipzig

Hunt JR (1908) Occupational neuritis of the deep palmar branch of the ulnar nerve. J Nerv Ment Dis 35:676–689

Inbal R, Devor M, Tuchendler O, Lieblick I (1980) Autotomy following nerve injury: genetic factors in the development of chronic pain. Pain 9:327–337

Jacobsen HJ (1963) Microsurgical technique in the repair of traumatized extremity. Clin Orthop 29:132–145

Keck C (1962) The tarsal tunnel syndrome. J Bone Joint Surg 44A:180–184

Kele H, Verheggen R, Bittermann HJ, Reimers CD (2003) The Potential value of ultrasonography in the evaluation of carpal tunnel syndrome. Neurology 61:389–391

Khalil H, Samii M, Penkert G, Kohmura E (1986) Ergebnisse der Nerventransplantation an der oberen Extremität. In: Kastenbauer E (ed) Das Transplantat in der Plastischen Chirurgie. Sasse, Rotenburg, pp 257–265

Kiloh LG, Nevin S (1952) Isolated neuritis of the anterior interosseus nerve. BMJ I:850–851

King T, Morgan FP (1959) Late results of removing the medial humeral epicondyle for traumatic ulnar neuritis. J Bone Joint Surg 41B:51

Kline DG, Hudson AR (1995) Nerve injuries. Saunders, Philadelphia

Koschorke GM, Meyer A, Tillman DB, Campbell JN (1991) Ectopic excitability of injured nerves in monkey: entrained responses to vibratory stimuli. J Neurophysiol 65:693–701

Lanz U (1977) Anatomical variations of the median nerve in the carpal tunnel. J Hand Surg 2:44–53

Lenz O, Fansa H, Schneider W, Feistner H (2001) Der Einsatz elektrophysiologischer Verfahren bei der Diagnostik peripherer Nervenkompressionssyndrome. Handchir Mikrochir Plast Chir 33:342–348

Lusk M, Kline DG, Garcia C (1987) Tumors of the brachial plexus. Neurosurg 21:439–453

Marinacci AA (1968) Neurological syndromes of the tarsal tunnels. Bull Los Angeles Neurol Soc 33:90–100

Maxion H, Samii M, Scheinpflug W, Wallenborn R (1972) Elektromyographische Verlaufsuntersuchungen nach Nervennaht und Nerventransplantation beim Kaninchen. EEG-EMG 2:89–94

Melzack R, Wall P (1965) Pain mechanisms: a new theory. Science 150:971–979

Merle d'Aubigné R, Lange P (1946) Transplantations tendineuses dans la traitement des paralysies radiales post-traumatiques. Sem Hôp Paris 22:1666–1680

Millesi H (2002) Brachial plexus surgery – is it still salvage surgery or can we reach a standardized treatment? Symposium, Hannover, 17–21 June 2002

Millesi H (1992) Chirurgie der peripheren Nerven. Urban & Schwarzenberg, München

Millesi H (1977) Interfascicular grafts for repair of peripheral nerves of the upper extremity. Orthop Clin North Am 8:387–404

Millesi H (1979) Nerve suture and grafting to restore the extratemporal facial nerve. Clin Plast Surg 6:333–341

Millesi H, Meissel G, Berger A (1976) Further experience with interfascicular grafting of the median ulnar and radial nerves. J Bone Joint Surg 58A:209–218

Millesi H, Meissel G, Berger A (1975) Repair of peripheral nerves by the use of autografts. Proceedings of the IX European Federation Congress, Amsterdam, June 29–July 4. In: Excerpta Med Int Congress Series 377:43–47

Millesi H, Walzer L (1981) Problems of direct neurotization. In: Freilinger G (ed) Muscle transplantation. Springer, Berlin Heidelberg New York, pp 279–282

Mirzai S, Sepehrnia A, El Azm M, Penkert G, Samii M (1993) Results of surgical treatment of meralgia paresthetica. In: Mirzai S, Sepehrnia A, Penkert G et al (eds) Advances in Neurosurgery 21. Springer, Berlin Heidelberg New York, pp 268–273

Mirzai S, Sepehrnia A, Penkert G et al (1993) Radial nerve lesions associated with fractures of the humerus or radius: results of surgical treatment. In: Mirzai S, Sepehrnia A, Penkert G et al (eds) Advances in Neurosurg 21. Springer, Berlin Heidelberg New York, pp 215–219

Mitchell SW (1872) Injuries to nerves and their consequences. Lippincott, Philadelphia

Moberg E (1987) The upper limb in tetraplegia. A new approach to surgical rehabilitation. Thieme, Stuttgart

Morton TG (1876) A peculiar and painful affection of the fourth metatarso-phanlangeal articulation. Am J Med Sci 71:37–45

Nicholson OR, Seddon HJ (1957) Nerve Repair in civil practice. results of treatment of median and ulnar nerve lesions. BMJ 9:83–91

Nigst H (1991) Motorische Ersatzoperationen der oberen Extremität. Vol 3: Operationen an Tetraplegikern. Hippokrates, Stuttgart

Noopdenbos W, Wall PD (1981) Implications of the failure of nerve resection and graft to cure chronic pain produced by nerve lesions. J Neurol Neurosurg Psychiat 44:1068–1073

Omer GE (1988) Timing of tendon transfers in peripheral nerve injury. Hand Clin 4:317–322

Peer S, Bodner G, Meirer R, Willeit J, Piza-Katzer H (2001) Examination of postoperative peripheral nerve lesions with high-resolution sonography. AJR 177:415–419
Penkert G, Bini W, Samii M (1988) Revascularization of nerve grafts: an experimental study. J Reconstr Microsurg 4:319–325
Penkert G, Carvalho GA, Nikkhah G, Tatagiba M, Matthies C (1999) Diagnosis and surgery of brachial plexus injuries. J Reconstr Microsurg 15:3–8
Phillipeaux JM, Vulpian A (1870) Note sur des essais de greffe d'un troncon de nerf lingual entre les deux bouts du nerf hypoglosse. Arch Physiol Norm Path 3:618–620
Phipps GJ, Hoffer MM (1995) Latissimus dorsi and teres major transfer to rotator cuff for Erb's palsy. J Shoulder Elbow Surg 4:124–129
Portilla Molinar AE, Bour C, Oberlin C, Nzeusseu A, Vanwijck R (1998) The posterior interosseous nerve and the radial tunnel syndrome: an anatomical study. Int. Orthopaed (Sicot) 22:102–106
Röttgen P, Wüllenweber R (1974) Die Chirurgie der peripheren Nerven. In: Olivecrona H, Tönnis W, Krenkel W (eds) Handbuch der Neurochirurgie. Springer, Berlin Heidelberg New York
Rudigier J (1991) Motorische Ersatzoperationen der oberen Extremität. vol 1. Schultergürtel Oberarm und Ellenbogen. Hippokrates, Stuttgart
Saha AK (1967) Surgery of the paralysed and flail shoulder. Acta Orthop Scand Suppl 97:5–90
Samii M (1981) Centrocentral anastomosis of peripheral nerves: a neurosurgical treatment of amputation neuromas. In: Siegfried J, Zimmerman M (eds) Phantom and stump pain. Springer, Berlin Heidelberg New York, pp 123–125
Samii M, Carvalho GA, Nikkhah G, Penkert G (1997) Surgical reconstruction of the musculocutaneous nerve in traumatic brachial plexus injuries. J Neurosurg 87:881–886
Samii M, Penkert G (1998) Traumatic disorders of the peripheral nervous system. In: Cruz J (ed) Neurologic and Neurosurgical emergencies. Saunders, Philadelphia, pp 349–362
Samii M, Wallenborn R (1972) Tierexperimentelle Untersuchungen über den Einfluss der Spannung auf den Regenerationserfolg nach Nervennaht. Acta Neurochir 27:87–110
Schottstaedt ER, Larsen LJ, Bost FC (1958) The surgical reconstruction of the upper extremity paralysed by poliomyelitis. J Bone Joint Surg 40A:633–643
Schröder JM (2001) Pathology of peripheral nerves: an atlas of structural and molecular pathological changes. Springer, Berlin Heidelberg New York
Schwartzmann JR, Crego CH (1948) Hamstring-tendon transplantation for the relief of quadriceps femoris paralysis in residual poliomyelitis: a follow-up study of 134 cases. J Bone Joint Surg 30A:541–552
Seddon HJ (1972) Surgical disorders of the peripheral nerves. Churchill Livingstone, Edinburgh
Seddon HJ (1943) Three types of nerve injury. Brain 66:237–288
Shetter AG, Racz GB, Lewis R, Heavner JE (1997) Peripheral nerve stimulation. In: North RB, Levy RM (eds) Neurosurgical management of pain. Springer, Berlin Heidelberg New York, pp 261–270
Smith RJ, Hastings H (1980) Principles of tendon transfers to the hand. American Academy of Orthopedic Surgeons Instructional Course Lectures 29:129–152
Smith JW (1966) Factors influencing nerve repair. I Blood supply of peripheral nerves. Arch Surg 93:335–341
Smith JW (1964) Microsurgery of peripheral nerves. Plast Reconstr Surg 33:317–329
Spinner RJ, O'Driscoll SW, Jupiter JB, Goldner RD (2000) Unrecognized dislocation of the medial portion of the triceps: another cause of failed ulnar nerve transposition. J Neurosurg 92:52–57
Steindler A (1930) Die poliomyelitischen Lähmungen der oberen Extremität. Verh Dtsch Ortop Ges 25:113–124
Stern PJ, Fassler PR (1991) Pronator syndrome. In: Gelbermann RH (ed) Operative nerve repair and reconstruction. Lippincott, Philadelphia, pp 995–1002
Struthers J (1854) Anatomical and physiological observations, Part I. Sutherland and Knox, Edinburgh
Sunderland S (1978) Nerves and nerve injuries. Churchill Livingstone, Edinburgh
Sunderland S (1951) A classification of peripheral nerve injuries producing loss of function. Brain 74:491–516
Sunderland S (1991) Nerve injuries and their repair. A critical appraisal. Churchill Livingstone, Edinburgh
Tatagiba M, Penkert G, Samii M (1992) Surgical treatment of peripheral nerve ganglion. Neurons III 1–2:61–64
Terzis JK, Papakonstantinou KC (2002) Outcomes of scapula stabilization in obstetrical brachial plexus palsy: a novel dynamic procedure for correction of the winged scapula. Plast Reonstr Surg 109:548–561
Tubiana R (1969) Anatomic and physiologic basis for the surgical treatment of paralyses of the hand. J Bone Joint Surg 51A:643–660
Vispo Seara JL, Krimmer H, Lanz U (1994) Monofaszikuläre Nervenrotation. Handchir Mikrochir Plast Chir 26:190–193
Viterbo F, Trindade JC, Hoshino K, Mazzoni Neto A (1994) End-to-side neurorrhaphy with removal of the epineurial sheath: an experimental study in rats. Plast Reconstr Surg 94:1038–1047
Wall PD, Melzack R (eds) (1994) Textbook of pain. Churchill Livingstone, Edinburgh
Wall PD, Sweet WH (1967) Temporary abolition of pain in man. Science 155:108–109
Wilhelm A (1976) Radialiskompressionssyndrome. Handchirurgie 8:113–116
Wintsch K (1972) Physiotherapie und Ergotherapie nach Sehnentranspositionen. Handchirurgie 4:17–20
Wright J (1945) The neurovascular syndrome produced by hyperabduction of the arm. Am Heart J 29:1–19
Yoemans W (1928) The relation of arthritis of the sacroiliac joint to sciatica. Lancet 2:1119–1122
Zachary RB (1946) Tendon transplantation for radial paralysis. Brit J Surg 33:358–364
Zancolli E, Mitre H (1973) Latissimus dorsi transfer to restore elbow flexion. J Bone Joint Surg 55A:1265–1275
Zancolli EA (ed) (1979) Structural and dynamic bases of hand surgery, 2nd edn. Lippincott, Philadelphia
Zuker RM, Goldberg CS, Manktelow RT (2000) Facial animation in children with Moebius syndrome after segmental gracilis muscle transplant. Plast Reconstr Surg 106:1–8

Subject Index

D

E

F

G

N

S

T

U

V

W

Z

MIX
Papier aus verantwortungsvollen Quellen
Paper from responsible sources
FSC® C105338

If you have any concerns about our products,
you can contact us on
ProductSafety@springernature.com

In case Publisher is established outside the EU,
the EU authorized representative is:
Springer Nature Customer Service Center GmbH
Europaplatz 3, 69115 Heidelberg, Germany

Printed by Libri Plureos GmbH
in Hamburg, Germany